Heart Disease: Advances in Cardiovascular Medicine

Heart Disease: Advances in Cardiovascular Medicine

Editor: Warren Lyde

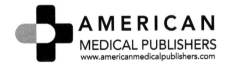

AMERICAN
MEDICAL PUBLISHERS
www.americanmedicalpublishers.com

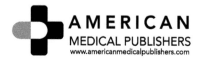

Cataloging-in-Publication Data

Heart disease : advances in cardiovascular medicine / edited by Warren Lyde.
   p. cm.
Includes bibliographical references and index.
ISBN 978-1-63927-691-2
1. Cardiovascular system--Diseases. 2. Heart--Diseases. 3. Cardiology. I. Lyde, Warren.
RC667 .H43 2023
616.1--dc23

American Medical Publishers,
41 Flatbush Avenue,
1st Floor, New York,
NY 11217, USA

ISBN 978-1-63927-691-2 (Hardback)

Contents

Preface

Every book is a source of knowledge and this one is no exception. The idea that led to the conceptualization of this book was the fact that the world is advancing rapidly; which makes it crucial to document the progress in every field. I am aware that a lot of data is already available, yet, there is a lot more to learn. Hence, I accepted the responsibility of editing this book and contributing my knowledge to the community.

The diseases which impact the blood or heart vessels fall under the category of heart diseases. It involves various conditions, which affect the normal heart function. Its types include arrhythmia, atherosclerosis, cardiomyopathy, coronary artery disease, congenital heart defects and heart infections. Symptoms of heart disease comprise chest pressure, chest pain, discomfort and tightness in chest. Its risk factors are a family history of heart disease, high blood pressure, diabetes, poor diet, high cholesterol, obesity, physical inactivity and stress. Treatment of heart diseases vary based on the type of disease and can be classified into three major categories, which are lifestyle changes, medications, and invasive procedures of surgery. Various advances in their treatment include genetic and stem cells techniques, which enable treatment at cellular and subcellular levels. Furthermore, highly sensitive and non-invasive imaging techniques are evolving in diagnostic imaging. The topics included in this book on heart diseases are of utmost significance and bound to provide incredible insights to readers. It will also provide interesting topics for research which interested readers can take up. The extensive content of this book provides the readers with a thorough understanding of these diseases.

While editing this book, I had multiple visions for it. Then I finally narrowed down to make every chapter a sole standing text explaining a particular topic, so that they can be used independently. However, the umbrella subject sinews them into a common theme. This makes the book a unique platform of knowledge.

I would like to give the major credit of this book to the experts from every corner of the world, who took the time to share their expertise with us. Also, I owe the completion of this book to the never-ending support of my family, who supported me throughout the project.

Editor

Pilot Study on the Role of Circulating miRNAs for the Improvement of the Predictive Ability of the 2MACE Score in Patients with Atrial Fibrillation

José Miguel Rivera-Caravaca [1],[†]●, Raúl Teruel-Montoya [2],[3],[†]●, Vanessa Roldán [2]●, Rosa Cifuentes-Riquelme [2], José Antonio Crespo-Matas [2], Ascensión María de los Reyes-García [2]●, Sonia Águila [2], María Piedad Fernández-Pérez [2], Laura Reguilón-Gallego [2], Laura Zapata-Martínez [2], Nuria García-Barberá [2], Vicente Vicente [2],[3]●, Francisco Marín [1], Constantino Martínez [2],[*],[‡]● and Rocío González-Conejero [2],[*],[‡]●

[1] Department of Cardiology, Hospital Clínico Universitario Virgen de la Arrixaca, University of Murcia, Instituto Murciano de Investigación Biosanitaria (IMIB-Arrixaca), CIBERCV, 30120 Murcia, Spain; jmrivera429@gmail.com (J.M.R.-C.); fcomarino@hotmail.com (F.M.)

[2] Department of Hematology and Medical Oncology, Hospital General Universitario Morales Meseguer, University of Murcia, Centro Regional de Hemodonación, Instituto Murciano de Investigación Biosanitaria (IMIB-Arrixaca), 30003 Murcia, Spain; raulteruelmontoya@hotmail.com (R.T.-M.); vroldans@gmail.com (V.R.); rcifuentesriquelme@gmail.com (R.C.-R.); jocresma@hotmail.com (J.A.C.-M.); sregapa@gmail.com (A.M.d.l.R.-G.); sonia.aguila@um.es (S.Á.); mpfernandezperez@gmail.com (M.P.F.-P.); reguilongallegolaura@gmail.com (L.R.-G.); laurazap97@gmail.com (L.Z.-M.); nurgarbar@gmail.com (N.G.-B.); vicente.vicente@carm.es (V.V.)

[3] CIBERER (U765), 30003 Murcia, Spain

[*] Correspondence: constant@um.es (C.M.); rocio.gonzalez@carm.es (R.G.-C.);

[†] Both authors contributed equally.

[‡] Joint senior authors.

Abstract: *Background.* Atrial fibrillation (AF) increases the risk for stroke but also for non-stroke major adverse cardiovascular events (MACE). The 2MACE score was recently proposed to predict these events. Since the interest of microRNAs (miRNAs) in cardiovascular diseases is increasing, we aimed to investigate whether miRNA levels may improve the predictive performance of the 2MACE score. *Methods.* We included consecutive AF patients stable on vitamin K antagonist therapy. Blood samples were drawn at baseline and plasma expression of miRNAs was assessed. During a median of 7.6 (interquartile range (IQR) 5.4–8.0) years, the occurrence of any MACE (nonfatal myocardial infarction/cardiac revascularization and cardiovascular death) was recorded. *Results.* We conducted a miRNA expression analysis in plasma from 19 patients with and without cardiovascular events. The miRNAs selected (miR-22-3p, miR-107, and miR-146a-5p) were later measured in 166 patients (47% male, median age 77 (IQR 70–81) years) and all were associated with a higher risk of MACE. The addition of miR-107 and miR-146a-5p to the 2MACE score significantly increased the predictive performance (c-indexes: 0.759 vs. 0.694, $p = 0.004$), and the model with three miRNAs also improved the predictive performance compared to the original score (c-indexes: 0.762 vs. 0.694, $p = 0.012$). 2MACE models with the addition of miRNAs presented higher net benefit and potential clinical usefulness. *Conclusions.* Higher miR-22-3p andmiR-107 and lower miR-146a-5p levels were associated with a higher risk of MACE. The addition of these miRNAs to the 2MACE score significantly increased the predictive performance for MACE, which may aid to some extent in the decision-making process about risk stratification in AF.

Keywords: miRNAs; atrial fibrillation; risk stratification; adverse cardiovascular event; 2MACE

1. Introduction

Atrial fibrillation (AF) is the most frequent cardiac arrhythmia and it implies a high morbidity and mortality [1,2]. There is evidence supporting the presence of a prothrombotic or hypercoagulable state in AF, which is associated with an increased risk of stroke and thromboembolism [3]. However, a non-negligible proportion of patients suffer from adverse cardiovascular events regardless of stroke, including myocardial infarction (MI) [4]. For this reason, the 2MACE score was proposed to predict major adverse cardiovascular events (MACE; MI, cardiac revascularization, and cardiovascular death) in AF patients [5], and external validations have shown promising results [6,7].

On the other hand, the study of biomarkers as prognostic or risk stratification markers has gained attention. In this context, microRNAs (miRNAs) are post-transcriptional regulators that have been widely recognized as active effectors of the cardiovascular system [8]. The recognition of miRNAs as plasma biomarkers of cardiovascular disease is being consolidated because their collect is minimally invasive, only a blood sample is required, and they are remarkably stable in the bloodstream, and sensitive to acute or chronic environmental alterations [9,10]. In addition to their great accessibility, circulating miRNAs are relatively easy to measure [11]. While a few works have reported profiles of circulating miRNAs as predictors for cardiovascular events in patients presenting MI [12], coronary artery disease [13], or acute coronary syndrome [14], their role as prognostic markers in AF is still unknown.

In the present study, we aimed to determine a profile of circulating miRNAs with the ability to predict MACE in AF, and to assess whether plasma miRNA levels can improve the predictive performance of the 2MACE score in a "real-world" cohort of AF patients under vitamin K antagonist (VKA) therapy.

2. Methods

We included a prospective cohort of permanent/paroxysmal AF patients from our outpatient anticoagulation clinic in a tertiary hospital (Murcia, southeast of Spain). All patients were on VKA therapy with stable international normalized ratios (INR 2.0–3.0) during at least the previous 6 months. This 6-month period of good anticoagulation control with VKA before inclusion was required to have a baseline homogeneity that would allow us to avoid the potential bias of poor anticoagulation control on clinical outcomes. Patients with prosthetic heart valves, rheumatic AF, or patients with acute coronary syndrome, stroke (ischemic or embolic), unstable chest pain, hemodynamic instability, hospital admission, or surgical intervention in the preceding 6 months were excluded.

The recruitment period was from May 2007 to December 2007. At inclusion, a complete medical history was recorded, and stroke risk (CHA_2DS_2-VASc) and bleeding risk (HAS-BLED) were estimated. The time in the therapeutic range at 6 months after entry was calculated using the Rosendaal method.

All subjects who met eligibility criteria were enrolled after providing written informed consent. The study was approved by the ethical committee of our institution (code: AVAL03/11) and performed in accordance with the ethical standards laid down in the 1964 Declaration of Helsinki and its subsequent amendments.

2.1. Assessment of the 2MACE Score

The baseline 2MACE score was retrospectively calculated in all patients as described by Pastori et al. [5]. This score was described as a simple risk score to identify AF patients with a high residual risk of cardiovascular events and to improve cardiovascular risk stratification. The 2MACE score includes 2 points for metabolic syndrome and age ≥75, and 1 point for MI/revascularization, congestive heart failure (ejection fraction ≤40%) and thromboembolism (stroke/transient ischemic attack). The original publication stated that the 2MACE score was proposed to predict MACE (i.e., any of the following: MI, cardiac revascularization, and cardiovascular death) in AF patients.

2.2. Blood Samples Collection and miRNome Analysis

Blood samples were atraumatically drawn at study entry and without stasis into syringes preloaded with trisodium citrate (0.011 mol/L), i.e., all patients were stable under VKA therapy for at least 6 months when the blood sample was collected. Samples were centrifuged at $2200\times g$ and 4 °C for 10 min, and the supernatants were stored in aliquots at −80 °C until further use. miRNAs from plasma were purified using the Nucleo Spin miRNA Plasma Kit (Macherey–Nagel) in accordance with the manufacturer's protocol. Plasma miRNAs were screened using the plasma/serum focus microRNA PCR Panel V4 (Exiqon) composed of 179 miRNAs as has been previously described [15]. Data were normalized by cycle threshold (Ct) mean value for miR-103a and miR-191-5p, which showed a high correlation (Pearson correlation) with both the global geometrical mean value and the top 20 expressed miRNA geometric mean values, resulting in an $r = 0.8607$ (p-value < 0.0001) and $r = 0.8902$ (p-value < 0.0001), respectively. Plasma expression of miRNAs was calculated using the $2^{-\Delta Ct}$ method.

2.3. Follow-Up and Endpoints

The primary endpoint was the occurrence of any MACE (the composite of nonfatal MI or cardiac revascularization and cardiovascular death (death caused by sudden death, progressive congestive heart failure, fatal MI, or procedure-related death), during the follow-up period. We excluded from MACE all embolic events; i.e., stroke, transient ischemic attack, and peripheral or systemic embolism.

The median follow-up was 7.6 (interquartile range (IQR) 5.4–8.0) years. Follow-up was performed through routine visits to the anticoagulation clinic, the hospital electronic medical records, or, when unavailable, by telephone interview. No specific visits were performed regarding the study. Of note, no patient was lost to follow-up. The investigators identified, confirmed, and recorded all adverse events and outcomes.

2.4. Statistical Analysis

Continuous variables were presented as mean±SD or median (interquartile range (IQR)), according to the Kolmogorov–Smirnov test. Categorical variables were presented as absolute frequencies and percentages. The Pearson $\chi2$ test was used to compare frequencies and comparisons of miRNA levels were analyzed using the Mann–Whitney U test or the Student t-test, as appropriate.

Cox regression analyses were performed to investigate the association of each miRNA with the risk of MACE.

Receiver operating characteristic curves were used to evaluate the predictive ability (expressed as c-indexes) of the original 2MACE score and the miRNA-modified ones. The cut-off point of each miRNA with the best combination of specificity and sensitivity was assessed by the Youden index. Comparisons of receiver operating characteristic curves were performed as described by DeLong et al. [16].

Discrimination and reclassification performances were evaluated by calculating the integrated discrimination improvement (IDI) and the net reclassification improvement (NRI), according to the methods of Pencina et al. [17].

The clinical usefulness and the net benefit of the original score in comparison with the miRNA-modified scores was estimated by using the decision curve analysis (DCA), as was proposed by Vickers et al. [18]. The DCA shows the clinical usefulness of each new model based on a continuum of potential thresholds for adverse events (x axis) and the net benefit of using the model to stratify patients at risk (y axis) relative to assuming that no patient will have an adverse event. Here, those models that are the farthest away from the slanted dashed line (i.e., assumes all MACEs) and the horizontal line (i.e., assumes no MACE) at a particular threshold probability demonstrate the higher net clinical benefit.

A p-value < 0.05 was accepted as statistically significant. Statistical analyses were performed using SPSS 21.0 (SPSS Inc., Chicago, IL, USA), MedCalc v. 16.4.3 (MedCalc Software bvba, Ostend, Belgium), STATA v. 12.0 (Stata Corp, College Station, TX, USA), and survIDINRI package for R v. 3.3.1 for Windows.

3. Results

3.1. Pilot Study

To test if miRNA levels were associated with the development of cardiovascular events, we firstly conducted a miRNA expression pattern analysis in plasma from 9 patients with and 10 patients without cardiovascular events. Since ischemic stroke is the classic main efficacy outcome in AF, we initially selected this endpoint to homogenize the samples. As shown in Supplementary Table S1, cases with stroke and controls without stroke were matched and no clinical differences between these two groups were observed. Of the 178 miRNAs on the panel, we selected those that were detected in all the samples (n = 110) for further analysis. Assuming the criteria of: (i) Fold change in log2 greater than 1.25 and (ii) a statistical significance level of 0.1, due to the limited number of samples; differences of plasma miRNA levels between cases and controls were found only for miR-22-3p and miR-107 (Figure 1). In addition to the two miRNAs selected from this pilot study, we also included miR-146a-5p in the validation study due to its role in the development of cardiovascular events in AF patients [19,20].

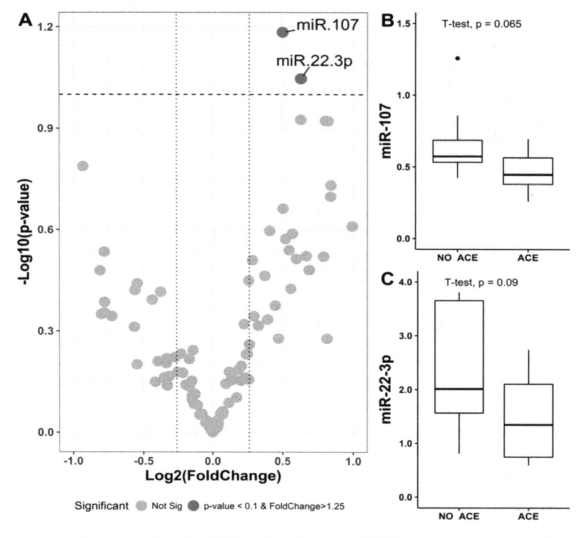

Figure 1. Levels and selection of miRNAs in the pilot study. (**A**) Volcano plot representing the fold change values in logarithm of base 2 (X-axis) and the *p*-values in logarithm of base 10 (Y-axis). (**B,C**) Box plots representing the miRNA levels selected for meeting the criteria of *p*-value less than 0.1 and fold change greater than 1.25. ACE = adverse cardiovascular events.

3.2. Validation Study

The three miRNAs selected were measured in 166 patients (47% male, median age 77 (IQR 70–81) years). The median CHA_2DS_2-VASc and HAS-BLED were 4 (IQR 3–5) and 2 (IQR 2–3), respectively, whereas the median 2MACE score was 2.5 (IQR 1–4). A summary of baseline clinical characteristics is shown in Table 1.

Table 1. Validation study cohort baseline clinical characteristics.

	Overall N = 166	Patients Without MACE N = 117	Patients with MACE N = 49	p
Demographic				
Male sex, n (%)	78 (47.0)	54 (46.2)	24 (49.0)	0.739
Age (years), median (IQR)	77 (70–81)	74 (68–79)	80 (77–84)	<0.001
Comorbidities, n (%)				
Hypertension	140 (84.3)	96 (82.1)	44 (89.8)	0.210
Diabetes mellitus	41 (24.7)	25 (21.4)	16 (32.7)	0.124
Heart failure	68 (41.0)	37 (31.6)	31 (63.3)	0.001
History of stroke/TIA/thromboembolism	32 (19.3)	17 (14.5)	15 (30.6)	0.016
Renal impairment	13 (7.8)	6 (5.1)	7 (14.3)	0.045
Coronary artery disease	36 (21.7)	22 (18.8)	14 (28.6)	0.163
Hypercholesterolemia	54 (32.5)	41 (35.0)	13 (26.5)	0.286
Current smoking habit	26 (15.7)	12 (10.3)	14 (28.6)	<0.01
Current alcohol consumption	3 (1.8)	3 (2.6)	0 (0.0)	0.622
History of previous bleeding	12 (7.2)	5 (4.3)	7 (14.3)	0.052
Concomitant treatment, n (%)				
Amiodarone	13 (7.8)	10 (8.5)	3 (6.1)	0.596
Digoxin	28 (16.9)	17 (14.5)	11 (22.4)	0.214
Calcium antagonist	41 (24.7)	24 (20.5)	17 (34.7)	0.053
Beta-blockers	53 (31.9)	39 (33.3)	14 (28.6)	0.548
Statins	35 (21.1)	27 (23.1)	8 (16.3)	0.331
Diuretics	81 (48.8)	52 (44.4)	29 (59.2)	0.083
Antiplatelet therapy	25 (15.1)	16 (13.7)	9 (18.4)	0.441
ACE inhibitors/ARBs	80 (48.2)	51 (43.6)	29 (59.2)	0.067
TTR at 6 months of entry, n (%)	80 (60–100)	80 (60–100)	80 (60–83)	0.250
CHA_2DS_2-VASc score, median (IQR)	4 (3–5)	4 (3–5)	5 (4–6)	<0.001
HAS-BLED score, median (IQR)	2 (2–3)	2 (2–3)	3 (2–3)	<0.001

ACE inhibitors = angiotensin-converting-enzyme inhibitors; ARBs = angiotensin II receptor blockers; IQR = interquartile range; TIA = transient ischemic attack; TTR = time in therapeutic range.

We first aimed to find an association between the levels of these three miRNAs and MACE in the cohort of 166 patients. During a median of 7.6 (IQR 5.4–8.0) years, 49 (29.5%; annual rate 3.88%/year) patients suffered a MACE. As shown in Table 2, all miRNAs were associated with the risk of MACE. Hence, miR-22-3p presented a hazard ratio (HR) of 1.07 (95% CI 1.02–1.14), miR-107 presented an HR of 3.66 (95% CI 1.19–11.24), and miR-146a-5p showed an inverse association with MACE, with an HR of 0.86 (95% CI 0.74–0.99).

Table 2. Crude risk of major adverse cardiovascular events (MACE) according to miRNAs.

	HR	95% CI	p-Value
miR-22-3p	1.07	1.02–1.14	0.013
miR-107	3.66	1.19–11.24	0.023
miR-146a-5p	0.86	0.74–0.99	0.042

HR = hazard ratio; CI = confidence interval.

When the predictive ability for MACE was tested, receiver operating characteristic (ROC)curve analyses demonstrated that miR-22-3p and miR-107 presented poor c-indexes (0.523; 95% CI 0.431–0.632 and 0.555; 95% CI 0.476–0.632, respectively) whereas miR-146a-5p exhibited a moderate c-index (0.656; 95% CI 0.578–0.728). In order to test if any of these miRNAs could enhance the predictive ability of the 2MACE score, we identified cut-off points with the best combination of sensitivity and specificity. The best cut-offs were 0.191, 0.137, and 1.979 for miR-22-3p, miR-107, and miR-146a-5p, respectively. Therefore, patients with miR-22-3p or miR-107 levels over the cut-off points and patients with miR-146a-5p levels under the cut-off point were categorized as being at "high risk" of MACE.

Combinations of miRNAs were then included in the 2MACE score, according to the previously established miRNA risk category. Thus, the addition of miR-107 and miR-146a-5p to the 2MACE significantly increased the predictive performance (c-indexes: 0.759 vs. 0.694, $p = 0.004$). Although miR-22-3p alone showed a poor c-index, we also tested a model with this miRNA in addition to miR-107 and miR-146a-5p into the 2MACE score. Similarly, this model also improved the predictive performance of the original 2MACE (0.762 vs. 0.694, $p = 0.012$). In both models of miRNAs, the sensitivity was also enhanced, as is shown by the results of IDI (Table 3, Figure 2).

Table 3. C-indexes, c-indexes comparison, integrated discrimination improvement (IDI), and net reclassification improvement (NRI) after the addition of miRNAs to the 2MACE score.

	C-index	95% CI	Z Score *	p *	IDI	95% CI	p	NRI	95% CI	p
2MACE	0.694	0.617–0.764								
+ miR-107 + miR-146a-5p	0.759	0.686–0.822	2.876	0.004	0.053	0.011/ 0.096	0.014	0.345	−0.327/ 0.518	0.736
+ miR-107 + miR-146a-5p+ miR-22-3p	0.762	0.689–0.825	2.518	0.012	0.056	0.012/ 0.101	0.015	0.047	−0.274/ 0.519	0.627

* for C-index comparison. CI = confidence interval; IDI = integrated discrimination improvement; NRI = net reclassification improvement.

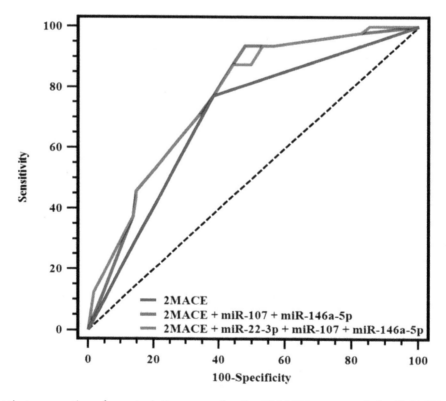

Figure 2. Receiver operating characteristic-curves for the 2MACE score and the 2MACE models with the addition of miRNAs.

Finally, a DCA was plotted, showing that both 2MACE models with the addition of miRNAs presented higher net benefit and clinical usefulness compared to the original 2MACE for a large threshold of probabilities (from 10 to 25% and 35 to 55%) (Figure 3).

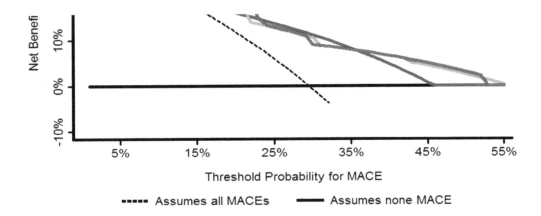

3. Decision curve analysis for the 2MACE score and the 2MACE models wi
ʼn of miRNAs. MACE = major adverse cardiovascular event.

Figure 3. Decision curve analysis for the 2MACE score and the 2MACE models with the addition of miRNAs. MACE = major adverse cardiovascular event.

4. Discussion

In this study including steadily anticoagulated AF patients taking VKAs, we observed that plasma levels of miR-22-3p, miR-107, and miR-146a-5p were associated with a higher risk of MACE. Importantly, the predictive ability of the 2MACE score for this event was enhanced with the addition of miRNAs.

During the last years, the interest of miRNAs in AF is increasing [21–23]. Despite most of the evidence suggesting a relationship of miRNAs with incident AF or recurrent AF after ablation [24–27], the therapeutic potential of miRNAs in AF has also emerged [28,29].

For example, miR-22-3p showed to play a role in several cardiovascular diseases [30]. Thus, a recent study has demonstrated that miR-22-3p plasma levels tend to be higher in patients with AF and a high CHA_2DS_2-VASc score. This suggests that this miRNA is more expressed in patients with high thromboembolic risk, which could provide some information about the pathophysiological conditions of AF patients [31]. Previously, elevated miR-22-3p serum levels have been shown in patients with heart failure, suggesting that high miR-22-3p circulating levels in serum may reflect intracellular levels in certain tissues and thus may explain the potential functional effect of the miRNA [32]. This is of particular importance since different in vivo models have shown that miR-22-3p overexpression promotes heart hypertrophy while downregulation protects mice from the pathology [33,34]. It is thus tempting to speculate that the higher levels of miR-22-3p in patients with MACE may induce a functional effect in tissues, still to be determined, and therefore may not act only as a mere biomarker of comorbidities.

In another recent study, miR-107 was investigated in AF patients undergoing catheter ablation. Although this miRNA was downregulated in sera from patients with AF recurrence compared to patients without AF recurrence, differences in expression were not significant [35]. However, the role of miR-107 in cardiovascular diseases is not well documented.

There is, however, more prognosis information regarding miR-146a-5p. A preliminary analysis of patients from this cohort at ~3 years of follow-up already showed an association of miR-146a-5p with adverse cardiovascular events (any of the following: Stroke/transient ischemic attack, systemic embolism, MI, and acute heart failure). In that study, lower levels of miR-146a-5p due to the presence of a functional single-nucleotide polymorphism rs2431697 were related to poor prognosis [20]. These data have been later confirmed at ~8 years, where miR-146a-5p was suggested as a regulator of neutrophil extracellular trap formation, and thus associated with cardiovascular risk [19]. Then, it could be hypothesized that dysregulation of miRNAs involved in inflammation may be associated with a higher risk of adverse events in patients with AF [36,37].

Nevertheless, the clinical usefulness of biomarkers when they are evaluated alone may be only limited. In fact, a common criticism of biomarkers is their high variability and lack of specificity in different clinical settings [38–40]. However, an advantage of miRNAs compared to other biomarkers is their plasma stability, which makes them less likely to be altered due to acute conditions [9,41], even though results from miRNAs levels should be interpreted with caution and contextualized according to clinical risk factors. In the present analysis, we considered this approach and included several miRNAs into the 2MACE score, which is a clinical score encompassing traditional risk factors for MI. In a similar way, a previous study also suggested that the use of a scoring system that would incorporate both circulating biomarkers and clinical factors might be more useful [42].

Limitations

There are some limitations that we aim to acknowledge. First, this study was performed in a single center, and it was composed of a Caucasian-based population. Second, all patients were hemodynamically stable and had good anticoagulation control during the previous 6 months after entry, in an attempt to homogenize the sample and avoid the potential impact of acute conditions or poor anticoagulation control in the development of adverse events. Therefore, our results might not be extrapolated to different clinically contexts. In addition, our study is limited only to AF patients treated with VKAs, since all patients were under this therapy at inclusion. Although VKAs are still the most commonly prescribed oral anticoagulants in Spain, the use of direct-acting oral anticoagulants (DOACs) is increasing worldwide. Thus, our results require further validation in AF patients under VKAs and DOACs in order to broaden their clinical usefulness. Finally, we only measured miRNAs at inclusion, and no other determinations have been performed throughout the follow-up. Comorbidities change over time and how miRNAs could evolve during the follow-up period has not been determined. For the above reason, further studies are warranted to confirm our results.

5. Conclusions

In this study including AF patients taking VKAs, we found that higher miR-22-3p and miR-107 and lower miR-146a-5p plasma levels were associated with higher risk of MACE at follow-up. The addition of these miRNAs to the 2MACE score significantly increased the predictive performance for MACE and enhanced its clinical usefulness. A combination of miRNAs and clinical risk factors could aid to some extent in the decision-making process about risk stratification in patients with AF.

Author Contributions: Data curation, J.M.R.-C. and R.T.-M.; formal analysis, J.M.R.-C. and R.T.-M.; funding acquisition, R.G.-C. and C.M.; investigation, A.M.d.l.R.-G., S.Á., and M.P.F.-P.; methodology, R.C.-R., J.A.C.-M., L.Ž.-M., and N.G.-B.; resources, L.R.-G.; supervision, R.G.-C. and C.M.; writing–original draft, J.M.R.-C. and R.T.-M.; writing–review and editing, V.R., V.V., F.M., R.G.-C., and C.M. All authors have read and agreed to the published version of the manuscript.

References

1. Lip, G.; Freedman, B.; de Caterina, R.; Potpara, T.S. Stroke prevention in atrial fibrillation: Past, present and future. Comparing the guidelines and practical decision-making. *Thromb. Haemost.* **2017**, *117*, 1230–1239. [CrossRef] [PubMed]

2. Hindricks, G.; Potpara, T.; Dagres, N.; Arbelo, E.; Bax, J.J.; Blomström-Lundqvist, C.; Boriani, G.; Castella, M.; Dan, G.A.; Dilaveris, P.E.; et al. 2020 ESC Guidelines for the diagnosis and management of atrial fibrillation developed in collaboration with the European Association of Cardio-Thoracic Surgery (EACTS). *Eur. Heart J.* **2020**. [CrossRef] [PubMed]

3. Khan, A.A.; Lip, G.Y.H. The prothrombotic state in atrial fibrillation: Pathophysiological and management implications. *Cardiovasc. Res.* **2019**, *115*, 31–45. [CrossRef] [PubMed]

4. Violi, F.; Soliman, E.Z.; Pignatelli, P.; Pastori, D. Atrial fibrillation and myocardial infarction: A systematic review and appraisal of pathophysiologic mechanisms. *J. Am. Heart Assoc.* **2016**, *5*, e003347. [CrossRef] [PubMed]

5. Pastori, D.; Farcomeni, A.; Poli, D.; Antonucci, E.; Angelico, F.; Del Ben, M.; Cangemi, R.; Tanzilli, G.; Lip, G.Y.; Pignatelli, P.; et al. Cardiovascular risk stratification in patients with non-valvular atrial fibrillation: The 2MACE score. *Intern. Emerg. Med.* **2016**, *11*, 199–204. [CrossRef] [PubMed]

6. Polovina, M.; Đikić, D.; Vlajković, A.; Vilotijević, M.; Milinković, I.; Ašanin, M.; Ostojić, M.; Coats, A.J.S.; Seferović, P.M. Adverse cardiovascular outcomes in atrial fibrillation: Validation of the new 2MACE risk score. *Int. J. Cardiol.* **2017**, *249*, 191–197. [CrossRef]

7. Rivera-Caravaca, J.M.; Marín, F.; Esteve-Pastor, M.A.; Raña-Míguez, P.; Anguita, M.; Muñiz, J.; Cequier, Á.; Bertomeu-Martínez, V.; Valdés, M.; Vicente, V.; et al. Usefulness of the 2MACE score to predicts adverse cardiovascular events in patients with atrial fibrillation. *Am. J. Cardiol.* **2017**, *120*, 2176–2181. [CrossRef]

8. Halushka, P.V.; Goodwin, A.J.; Halushka, M.K. Opportunities for microRNAs in the crowded field of cardiovascular biomarkers. *Annu. Rev. Pathol.* **2019**, *14*, 211–238. [CrossRef]

9. Viereck, J.; Thum, T. Circulating Noncoding RNAs as Biomarkers of Cardiovascular Disease and Injury. *Circ. Res.* **2017**, *120*, 381–399. [CrossRef]

10. Vrijens, K.; Bollati, V.; Nawrot, T.S. MicroRNAs as potential signatures of environmental exposure or effect: A systematic review. *Environ. Health Perspect.* **2015**, *123*, 399–411. [CrossRef]

11. Mitchell, P.S.; Parkin, R.K.; Kroh, E.M.; Fritz, B.R.; Wyman, S.K.; Pogosova-Agadjanyan, E.L.; Peterson, A.; Noteboom, J.; O'Briant, K.C.; Allen, A.; et al. Circulating microRNAs as stable blood-based markers for cancer detection. *Proc. Natl. Acad. Sci. USA* **2008**, *105*, 10513–10518. [CrossRef] [PubMed]

12. Jakob, P.; Kacprowski, T.; Briand-Schumacher, S.; Heg, D.; Klingenberg, R.; Stähli, B.E.; Jaguszewski, M.; Rodondi, N.; Nanchen, D.; Räber, L.; et al. Profiling and validation of circulating microRNAs for cardiovascular events in patients presenting with ST-segment elevation myocardial infarction. *Eur. Heart J.* **2017**, *38*, 511–515. [CrossRef] [PubMed]

13. Rizzacasa, B.; Morini, E.; Mango, R.; Vancheri, C.; Budassi, S.; Massaro, G.; Maletta, S.; Macrini, M.; D'Annibale, S.; Romeo, F.; et al. MiR-423 is differentially expressed in patients with stable and unstable coronary artery disease: A pilot study. *PLoS ONE* **2019**, *14*, e0216363. [CrossRef] [PubMed]

14. Barraclough, J.Y.; Joan, M.; Joglekar, M.V.; Hardikar, A.A.; Patel, S. MicroRNAs as prognostic markers in acute coronary syndrome patients—A systematic review. *Cells* **2019**, *8*, 1572. [CrossRef]

15. Manna, I.; Iaccino, E.; Dattilo, V.; Barone, S.; Vecchio, E.; Mimmi, S.; Filippelli, E.; Demonte, G.; Polidoro, S.; Granata, A.; et al. Exosome-associated miRNA profile as a prognostic tool for therapy response monitoring in multiple sclerosis patients. *FASEB J.* **2018**, *32*, 4241–4246. [CrossRef] [PubMed]

16. DeLong, E.R.; DeLong, D.M.; Clarke-Pearson, D.L. Comparing the areas under two or more correlated receiver operating characteristic curves: A nonparametric approach. *Biometrics* **1988**, *44*, 837–845. [CrossRef]

17. Pencina, M.J.; D'Agostino, R.B., Sr.; D'Agostino, R.B., Jr.; Vasan, R.S. Evaluating the added predictive ability of a new marker: From area under the ROC curve to reclassification and beyond. *Stat. Med.* **2008**, *27*, 157–172. [CrossRef]

18. Vickers, A.J.; Elkin, E.B. Decision curve analysis: A novel method for evaluating prediction models. *Med. Decis. Mak.* **2006**, *26*, 565–574. [CrossRef]

19. Arroyo, A.B.; de Los Reyes-García, A.M.; Rivera-Caravaca, J.M.; Valledor, P.; García-Barberá, N.; Roldán, V.; Vicente, V.; Martínez, C.; González-Conejero, R. MiR-146a regulates neutrophil extracellular trap formation that predicts adverse cardiovascular events in patients with atrial fibrillation. *Arterioscler. Thromb. Vasc. Biol.* **2018**, *38*, 892–902. [CrossRef]

20. Roldán, V.; Arroyo, A.B.; Salloum-Asfar, S.; Manzano-Fernández, S.; García-Barberá, N.; Marín, F.; Vicente, V.; González-Conejero, R.; Martínez, C. Prognostic role of MIR146A polymorphisms for cardiovascular events in atrial fibrillation. *Thromb. Haemost.* **2014**, *112*, 781–788. [CrossRef]

21. Komal, S.; Yin, J.J.; Wang, S.H.; Huang, C.Z.; Tao, H.L.; Dong, J.Z.; Han, S.N.; Zhang, L.R. MicroRNAs: Emerging biomarkers for atrial fibrillation. *J. Cardiol.* **2019**, *74*, 475–482. [CrossRef] [PubMed]

22. Franco, D.; Aranega, A.; Dominguez, J.N. Non-coding RNAs and atrial fibrillation. *Adv. Exp. Med. Biol.* **2020**, *1229*, 311–325. [CrossRef] [PubMed]

23. Jiang, S.; Guo, C.; Zhang, W.; Che, W.; Zhang, J.; Zhuang, S.; Wang, Y.; Zhang, Y.; Liu, B. The integrative regulatory network of circRNA, microRNA, and mRNA in Atrial Fibrillation. *Front. Genet.* **2019**, *10*, 526. [CrossRef] [PubMed]

24. Briasoulis, A.; Sharma, S.; Telila, T.; Mallikethi-Reddy, S.; Papageorgiou, N.; Oikonomou, E.; Tousoulis, D. MicroRNAs in Atrial Fibrillation. *Curr. Med. Chem.* **2019**, *26*, 855–863. [CrossRef]

25. da Silva, A.M.; de Araújo, J.N.; de Freitas, R.C.; Silbiger, V.N. Circulating MicroRNAs as potential biomarkers of atrial fibrillation. *BioMed. Res. Int.* **2017**, *2017*, 7804763. [CrossRef]

26. Kapodistrias, N.; Theocharopoulou, G.; Vlamos, P. A hypothesis of circulating MicroRNAs' implication in high incidence of atrial fibrillation and other electrocardiographic abnormalities in cancer patients. *Adv. Exp. Med. Biol.* **2020**, *1196*, 1–9. [CrossRef]

27. Zhang, P.P.; Sun, J.; Li, W. Genome-wide profiling reveals atrial fibrillation-related circular RNAs in atrial appendages. *Gene* **2020**, *728*, 144286. [CrossRef]

28. Xu, X.; Zhao, Z.; Li, G. The therapeutic potential of MicroRNAs in Atrial Fibrillation. *Mediat. Inflamm.* **2020**, *2020*, 3053520. [CrossRef]

29. Lozano-Velasco, E.; Garcia-Padilla, C.; Aránega, A.E.; Franco, D. Genetics of Atrial Fibrilation: In search of novel therapeutic targets. *Cardiovasc. Hematol. Disord. Drug Targets* **2019**, *19*, 183–194. [CrossRef]

30. Huang, Z.P.; Wang, D.Z. miR-22 in cardiac remodeling and disease. *Trends Cardiovasc. Med.* **2014**, *24*, 267–272. [CrossRef]

31. Kiyosawa, N.; Watanabe, K.; Morishima, Y.; Yamashita, T.; Yagi, N.; Arita, T.; Otsuka, T.; Suzuki, S. Exploratory analysis of circulating miRNA signatures in Atrial Fibrillation patients determining potential biomarkers to support decision-making in anticoagulation and catheter ablation. *Int. J. Mol. Sci.* **2020**, *21*, 2444. [CrossRef] [PubMed]

32. Goren, Y.; Kushnir, M.; Zafrir, B.; Tabak, S.; Lewis, B.S.; Amir, O. Serum levels of microRNAs in patients with heart failure. *Eur. J. Heart Fail.* **2012**, *14*, 147–154. [CrossRef] [PubMed]

33. Huang, Z.P.; Chen, J.; Seok, H.Y.; Zhang, Z.; Kataoka, M.; Hu, X.; Wang, D.Z. MicroRNA-22 regulates cardiac hypertrophy and remodeling in response to stress. *Circ. Res.* **2013**, *112*, 1234–1243. [CrossRef] [PubMed]

34. Xu, X.D.; Song, X.W.; Li, Q.; Wang, G.K.; Jing, Q.; Qin, Y.W. Attenuation of microRNA-22 derepressed PTEN to effectively protect rat cardiomyocytes from hypertrophy. *J. Cell. Physiol.* **2012**, *227*, 1391–1398. [CrossRef] [PubMed]

35. Kiliszek, M.; Maciak, K.; Maciejak, A.; Krzyżanowski, K.; Wierzbowski, R.; Gora, M.; Burzynska, B.; Segiet, A.; Skrobowski, A. Serum microRNA in patients undergoing atrial fibrillation ablation. *Sci. Rep.* **2020**, *10*, 4424. [CrossRef]

36. Li, Y.; Tan, W.; Ye, F.; Wen, S.; Hu, R.; Cai, X.; Wang, K.; Wang, Z. Inflammation as a risk factor for stroke in atrial fibrillation: Data from a microarray data analysis. *J. Int. Med Res.* **2020**, *48*. [CrossRef]

37. Zhang, Y.; Shen, H.; Wang, P.; Min, J.; Yu, Y.; Wang, Q.; Wang, S.; Xi, W.; Nguyen, Q.M.; Xiao, J.; et al. Identification and characterization of circular RNAs in atrial appendage of patients with atrial fibrillation. *Exp. Cell Res.* **2020**, *389*, 111821. [CrossRef]

38. Camelo-Castillo, A.; Rivera-Caravaca, J.M.; Marín, F.; Vicente, V.; Lip, G.Y.H.; Roldán, V. Predicting adverse events beyond stroke and bleeding with the ABC-stroke and ABC-bleeding scores in patients with atrial fibrillation: The murcia AF project. *Thromb. Haemost.* **2020**, *120*, 1200–1207. [CrossRef]

39. Rivera-Caravaca, J.M.; Esteve-Pastor, M.A. Heart failure and cardiac events: Is a consecutive measurement of biomarkers a simple and practical approach? *Thromb. Haemost.* **2019**, *119*, 1891–1893. [CrossRef]

40. Esteve-Pastor, M.A.; Roldán, V.; Rivera-Caravaca, J.M.; Ramírez-Macías, I.; Lip, G.Y.H.; Marín, F. The use of biomarkers in clinical management guidelines: A critical appraisal. *Thromb. Haemost.* **2019**, *119*, 1901–1919. [CrossRef]

41. Wang, Y.; Liu, B. Circular RNA in diseased heart. *Cells* **2020**, *9*, 1240. [CrossRef] [PubMed]

42. Ioannou, A.; Papageorgiou, N.; Falconer, D.; Rehal, O.; Sewart, E.; Zacharia, E.; Toutouzas, K.; Vlachopoulos, C.; Siasos, G.; Tsioufis, C.; et al. Biomarkers associated with stroke risk in Atrial Fibrillation. *Curr. Med. Chem.* **2019**, *26*, 803–823. [CrossRef] [PubMed]

2

Accuracy of Commonly-Used Imaging Modalities in Assessing Left Atrial Appendage for Interventional Closure

Ramez Morcos [1], Haider Al Taii [2], Priya Bansal [2], Joel Casale [1], Rupesh Manam [1], Vikram Patel [1], Anthony Cioci [3], Michael Kucharik [3], Arjun Malhotra [4] and Brijeshwar Maini [5,*]

[1]   Department of Internal Medicine, Florida Atlantic University, Boca Raton, FL 33431, USA; morcos.ramez@gmail.com (R.M.); jcasale3@health.fau.edu (J.C.); rmanam@health.fau.edu (R.M.); patelv@health.fau.edu (V.P.)

[2]   Department of Cardiovascular Diseases, Florida Atlantic University, Boca Raton, FL 33431, USA; haltaii@health.fau.edu (H.A.T.); Pbansal@health.fau.edu (P.B.)

[3]   College of Medicine, Florida Atlantic University, Boca Raton, FL 33431, USA; acioci@health.fau.edu (A.C.); mkucharik2016@health.fau.edu (M.K.)

[4]   University of Miami, Coral Gables, FL 33124, USA; a.malhotra2@umiami.edu

[5]   Tenet Florida & Department of Cardiovascular Diseases, Florida Atlantic University, Boca Raton, FL 33431, USA

*   Correspondence: brijmaini1@gmail.com;

Abstract: Periprocedural imaging assessment for percutaneous Left Atrial Appendage (LAA) transcatheter occlusion can be obtained by utilizing different imaging modalities including fluoroscopy, magnetic resonance imaging (MRI), computed tomography (CT), and ultrasound imaging. Given the complex and variable morphology of the left atrial appendage, it is crucial to obtain the most accurate LAA dimensions to prevent intra-procedural device changes, recapture maneuvers, and prolonged procedure time. We therefore sought to examine the accuracy of the most commonly utilized imaging modalities in LAA occlusion. Institutional Review Board (IRB) approval was waived as we only reviewed published data. By utilizing PUBMED which is an integrated online website to list the published literature based on its relevance, we retrieved thirty-two articles on the accuracy of most commonly used imaging modalities for pre-procedural assessment of the left atrial appendage morphology, namely, two-dimensional transesophageal echocardiography, three-dimensional transesophageal echocardiography, computed tomography, and three-dimensional printing. There is strong evidence that real-time three-dimensional transesophageal echocardiography is more accurate than two-dimensional transesophageal echocardiography. Three-dimensional computed tomography has recently emerged as an imaging modality and it showed exceptional accuracy when merged with three-dimensional printing technology. However, real time three-dimensional transesophageal echocardiography may be considered the preferred imaging modality as it can provide accurate measurements without requiring radiation exposure or contrast administration. We will present the most common imaging modality used for LAA assessment and will provide an algorithmic approach including preprocedural, periprocedural, intraprocedural, and postprocedural.

Keywords: left atrial appendage; WATCHMAN occlusive device; 2D transesophageal echocardiography; 3D transesophageal echocardiography; computerized tomography

1. Introduction

Atrial Fibrillation (AF) is a major burden on public health, it is estimated to be the cause of $\geq 15\%$ of all strokes in the United States, and >100,000–125,000 embolic strokes per year, of which >20% are fatal [1]. AF risk factors, pathogenesis, prevention, and treatment are beyond the scope of this review. We will focus on the classification when patients may or may not have valvular heart disease. The distinction still an area of debate. Valvular AF is the terminology used in those patients who have heart valve disorder or a prosthetic heart valve. Nonvalvular AF is generally referred in those patients who have other etiology causing the AF. The rapid and chaotic heartbeats restrict the left atrium from pumping the blood properly, which may cause it to pool and form a clot. More than 90% of thrombi in AF is formed in the left atrial appendage (LAA) [2]. The standard treatment for AF is heart rate or rhythm control and stroke prevention. Prophylactic anticoagulation is the gold standard to prevent embolic strokes in AF patients with CHADS-VASC score greater than or equal to two. For many years there has been no alternative treatment available to prevent strokes in AF patients who have high risk of bleeding and only 50–60% are therapeutically anticoagulated which make the effective long-term anticoagulation very challenging [3].

In 2001 a successful percutaneous implantation of a device to occlude the LAA cavity was done in a patient with non-valvular AF to prevent embolism [4]. Interventional closure of the LAA employing the Watchman device (Boston Scientific) was shown to be non-inferior to Oral anticoagulation (OAC) in randomized trials and has since been approved in the United States and Europe [5]. The LAA exhibits complex anatomy that commonly varies morphologically among different individuals. Post-mortem analysis of 100 left atrial appendages has demonstrated significant variability in appendage shape, dimensions, and the number of lobes presents [6]. Therefore, accurate visualization of the LAA and appreciation of its morphological considerations is an essential step in occlusion procedures. Specifically, accurately measuring the dimensions of the LAA ostium, landing zone, and maximum length of the main anchoring lobe is necessary for selecting an adequately sized occlusion device successful device placement [4]. Choosing a device that is too small increases the risk of device instability and peri-device leakage, whereas selecting a device that is too large increases the risk of LAA perforation and cardiac tamponade [7,8]. Additionally, improper device selection can result in intra-procedural device changes and recapture maneuvers and increasing length of the procedure [9].

We present a review on the most commonly used imaging modality for pre-procedural planning and assessment of the LAA morphology, which include 2D Transesophageal echocardiography (2D TEE), 3D Transesophageal echocardiography (3D TEE), Computed tomography (CT), and 3D Printing (3DP).

1.1. 3D TEE Modality Is Superior to 2D TEE

2D TEE has been the most commonly used imaging modality for pre-procedural planning. However, three-dimensional multiplanar transesophageal electrocardiography is a more accurate alternative to 2D TEE in the assessment of the LAA morphology. Advantages of 3D TEE vs. 2D TEE are illustrated in (Table 1), and comparative studies using 3D TEE are illustrated in (Table 2).

Zhou et al. found 3D TEE to be more accurate than 2D TEE for measuring the LAA Landing zone, LAA depth, and LAA ostial dimensions, LAA morphology after the occlusion device deployment, and visualizing any residual shunts around the entire device in one more view. In the Zhou et al. study, a residual shunt of less than 1mm was identified in three cases by 3D TEE and only once by 2D TEE [7]. Salzman et al. determined that area-derived diameter (ADD) and perimeter-derived diameter (PDD) measurements obtained via 3D TEE correlated well with the occlusion device size chosen in the procedure. Furthermore, the 3D landing zone measurements demonstrated a higher reproducibility relative to 2D TEE [8].

Yosefi et al. found that RT3DTEE provides more accurate measurements of the maximal LAA orifice than 2D TEE. 2D TEE significantly undersized the diameter of the LAA orifice relative to RT3DTEE, when compared to CT [10]. Nucifora et al. found that RT3DTEE is in more significant agreement with the dimensions obtained from CT as demonstrated by smaller bias and narrower limits of agreement with CT. Therefore, these authors believe that RT3DTEE may be the preferred imaging modality to assess LAA dimensions as it can provide accurate measurements of the LAA without requiring radiation exposure or contrast administration [11].

The real-time 3DTEE method is a feasible, fast way to assess the LAA number of lobes, the area of the orifice, maximal LAA diameter, minimum LAA diameter, and LAA depth with similar accuracy to RT3DTEE and CT according to a study published by Yosefy et al. Real-time 3DTEE consists of converting a 3DTEE image into three 2D planes (X,Y,Z), at which time a 360 degree rotational in the sagittal plane creates a single "stop shop" image that displays all aspects of the LAA morphology including number of lobes, orifice area, and maximal and minimal diameter [12]. Nakajima et al. determined that 3D TEE could accurately visualize LAA morphological variations. They studied 55 patients in normal sinus rhythm and 52 patients with atrial fibrillation. 3D TEE provides adequate 3D full volume images of all patients in NSR, whereas sufficient images were obtained in 94.6% of patients with AF using zoom mode. Excellent correlation was found between full volume mode and zoom mode [13].

Table 1. Advantages of 3D TEE vs. 2D TEE.

Author	Advantages of 3D TEE vs. 2D TEE	Study
Zhou et al.	-More accurate measuring of Landing zone and depth -More significant association between the closure device -Displaying cross-sectional images from any angle using Flexi Slice mode -Useful in displaying the LAA morphology after the occlusion device deployed -Visualizing any residual shunts around the entire device in one more view	[7]
Salzman et al.	-Producing (ADD) and (PDD) measurements of the LAA ostium -3D landing zone measurements demonstrated a higher reproducibility	[8]
Yosefi et al.	-3DTEE is a feasible, fast way to assess LAA morphology with similar accuracy to RT3DTEE and CT	[10]
Nucifora et al.	-RT3DTEE more significant agreement with the dimensions obtained from CT -RT3DTEE Provide accurate measurements without radiation exposure or contrast	[11]
Yosefi et al.	-RT3DTEE provides more accurate measurements of the maximal LAA orifice	[12]
Nakajima et al.	-Accurately visualize LAA morphological variations -Excellent correlation was found between full volume mode and zoom mode	[13]

Table 2. Literature review summary table for 3D TEE vs. 2D TEE in the preprocedural assessment of the left atrial appendage.

Ref	Author	Country	Date (mm/dd)	Objective	Study	Result/Outcome	Conclusion
[7]	Zhou et al.	China	01/17	To determine the clinical values of RT-3D TEE in the peri-procedure of LAA closure.	Observational study, of 38 patients conducted real-time 3D TEE (3D TEE) of the LAA for all subjects	-The landing zone dimension of LAA revealed by 2D TEE, showed statistical difference compared with the dimensions obtained from the 3D TEE -No statistical difference was noticed in the landing zone values of 3D TEE compared with that of X-ray -No statistical difference was noticed in the landing zone values of 3D TEE compared with that of X-ray	RT-3D TEE has better visualization of the LAA compared with 2D TEE.
[8]	Salzman et al.	Germany	07/17	To establish measurements based on 3D TEE imaging that would be most helpful in achieving successful cardiovascular intervention	Retrospective study analyzed 55 patient who underwent LAA occlusion using Watchman	ADD) and perimeter-derived diameter (PDD) from 3D TEE can reduce intra-procedural recapture maneuvers, peridevice leakage, and device size changes compared with two-dimensional (2D) measurements.	3D ADD and PDD may help with reducing intraprocedural recapture maneuvers, device size changes, and peridevice leakage.
[10]	Yosefi et al.	Israel	01/16	Compared RT3DTEE and 2DTEE versus CT when measuring LAA dimensions	Prospective study of 30 patients compared RT 3D TEE and 2D TEE versus 64 slice CT for measuring LAA dimensions	No difference was found between LAA depth using RT 3D TEE (19.5 ± 2.3 mm) vs. CT (19.6 ± 2.3, P = NS) and 2D TEE (19.4 ± 2.2 mm) vs. CT (P = NS). However, RT 3D TEE (24.5 ± 4.7 mm) vs. CT (24.6 ± 5, P = NS) was more accurate in measuring maximal LAA diameter compared to 2D TEE (23.5 ± 3.9 mm) vs. CT ($P < 0.01$).	RT3DTEE provides more accurate measurements of the maximal LAA orifice than 2D TEE.
[11]	Nucifora et al.	Switzerland	09/11	The accuracy of the measurements obtained via 2DTEE and RT3DTEE were subsequently compared against measurements obtained via CT.	Prospective study of 137 patients who underwent 2DTEE, RT3DTEE, and CT to measure the dimensions of the LAA orifice	-Compared to CT, both 2DTEE and RT3DTEE underestimated LAA dimensions. -RT3DTEE was found to be in greater agreement with the dimensions obtained from CT as demonstrated by smaller bias and narrower limits of agreement with CT	RT3DTEE may be the preferable imaging modality to assess LAA dimensions.

Table 2. *Cont.*

Ref	Author	Country	Date (mm/dd)	Objective	Study	Result/Outcome	Conclusion
[12]	Yosefi et al.	Israel	09/16	To validate the accuracy of Rotational 3DTEE versus RT3DTEE when assessing LAA	Prospective study of 41 patients who underwent a rotational 3D TEE	Rotational 3D TEE measurements of LAA were not statistically different from RT3DTEE and from 64-slice CT regarding Rotational 3D TEE is achieved by rotating the sagittal plane (in the green box, x-plane) 360° and allows for a faster method of achieving necessary LAA measurements.	Choosing the appropriate device size for LAA closure can be achieved by Rotational 3DTEE ("Yosefy rotation").
[13]	Nakajima et al.	Japan	09/10	To determined if 3D TEE could accurately visualize LAA morphological variations	Prospective od 107 patients, 55 were in SR in whom 3DTEE. 52 were in Afib, zoom-mode imaging was used.	3D TEE proviced adequate 3D full volume images of all patients in NSR, whereas adequate images were obtained in 94.6% of patients with AF using zoom mode. Excellent correlation was found between full volume mode and zoom mode.	3D TEE is a reliable modality when evaluating LAA geometry and LAA characteristics.

1.2. CT Is More Accurate Than TEE

CT has been considered the gold standard for visualizing the LAA for its ability to acquire 3D volumetric data of the LAA at various points in the cardiac cycle [4]. However, it has only recently emerged as an imaging modality for sizing the LAA before occlusion and for post-procedural evaluation of residual peri-device shunts. Although TEE remains the most commonly used imaging modality for sizing the LAA, CT may be the most accurate imaging modality. Yosefy et al. compared 2D TEE to CT and found 2D TEE to be non-inferior to CT for determining LAA area and volume. Additionally, Yosefy et al. found that of 30 patients who underwent routine TEE examination and CT in the workup of PE, RT3DTEE was found to yield measurements not significantly different than CT for the number of LAA lobes, LAA depth, LAA internal area, and LAA maximal and minimal diameter. They concluded that 3DTEE might be more practical for sizing the LAA due to its accuracy, lack of radiation, and bedside capabilities [10]. In contrast, other studies have demonstrated that measurements obtained via TEE and CT are not interchangeable and may result in clinically significant consequences. One such study by Sievert et al. showed that LAA sizing by 2D TEE alone might result in the selection of a closure device that is undersized by 20–40% [2]. Advantages of CT are illustrated in (Table 3), and comparative studies using CT are illustrated in (Table 4).

MSCT is a more accurate tool in selecting proper LAA closure device size than the conventionally used TEE according to the study by Chow et al. [14] 2D-TEE measurements of orifice size are not interchangeable with those obtained via CT according to a study by Rawjani et al. The researchers concluded that due to the irregular and eccentric nature of the LAA orifice, obtaining mean orifice diameter measurements may be more accurate than planar maximal diameters for sizing circular occluder devices [15].

In the study by Wang et al. patients who underwent advanced CT imaging at this site required 1.245 devices per implantation attempt with 100% success rate, compared to patients in the first half of the PROTECT AF study who averaged 1.8 devices used per implantation attempt with an 82% success rate. Accurate sizing of the LAA landing zone is critical in successful implantation of the WATCHMAN, and this study suggests high-resolution volumetric imaging with CT should be preferred over TEE [9].

Budge et al. determined that measurements obtained via CTsb, CTp, and TEE are not interchangeable. CTsb was found to yield larger mean orifice diameters than both TEE and CTp, which produced similar mean orifice diameters. It was speculated that this was due to foreshortening associated with 2D modalities. Furthermore, when compared to TEE, both CT modalities yielded larger ostial measurements for small LAA orifices and smaller ostial measurements for larger LAA orifices within this cohort [16].

Table 3. Advantages of CT when assessing the left atrial appendage.

Author	Advantages of CT	Study
Chow et al.	-Allows more accurate assessment of the LAA ostium and landing zone. -Allows higher appreciation for the morphology of the LAA and surrounding structures	[14]
Rawjani et al.	-device sizing by CT-derived mean diameter was in most agreement with the actual device implanted -Better in detection and avoidance of sizing error by 2D TOE	[15]
Wang et al.	-WATCHMAN device selection was 100% accurate when selected by CT imaging -Provides a comprehensive assessment for LAA which is accurate	[9]
Budge et al.	-Provides accurate sizing of LAA occlusion devices	[16]

Table 4. Literature review summary table of CT imaging in the preprocedural assessment of the left atrial appendage.

Ref	Author	Country	Date (mm/dd)	Objective	Study	Result/Outcome	Conclusion
[14]	Chow et al.	Denmark	06/17	To compare available LAA imaging and sizing modalities which lead to successful LAA closure	Retrospective, 67 patients who underwent preprocedural MSCT and 2D TEE for LAA closure device sizing from 2014 to 2016	MSCT resulted in correct LAA sizing in 83% of patients, whereas 2D TEE would have produced in only 57% proper sizing	CT derived PD mean diameter may be the optimal measurement for sizing 'closed-ended' devices (Amulet and WATCHMANFLX) whereas CT derived maximal diameter is more accurate for sizing 'open-ended' devices (WATCHMAN)
[15]	Rawjani et al.	Australia	12/17	To evaluate the use of CT, procedural safety, and outcomes for percutaneous LAA closure	A registry between July 2010 and December 2015 was prospectively established for individuals undergoing LAA closure	2D TEE sizing resulted in gross sizing errors in 3.4% of cases. 2D-TEE measurements resulted in device selection that was 3mm smaller than those from CT measurements	CT has excellent outcomes for procedural safety with absence of major residual leak
[9]	Wang et al.	USA	11/16	To determine the role of 3DCT guided planning for LAA occlusion on the early operator WATCHMAN learning curve	Prospective study studied 53 patients who underwent 2D TEE, 3D TEE, and 3DCT for Watchman device qualification and sizing	53 patients underwent successful device implantation. Compared with 2D and 3D TEE sizing, 3D CT maximal width of the LAA landing zone was larger ($p \leq 0.0001$). Pearson correlation coefficient showed a significant difference when sizing by CT against TEE ($r < 0.001$)	3D CT is an excellent tool in advanced case planning for precise WATCHMAN device size selection in LAA closure procedures compared to standard 2D TEE
[16]	Budge et al.	USA	11/08	To compare multiple different imaging modalities to assess the morphology of the LAA in AF patients	Prospective study of 66 patients where measurement relationships of TEE to planar CT (CTp), CTp to 3D cardiac segmented CT (CTsg), and CTsg to TEE were compared	Similar to CTp, CTsg orifice values were usually slightly smaller than TEE for large orifices, and larger than TEE for smaller orifices. LAA orifice measurements among CTsg, CTp, and TEE are not interchangeable which is clinically significant because of the need of accurate sizing of LAA occlusion devices	CTsg, either alone or in conjunction with TEE measurements, could allow for more accurate initial device sizing

1.3. The Use of 3D Printing Can Facilitate LAA Occlusion

As more LAA occlusion procedures have been conducted, physicians have recognized the unique and diverse morphology of the LAA [17]. This anatomical intricacy may be deceptively portrayed in standardized diagnostic modalities such as 2D and 3D transesophageal echocardiography (TEE), which are the conventional pre-procedural image technique. 3D CT characterization may provide exceptional accuracy when merged with 3D printing technology. By creating a model customized to each patient's anatomy, a physical Watchman device (Boston Scientific, Marlborough, MA, USA) can be implanted ex vivo so that spatial navigation and geographic accuracy of the left atrium may be established before the cardiac catheterization procedure commences. The following findings show this modality technology applied and successively replicated. They also suggest 3D CT as the best imaging technique when establishing device size. Hell et al. [18] and Li et al. [19] supported the use of 3D printing while, Goiten et al. did not support it [20] (Table 5).

Hell et al. and Li et al. in prospective studies both found that 3D printing of LAA was a feasible mechanism of predicting correct Watchman devices. In the study conducted by Hell et al. Mean LAA ostium diameter based on TEE was 22 ± 4 mm and based on CT 25 ± 3 mm ($p = 0.014$) [18]. Similarly, Li et al. performed successful Watchman implantation in 21 patients based on 3D model printing (3DP). In this study, although all patients in both groups underwent successful device implantation, significant differences did occur. After the occlusion, TOE showed that three patients in the control group had mild residual shunting (two patients with a 2 mm residual shunt, one patient with a 4 mm residual shunt). No residual shunt was observed in the 3DP group. The procedure times, contrast agent volumes, and costs were 96.4 ± 12.5 vs. 101.2 ± 13.6 min, 22.6 ± 3.0 vs. 26.9 ± 6.2 mL, and 12,676.1 vs. 12,088.6 USD for the 3DP and control groups, respectively. Compared with the control group, the radiographic exposure was significantly reduced in the 3DP group (561.4 ± 25.3 vs. 651.6 ± 32.1 mGy, $p = 0.05$) [19].

Goiten et al. found that LAA printed 3D models were accurate for prediction of LAA device size for the Amulet device but not for the Watchman device. Two procedures were aborted due to mismatch between LAA and any Watchman device dimensions in which all three interventional cardiology physicians that were involved in the study predicted the failures using the printed 3D model. Although 3D prints were found to be more accurate for Amulet compared to Watchman, strong agreement among physicians was demonstrated for both devices (average intra-class correlation of 0.915 for Amulet and 0.816 for Watchman) [20].

Table 5. Literature review summary table of CT 3D printing in the preprocedural assessment of the left atrial appendage.

Ref	Author	Country	Date (mm/dd)	Objective	Study	Result/Outcome	Conclusion
[17]	Hell et al.	Europe	11/17	To determine If using 3D-printed LAA models based on CT will permit accurate device sizing	Prospective study of 22 patients who underwent pre-procedure TEE and CT examinations in which a 3D printed model was created based on the CT images and CT measurements recorded.	-Implantation was successful in all patients -In 95% of the patients (21/22), predicted device size based on simulated implantation in the 3D model was equal to the device ultimately implanted. TEE would have undersized the device in 45% of the patients (10/22) and device compression determined in the 3D-CT model corresponded closely with compression upon implantation of Watchman device ($r = 0.622$, $p = 0.003$).	CT 3D-printing models may assist with device selection and the prediction of device compression.
[18]	Li et al.	China	03/17	To assess 3DP feasibility using CT for LAA closure	Prospective study for 42 patients were randomly split into 2 groups, one that had 3D LAA model printing and a control group. For the control group, device size was was based on TEE, cardiac CT angiogram, and intraoperative LAA angiography only	The diameter of the occlusion devices used in the 3DP group and control group were 27.6 ± 2.4 mm (21–33 mm) and 26.3 ± 3.4 mm (21–33 mm), respectively. TOE showed that the compression ratios of the occlusion devices were $19.7\% \pm 0.8\%$ and $19.3 \pm 1.0\%$ ($p = 0.05$), respectively.	3DP enhance the work efficiency for LAA closure which is valuable for clinical application.
[19]	Goiten et al.	Israel	10/17	To determine the feasibility of MDCT when predicting the accurate size of device for LAA closure	Prospective study including 29 patients compared 3D LAA model printing for predicting occlusion device size based on pre-procedure CT scan Amplatzer Amulet (St. Jude Medical/Abbott) was deployed in 12 patients and the other 17 received the Watchman device	Two procedures were aborted due to mismatch between LAA and any Watchman device dimensions in which all three interventional cardiology physicians that were involved in the study predicted the failures using the printed 3D model According to Bland-Altman analysis, the average difference between the predicted Amulet size using the 3D LAA printed model and the inserted Amulet was 0.848 mm (95% limit of agreement (LOA): −4.215, 5.912). The average difference between the predicted Watchman size using the 3D print and the inserted Watchman was 0.956 mm (95% LOA: −6.534, 8.445)	LAA 3DP model is not accurate for prediction of LAA using WATCHMAN devi.

2. Algorithmic Approach for the WATCHMAN Procedural

Here, we will provide an algorithmic approach including preprocedural, periprocedural, intraprocedural, and postprocedural. (Figures 1 and 2) [21].

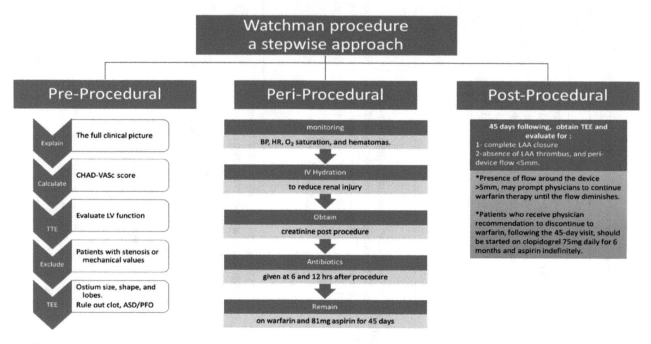

Figure 1. A stepwise approach for pre-, peri-, and post-procedure for the successful implantation of WATCHMAN device.

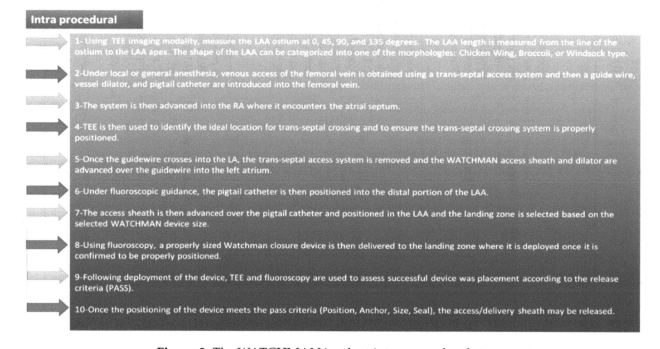

Figure 2. The WATCHMAN implant intra-procedural steps.

3. Pre-Procedural Assessment of the LAA

Here, we will provide the pre-procedural assessment of the LAA on 2D TEE, 3D TEE, and MDCT (Figure 3).

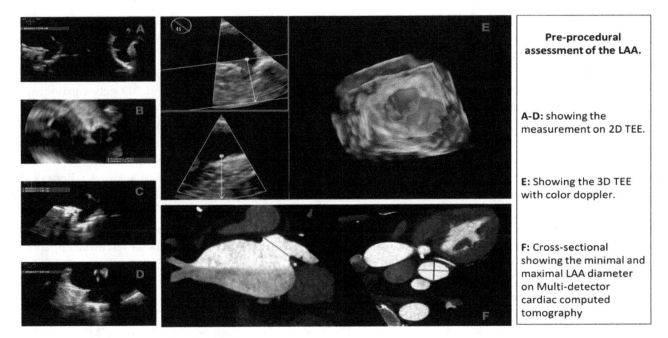

Figure 3. Pre-procedural assessment of the LAA using different imaging modalities.

4. Conclusions

Rotational three-dimensional transesophageal echocardiography is a more accurate alternative to two-dimensional transesophageal echocardiography in the assessment of the left atrial appendage morphology and has been the most commonly used imaging modality for sizing the left atrial appendage. Three-dimensional computed tomography has recently emerged as an imaging modality and it has showed exceptional accuracy when merged with three-dimensional printing technology. However, real-time three-dimensional transesophageal echocardiography may be considered the preferred imaging modality to assess left atrial appendage dimensions as it can provide accurate measurements without requiring radiation exposure or contrast administration (Table 6).

Table 6. Preprocedural imaging impact on predicting the correct size of the WATCHMAN device.

Imaging Modality	Impact on Implantation Success
2D TEE	Less accurate
3D TEE	Accurate without requiring radiation exposure or contrast administration
3D CT	Exceptional accuracy when merged with three-dimensional printing technology

Author Contributions: All authors contributed extensively to the work presented in this literature review. R.M. (Ramez Morcos) did the literature search, created the tables & the figures, and drafted the manuscript. H.T. & P.B. drafted the manuscript and provided revision. J.C., R.M. (Rupesh Manam) & V.P. drafted the manuscript. A.C., M.K. & A.M. collected the data, drafted the manuscript, and provided revisions. B.M. reviewed the manuscript and provided critical Revision.

References

1. Reiffel, J.A. Atrial fibrillation and stroke: Epidemiology. *Am. J. Med.* **2014**, *127*, e15–e16. [CrossRef] [PubMed]
2. Sievert, H.; Lesh, M.D.; Trepels, T.; Omran, H.; Bartorelli, A.; Della Bella, P.; Nakai, T.; Reisman, M.; DiMario, C.; Block, P.; et al. Percutaneous left atrial appendage transcatheter occlusion to prevent stroke in high-risk patients with atrial fibrillation: Early clinical experience. *Circulation* **2002**, *105*, 1887–1889. [CrossRef] [PubMed]

3. Go, A.S.; Hylek, E.M.; Borowsky, L.H.; Phillips, K.A.; Selby, J.V.; Singer, D.E. Warfarin use among ambulatory patients with nonvalvular atrial fibrillation: The anticoagulation and risk factors in atrial fibrillation (ATRIA) study. *Ann. Intern. Med.* **1999**, *131*, 927–934. [CrossRef] [PubMed]

4. Wunderlich, N.C.; Beigel, R.; Swaans, M.J.; Ho, S.Y.; Siegel, R.J. Percutaneous interventions for left atrial appendage exclusion: Options, assessment, and imaging using 2D and 3D echocardiography. *JACC Cardiovasc. Imaging* **2015**, *8*, 472–488. [CrossRef] [PubMed]

5. Holmes, D.R.; Reddy, V.Y.; Turi, Z.G.; Doshi, S.K.; Sievert, H.; Buchbinder, M.; Mulli, M.; Sick, P. Percutaneous closure of the left atrial appendage versus warfarin therapy for prevention of stroke in patients with atrial fibrillation: A randomised non-inferiority trial. *Lancet* **2009**, *374*, 534–542. [CrossRef]

6. Kamiński, R.; Kosiński, A.; Brala, M.; Piwko, G.; Lewicka, E.; Dąbrowska-Kugacka, A.; Raczak, G.; Kozłowski, D.; Grzybiak, M. Variability of the Left Atrial Appendage in Human Hearts. *PLoS ONE* **2015**, *10*, e0141901. [CrossRef] [PubMed]

7. Zhou, Q.; Song, H.; Zhang, L.; Deng, Q.; Chen, J.; Hu, B.; Wang, Y.; Guo, R. Roles of real-time three-dimensional transesophageal echocardiography in peri-operation of transcatheter left atrial appendage closure. *Medicine* **2017**, *96*, e5637. [CrossRef] [PubMed]

8. Schmidt-Salzmann, M.; Meincke, F.; Kreidel, F.; Spangenberg, T.; Ghanem, A.; Kuck, K.H.; Bergmann, M.W. Improved Algorithm for Ostium Size Assessment in Watchman Left Atrial Appendage Occlusion Using Three-Dimensional Echocardiography. *J. Invasive Cardiol.* **2017**, *29*, 232–238. [PubMed]

9. Wang, D.D.; Eng, M.; Kupsky, D.; Myers, E.; Forbes, M.; Rahman, M.; Zaidan, M.; Parikh, S.; Wyman, J.; Pantelic, M.; et al. Application of 3-Dimensional Computed Tomographic Image Guidance to WATCHMAN Implantation and Impact on Early Operator Learning Curve: Single-Center Experience. *JACC Cardiovasc. Interv.* **2016**, *9*, 2329–2340. [CrossRef] [PubMed]

10. Yosefy, C.; Laish-Farkash, A.; Azhibekov, Y.; Khalameizer, V.; Brodkin, B.; Katz, A. A New Method for Direct Three-Dimensional Measurement of Left Atrial Appendage Dimensions during Transesophageal Echocardiography. *Echocardiography* **2016**, *33*, 69–76. [CrossRef] [PubMed]

11. Nucifora, G.; Faletra, F.F.; Regoli, F.; Pasotti, E.; Pedrazzini, G.; Moccetti, T.; Auricchio, A. Evaluation of the left atrial appendage with real-time 3-dimensional transesophageal echocardiography: Implications for catheter-based left atrial appendage closure. *Circ. Cardiovasc. Imaging* **2011**, *4*, 514–523. [CrossRef] [PubMed]

12. Yosefy, C.; Azhibekov, Y.; Brodkin, B.; Khalameizer, V.; Katz, A.; Laish-Farkash, A. Rotational method simplifies 3-dimensional measurement of left atrial appendage dimensions during transesophageal echocardiography. *Cardiovasc. Ultrasound* **2016**, *14*, 36. [CrossRef] [PubMed]

13. Nakajima, H.; Seo, Y.; Ishizu, T.; Yamamoto, M.; Machino, T.; Harimura, Y.; RyoKawamura, R.; Sekiguchi, Y.; Tada, H.; Aonuma, K. Analysis of the left atrial appendage by three-dimensional transesophageal echocardiography. *Am. J. Cardiol.* **2010**, *106*, 885–892. [CrossRef] [PubMed]

14. Chow, D.H.; Bieliauskas, G.; Sawaya, F.J.; Millan-Iturbe, O.; Kofoed, K.F.; Søndergaard, L.; De Backer, O. A comparative study of different imaging modalities for successful percutaneous left atrial appendage closure. *Open Heart* **2017**, *4*, e000627. [CrossRef] [PubMed]

15. Rajwani, A.; Nelson, A.J.; Shirazi, M.G.; Disney, P.J.; Teo, K.S.; Wong, D.T.; Young, G.D.; Worthley, S.G. CT sizing for left atrial appendage closure is associated with favourable outcomes for procedural safety. *Eur. Heart J. Cardiovasc. Imaging* **2017**, *18*, 1361–1368. [CrossRef] [PubMed]

16. Budge, L.P.; Shaffer, K.M.; Moorman, J.R.; Lake, D.E.; Ferguson, J.D.; Mangrum, J.M. Analysis of in vivo left atrial appendage morphology in patients with atrial fibrillation: A direct comparison of transesophageal echocardiography, planar cardiac CT, and segmented three-dimensional cardiac CT. *J. Interv. Card. Electrophysiol.* **2008**, *23*, 87–93. [CrossRef] [PubMed]

17. Wang, Y.A.N.; Di Biase, L.; Horton, R.P.; Nguyen, T.; Morhanty, P.; Natale, A. Left atrial appendage studied by computed tomography to help planning for appendage closure device placement. *J. Cardiovasc. Electrophysiol.* **2010**, *21*, 973–982. [CrossRef] [PubMed]

18. Hell, M.M.; Achenbach, S.; Yoo, I.S.; Franke, J.; Blachutzik, F.; Roether, J.; Graf, V.; Raaz-Schrauder, D.; Marwan, D.; Schlundt, C. 3D printing for sizing left atrial appendage closure device: Head-to-head comparison with computed tomography and transoesophageal echocardiography. *EuroIntervention* **2017**, *13*, 1234–1241. [CrossRef] [PubMed]

19. Li, H.; Shu, M.; Wang, X.; Song, Z. Application of 3D printing technology to left atrial appendage occlusion. *Int. J. Cardiol.* **2017**, *231*, 258–263. [CrossRef] [PubMed]

20. Goitein, O.; Fink, N.; Guetta, V.; Beinart, R.; Brodov, Y.; Konen, E.; Goitein, D.; Di Segni, E.; Grupper, A.; Glikson, M. Printed MDCT 3D models for prediction of left atrial appendage (LAA) occluder device size: A feasibility study. *EuroIntervention* **2017**, *13*, e1076–e1079. [CrossRef] [PubMed]
21. Möbius-Winkler, S.; Sandri, M.; Mangner, N.; Lurz, P.; Dähnert, I.; Schuler, G. The WATCHMAN left atrial appendage closure device for atrial fibrillation. *J. Vis. Exp.* **2012**. [CrossRef] [PubMed]

3

Major Bleeding Predictors in Patients with Left Atrial Appendage Closure: The Iberian Registry II

José Ramón López-Mínguez [1,*], Juan Manuel Nogales-Asensio [1], Eduardo Infante De Oliveira [2], Lino Santos [3], Rafael Ruiz-Salmerón [4], Dabit Arzamendi-Aizpurua [5], Marco Costa [6], Hipólito Gutiérrez-García [7], Jose Antonio Fernández-Díaz [8], Xavier Freixa [9], Ignacio Cruz-González [10], Raúl Moreno [11], Andrés Íñiguez-Romo [12] and Fernando Alfonso-Manterola [13]

[1] Cardiology Department, Interventional Cardiology Section, Hospital Universitario de Badajoz, 06080 Badajoz, Spain; juanmanogales@yahoo.es

[2] Cardiology Department, Interventional Cardiology Section, Hospital de Santa María, 1649-028 Lisbon, Portugal; e.infante.de.oliveira@gmail.com

[3] Cardiology Department, Interventional Cardiology Section, Centro Hospitalario de Vila Nova de Gaia, 4430-999 Vila Nova de Gaia Oporto, Portugal; ljsantos30@gmail.com

[4] Cardiology Department, Interventional Cardiology Section, Hospital Virgen de la Macarena, 41009 Seville, Spain; rjruizsalmeron@yahoo.es

[5] Cardiology Department, Interventional Cardiology Section, Hospital Santa Creu i San Pau, 08041 Barcelona, Spain; dabitarza@gmail.com

[6] Cardiology Department, Interventional Cardiology Section, Centro Hospitalar e Universitário de Coimbra, 3004-561 Coimbra, Portugal; marcocostacard@sapo.pt

[7] Cardiology Department, Interventional Cardiology Section, Hospital Clínico de Valladolid, 47003 Valladolid, Spain; hggmaire@gmail.com

[8] Cardiology Department, Interventional Cardiology Section, Hospital Puerta de Hierro, Majadahona, 28222 Madrid, Spain; joseantoniofer@gmail.com

[9] Cardiology Department, Interventional Cardiology Section, Hospital Clínic de Barcelona, 08036 Barcelona, Spain; xavierfreixa@hotmail.com

[10] Cardiology Department, Interventional Cardiology Section, Hospital Universitario de Salamanca, 37007 Salamanca, Spain; cruzgonzalez.ignacio@gmail.com

[11] Cardiology Department, Interventional Cardiology Section, Hospital La Paz, 28046 Madrid, Spain; raulmorenog@hotmail.com

[12] Cardiology Department, Interventional Cardiology Section, Hospital Álvaro Cunqueiro, 36213 Vigo, Pontevedra, Spain; Andres.Iniguez.Romo@sergas.es

[13] Cardiology Department, Interventional Cardiology Section, Hospital La Princesa, IIS-IP, CIBER-CV, Universidad Autónoma de Madrid, 28006 Madrid, Spain; falf@hotmail.com

* Correspondence: lopez-minguez@hotmail.com

Abstract: Introduction and objective: Major bleeding events in patients undergoing left atrial appendage closure (LAAC) range from 2.2 to 10.3 per 100 patient-years in different series. This study aimed to clarify the bleeding predictive factors that could influence these differences. **Methods:** LAAC was performed in 598 patients from the Iberian Registry II (1093 patient-years; median, 75.4 years). We conducted a multivariate analysis to identify predictive risk factors for major bleeding events. The occurrence of thromboembolic and bleeding events was compared to rates expected from CHA2DS2-VASc (congestive heart failure, hypertension, age, diabetes, stroke history, vascular disease, sex) and HAS-BLED (hypertension, abnormal renal and liver function, stroke, bleeding, labile INR, elderly, drugs or alcohol) scores. **Results:** Cox regression analysis revealed that age ≥75 years (HR: 2.5; 95% CI: 1.3 to 4.8; $p = 0.004$) and a history of gastrointestinal bleeding (GIB) (HR: 2.1; 95% CI: 1.1 to 3.9; $p = 0.020$) were two factors independently associated with major bleeding during follow-up. Patients aged <75 or ≥75 years had median CHA2DS2-VASc scores of 4 (IQR: 2) and 5

(IQR: 2), respectively ($p < 0.001$) and HAS-BLED scores were 3 (IQR: 1) and 3 (IQR: 1) for each group ($p = 0.007$). Events presented as follow-up adjusted rates according to age groups were stroke (1.2% vs. 2.9%; HR: 2.4, $p = 0.12$) and major bleeding (3.7 vs. 9.0 per 100 patient-years; HR: 2.4, $p = 0.002$). Expected major bleedings according to HAS-BLED scores were 6.2% vs. 6.6%, respectively. In patients with GIB history, major bleeding events were 6.1% patient-years (HAS-BLED score was 3.8 ± 1.1) compared to 2.7% patients-year in patients with no previous GIB history (HAS-BLED score was 3.4 ± 1.2; $p = 0.029$). **Conclusions:** In this high-risk population, GIB history and age ≥ 75 years are the main predictors of major bleeding events after LAAC, especially during the first year. Age seems to have a greater influence on major bleeding events than on thromboembolic risk in these patients.

Keywords: atrial fibrillation; bleeding risk; age; left atrial appendage closure

---

1. Introduction

Left atrial appendage closure (LAAC) is a therapeutic option for patients with a high bleeding risk even in the absence of anticoagulant (AC) treatment after LAAC, and its use has been supported by the increasing body of evidence obtained from several studies and registries [1].

Comparison of results from the series of patients who underwent LAAC may show variations in the percentage of events during follow-up. In spite of some consistency in the relative reduction of stroke (60–80% of CHA2DS2-VASc (congestive heart failure, hypertension, age, diabetes, stroke history, vascular disease, sex) scores), there was a higher variability in bleeding events among the series from the first year of follow-up, with major bleeding events ranging from 2.2% to 10% per year [2–4].

We searched for variables that might be independent predictors for major bleeding events at follow-up. We based our analysis on the Iberian Registry II [5].

2. Methods

Patients and Procedures

Five hundred and ninety-eight patients from the Iberian Registry II referred for LAAC were recruited from 13 hospitals across the Iberian Peninsula (10 from Spain and 3 from Portugal) between 2 March 2009 and 18 December 2015 [5]. These were the set of patients prospectively included in the Iberian Registry I who are continuing long-term follow-up, plus additional patients successively included up to the end of the date set for end of recruitment. Inclusion criteria were one or more of the following conditions: serious hemorrhage during anticoagulant therapy, prior disease or clinical event that contraindicated oral anticoagulants (OACs) or repeated failure to adequately control INR, and hematologist indication to suspend anticoagulation therapy. Exclusion criteria were malignancy, life expectancy less than one year and refusal to provide informed consent for this study.

LAAC indication was as follows: stroke under OAC therapy 6.2%, previous bleeding 73.7%, high risk of bleeding 14.2% and other (poorly controlled INR, patient decision, etc.) 5.9%. Before LAAC, 74.8% and 25.2% of the patients were under OAC and antiplatelet therapy respectively.

The devices used were the Amplatzer® Cardiac Plug (ACP) and its subsequent version, the Amulet® (both from St. Jude Medical; Minneapolis, MN, USA), and the Watchman® (Boston Scientific; Boston, MA, USA).

Thromboembolic and bleeding events were compared with those expected from CHA2DS2-VASc (congestive heart failure, hypertension, age, diabetes, stroke history, vascular disease, sex) and HAS-BLED (hypertension, abnormal renal and liver function, stroke, bleeding, labile INR, elderly, drugs or alcohol) scores in the overall sample [6,7]. Major bleeding events were defined according to VARC-2 classification [8].

The observed incidence of events (number of events during the follow-up period divided by the number of patients per year of follow-up) was calculated per patient and year of follow-up (number of patients at the beginning of the follow-up period multiplied by the mean time of follow-up of those patients expressed in years). The expected incidence of events in the sample was calculated as the mean of the individual risk of each patient. Each patient was assigned an individual risk according to a score of bleeding and ictus risk depending on his or her CHADS2 and HAS-BLED score, as indicated in the work by Friberg and colleagues in the Swedish Atrial Fibrillation cohort study.

All subjects gave their informed consent for inclusion before they participated in the study. The study was conducted in accordance with the Declaration of Helsinki, and the protocol was approved by the Ethics Committee of Hospital Universitario de Badajoz (Project identification 5517).

3. Statistical Analysis

Quantitative variables are expressed as mean (±standard deviation (SD)) or median (interquartile range (IQR)). Categorical variables are expressed as absolute frequency and percentage. Categorical variables were compared using the $\chi 2$ test or Fisher's exact test, and quantitative variables using the Student t-test or Wilcoxon test. Comparisons between rates of observed and expected events were evaluated using binomial tests. Event-free survival analysis was performed using the Kaplan–Meier method and Cox regression. Multivariate analysis (Cox regression) was performed to identify which variables might be independent predictors for bleeding events. Proportional-hazard assumption for Cox Regression was checked by use of Cox proportional hazards regression test with time-dependent covariates. All analyses were carried out using the SPSS statistical package, version 19.0.

All patients gave their consent authorizing the intervention and subsequent follow-up. The study protocol was approved by the hospital ethics committee and conforms to the ethical guidelines of the 1975 Declaration of Helsinki. More details of patients, work methods, variable definitions and statistical analyses were previously reported [5].

4. Results

In the Iberian Registry II, during a mean follow-up of 22.9 months, the observed events for stroke and major bleeding events according to CHA2DS2-VASc and HAS-BLED scores in the total population were 1.6% (vs. expected 8.5%) and 3.9% (vs. expected 6.4%), with a relative risk reduction (RRR) of 81% for stroke and 39% for major bleeding events. In patients monitored for more than 24 months (683 patient-years), stroke and bleeding frequencies were 1.5% and 2.6%, with RRRs of 82% and 59%, respectively.

In the univariate analysis, the variables that were associated with a higher rate of "major bleeding events" at follow-up were: age $\geq$ 75 years (HR: 2.8; 95% CI: 1.5–5.2; $p = 0.002$), gastrointestinal bleeding (GIB) history (HR: 2.3; 95% CI95: 1.2–4.3; $p = 0.007$) and the antecedent of hypertension (HR: 0.5; 95% CI: 0.3–1; $p = 0.047$). Multivariate analysis (Cox regression analysis) showed that the variables associated with "major bleeding events" during follow-up were only age $\geq$ 75 years (HR: 2.5; 95% CI: 1.3 to 4.8; $p = 0.004$) and GIB history (HR: 2.1; 95% CI: 1.1 to 3.9; $p = 0.020$).

In patients with previous bleeding, these occurred in 82.1% and 17.9% of patients under OAC and antiplatelet therapy, respectively. GIB accounted for 55% of previous major bleeding events and 82% of major bleeding events during follow-up. Most of GIB (28 of 35) took place during the first 12 months (25 of them in the first 6 months).

Patients were then divided into two different populations according to their age: <75 or $\geq$ 75years (326 vs. 272 patients). Table 1 shows the main clinical variables between the two groups. The percentage of patients aged $\geq$75 years with a previous history of bleeding was 81.3%. In general, the percentage of patients with a history of intracranial hemorrhage (ICH) was lower (23.9% and 29.1% in older and younger groups; $p = 0.14$) compared to the percentage with a history of GIB or major bleeding events, which was even significantly higher in patients $\geq$ 75 years (GIB: 48.5% vs. 32.5%; $p < 0.001$; major bleeding: 53.3% vs. 39.9%; $p = 0.001$). There was also a higher percentage of patients with anemia and renal failure in the elderly group (Table 1). There were no significant differences with regard to the implant used in the procedure or in complications. Table 2 shows the following events presented as follow-up adjusted rates according to age group (<75 or ≥75 years): deaths, 3.9% vs. 11.8% (HR: 3; $p < 0.001$); stroke, 1.2% vs. 2.9% (HR: 2.4; $p = 0.12$); ICH, 1.2% vs. 0.2% (HR: 0.2; $p = 0.09$); GIB, 1.5% vs. 6.9% (OR: 4.6; $p < 0.001$) and major bleeding, 3.7 vs. 9.0 (HR: 2.4; $p = 0.002$) per 100 patient-years (corresponding to patients <75 vs. ≥75 years, respectively). A significant decrease in bleeding events occurred after 1 year of follow-up in both groups (0.5 and 2.9 per 100 patient-years for GIB ($p = 0.045$), and 0.4, and 1.9 per 100 patient-years ($p = 0.018$) for major bleeding, in younger and older patients, although patients aged ≥75 years continued to have more bleeding events) (Figure 1A,B). Figure 2 shows that survival rate with no GIB was significantly higher in patients aged <75 years compared to the elderly group.

Table 1. Clinical variables in the populations aged <75 and ≥75 years.

	<75 ($n = 326$)	≥75 ($n = 272$)	p-Value
Age	67.3 ± 5.8	80.3 ± 3.5	<0.001
Female	112 (34.4%)	116 (42.6%)	0.038
Hypertension	255 (78.2%)	213 (78.3%)	0.979
Diabetes	106 (32.5%)	98 (36.0%)	0.367
Permanent AF	149 (45.7%)	159 (58.5%)	0.002
Previous stroke	111 (34.0%)	77 (28.3%)	0.132
Previous bleeding	170 (52.1%)	221 (81.3%)	<0.001
Previous ICH	95 (29.1%)	65 (23.9%)	0.149
Previous GI bleeding	106 (32.5%)	132 (48.5%)	<0.001
Previous major bleeding	130 (39.9%)	145 (53.3%)	0.001
CHA_2DS_2-VASc *	4 [2]	5 [2]	<0.001
HAS-BLED *	3 [1]	3 [1]	0.007
Anemia	63 (19.3%)	102 (37.5%)	<0.001
Renal failure	42 (12.9%)	85 (31.3%)	<0.001

AF: atrial fibrillation; GI: gastrointestinal; ICH: intracranial hemorrhage. * Median (IQR).

Table 2. Adjusted event rates per 100 patient-years.

	<75 ($n = 326$)	≥75 ($n = 272$)	HR (<75 vs. ≥75)	p-Value
Death	3.9	11.8	3.0	<0.001
Stroke	1.2	2.9	2.4	0.120
ICH	1.2	0.2	0.2	0.099
GI bleeding	1.5	6.9	4.6	<0.001
Major bleeding	3.7	9.0	2.4	0.002

GI: gastrointestinal; ICH: intracranial hemorrhage.

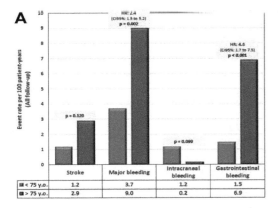 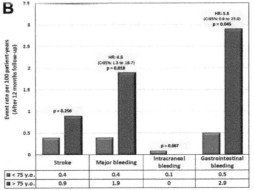

Figure 1. (**A**) Rate of events in patient-years according to age < or ≥75 years. (**B**) Rate of events in patients who completed the first year with no events. HR: hazard ratio; CI: confidence interval.

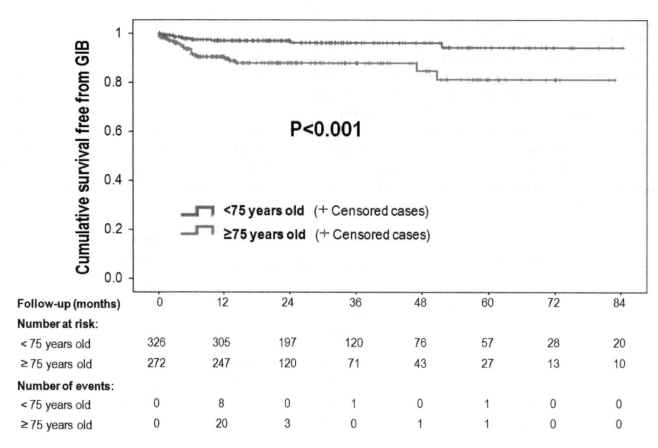

Follow-up (months)	0	12	24	36	48	60	72	84
Number at risk:								
< 75 years old	326	305	197	120	76	57	28	20
≥ 75 years old	272	247	120	71	43	27	13	10
Number of events:								
< 75 years old	0	8	0	1	0	1	0	0
≥ 75 years old	0	20	3	0	1	1	0	0

Figure 2. Cumulative survival free from gastrointestinal bleeding (GIB) is significantly higher in patients <75 years compared to patients ≥75 years.

Table 3 shows the rate of events per patient-year in patients aged ≥75 years compared to the rate expected by the risk scores. There were only small differences in stroke and ICH per patient-year between patients aged ≥75 or <75 years. In contrast, there was an increase in major bleeding events in patients aged ≥75 years, which did not occur for the group aged <75 years, in whom bleeding reduction was 40.3%. Most GIB events occurred in the first 6 months of follow-up in both groups. The two variables that were independently associated with the event "gastrointestinal bleeding" after multivariate analysis (Cox regression) were: age ≥75 years (HR: 3.0; 95% CI: 1.4 to 6,3; $p = 0.004$) and gastrointestinal bleeding (GIB) history (HR: 4.3; 95% CI: 2.0 to 9.4; $p < 0.001$).

Table 3. Overall event outcomes in patients aged <75 and ≥75 years.

	Expected events (×100 patient-years) in ≥75 years	Observed events (×100 patient-years) in ≥75 years	Expected events (×100 patient-years) in <75 years	Observed events (×100 patient-years) in <75 years
Ischemic stroke	7.2 CHADs-VASc score	2.9 Reduction, 59.7% $p \le 0.001$	5.1 CHADs-VASc score	1.2 Reduction, 76.5% $p \le 0.001$
ICH	1.0 HAS-BLED score	0.3 Reduction, 70.8% $p = 0.220$	0.9 HAS-BLED score	1.2 Increase, 33.3% $p = 0.642$
GI bleeding		6.9		1.5
Major bleeding	6.6 HAS-BLED score (Friberg Registry)	9.0 Increase, 26.7% $p < 0.001$	6.2 HAS-BLED score (Friberg Registry)	3.7 Reduction, 40.3%) $p = 0.007$

GI: gastrointestinal; HT: hypertension; ICH: intracranial hemorrhage.

Table 4 compares treatments at discharge between both age groups of patients, showing no significant differences. Table 5 divides patients in two groups based on new GIB or no new GIB events during follow-up and compares the main variables between the two subpopulations. We found significant differences in GIB history (74.3% vs. 37.7%, $p < 0.001$), HAS-BLED scores (3.8 ± 1.1 vs. 3.4 ± 1.2, $p = 0.029$), ICH (11.4% vs. 27.7%, $p = 0.035$) and death (25.7% vs. 12.6%, $p = 0.027$). Although patients with GIB history showed a higher death rate, multivariate analysis results showed that only age (HR: 1.08; 95% CI: 1.05 to 1.13; $p < 0.001$) and previous stroke (HR: 3.22; 95% CI: 1.64 to 6.34; $p = 0.001$) were predictive factors for death during follow-up.

Table 4. Treatment at discharge according to age group.

	<75 ($n = 326$)	≥75 ($n = 272$)	p-Value
AAS	208 (63.8%)	166 (61.0%)	0.485
Clopidogrel	207 (63.5%)	164 (60.3%)	0.422
AAS + Clopidogrel	185 (56.7%)	138 (50.7%)	0.142
Anticoagulants (acenocumarol or LMWH)	45 (13.8%)	40 (14.7%)	0.753
NOAC	9 (2.8%)	9 (3.3%)	0.696

AAS: acetylsalicylic acid; LMWH: low molecular weight heparin; NOAC: non-vitamin K antagonist oral anticoagulant.

Table 5. Comparison of the main variables in patients presenting GIB events or no GIB events during follow-up.

	GIB ($n = 35$)	No GIB ($n = 563$)	p-Value
Age	77.0 ± 8.2	74.0 ± 8.0	0.029
Female	15 (42.9%)	213 (37.8%)	0.553
Hypertension	23 (65.7%)	445 (79.0%)	0.064
Diabetes	14 (40.0%)	190 (33.7%)	0.449
Permanent AF	19 (54.3%)	289 (51.3%)	0.734
Previous stroke	7 (20.0%)	181 (32.1%)	0.133
Previous bleeding	26 (74.3%)	365 (64.8%)	0.254
Previous ICH	4 (11.4%)	156 (27.7%)	0.035
Previous GI bleeding	26 (74.3%)	212 (37.7%)	<0.001
Previous major bleeding	16 (45.7%)	259 (56.0%)	0.973
CHA$_2$DS$_2$-VASc *	5 [1]	4 [2]	0.390
HAS-BLED *	4 [2]	3 [1]	0.016
Anemia	13 (37.1%)	152 (27.0%)	0.269
Renal failure	10 (28.6%)	117 (20.8%)	0.766
AAS at discharge	23 (65.7%)	352 (62.3%)	0.689
Clopidogrel at discharge	21 (60.0%)	350 (62.2%)	0.798
AAS + Clopidogrel at discharge	19 (54.3%)	304 (54.0%)	0.973
Acenocumarol at discharge	1 (2.9%)	28 (5.0%)	0.572
LMWH at discharge	2 (5.7%)	54 (9.6%)	0.445
NOAC	1 (2.9%)	17 (3.0%)	0.956
Death in follow-up	9 (25.7%)	71 (12.6%)	0.027

AAS: acetylsalicylic acid; AF: atrial fibrillation; GI: gastrointestinal; ICH: intracranial hemorrhage; LMWH: low molecular weight heparin; NOAC: non-vitamin K antagonist oral anticoagulant. * Median (IQR).

Table 6 presents the main variables of LAAC patients with contraindications for OAC treatment, collected from different registries (data from > 500 patients).

Table 6. Mean variables of patients with contraindication for OAC treatment reported in different registries.

Registry	EWOLUTION Registry	Multicenter Amplatzer	Amulet Registry	Ii Iberian Registry	Italian Registry
Population (n)	$n = 1025$	$n = 1047$	$n = 1088$	$n = 598$	$n = 613$
Mean age	73.4 ± 8.9	75 ± 8	74 ± 8	75.4 ± 8.6	75.1 ± 8.0
Follow up (months)	12	13	12	22.9	20
CHA$_2$DS$_2$-VASc score (mean ± SD)	4.5 ± 1.6	4.5 ± 1.6	4.5 ± 1.6	4.4 ± 1.5	4.2 ± 1.5

Table 6. *Cont.*

Registry	EWOLUTION Registry	Multicenter Amplatzer	Amulet Registry	Ii Iberian Registry	Italian Registry
Population (*n*)	*n* = 1025	*n* = 1047	*n* = 1088	*n* = 598	*n* = 613
HAS-BLED score (mean ± SD)	2.3 ± 1.2	3.1 ± 1.2	3.3 ± 1.1	3.4 ± 1.2	3.2 ± 1.1
Rate of events per 100 patient-years					
Deaths	9.8%	4.3%	8.4%	7%	7.4%
History of Stroke	30.5%	39%	28%	39%	36.3%
History of major Bleeding	31%	47.7%	72%	46%	41.6%
Observed vs. Expected					
Stroke	1.1% vs. 7.2% (CHA$_2$DS$_2$-VASc) RRR, 83%	1.8% vs. 5.62% (CHA$_2$DS$_2$-VASc) RRR, 59%	2.9 vs. 6.7% (CHA$_2$DS$_2$-VASc) RRR, 57%	1.6% vs. 8.5% (CHA$_2$DS$_2$-VASc) RRR, 81%	2.9% vs. 8.6% (CHA$_2$DS$_2$-VASc) RRR, 66%
Major bleeding	2.7% vs. 5% (HAS-BLED) RRR, 46%	2.1% vs. 5.34% (HAS-BLED) RRR, 46%	7.1% vs. 10.3%	3.9% vs. 6.4% (HAS-BLED) RRR, 39%	4.5% vs. 6.3% (HAS-BLED) RRR, 29%

OAC: Oral anticoagulants; RRR: relative risk reduction; SD: standard deviation.

5. Discussion

Our study shows that during follow-up, both age and major GIB history are the main predictors of major bleeding events and therefore both variables should be taken into account when making comparisons between bleeding percentages in the different series of patients. It is also important that results are interpreted according to the follow-up time, as bleeding rates are higher during the first year [9].

5.1. The Importance of GIB, Major Bleeding History and Follow-up Time

Only around 16%-17% of patients included in randomized trials of both non-vitamin K antagonist oral anticoagulant (NOAC) and LAAC with warfarin therapies have a previous history of bleeding [10]; conversely, in LAAC registries, major bleeding events range from 31% in the EWOLUTION Registry to 72% in the Amulet Registry, with the remainder having conditions associated with a high bleeding risk, such as severe anemia [2,5,11–13].

We show in Table 2 that GIBs represent a higher percentage of severe bleedings in older patients (≥75 years).

In the Amulet and II Iberian Registries, where we find higher HAS-BLED scores and higher percentages of patients with major bleeding history, major bleeding during follow-up rises to 10.3% and 5.4%, respectively, during the first year, in contrast to the results of the Multicentre and EWOLUTION studies, that range from 2.1% to 2.7% [2,9,11,12].

However, in the Iberian Registry II, bleeding events were reduced to 3.9% after two years of follow-up and to 2.6% after more than two years, which corresponded to a relative reduction of more than 21% (39% after two years and 58.7% after more than two years) [5].

Bleeding events, especially GIB, were higher during the first 6 months post-procedure, which is the time window when a higher percentage of patients were receiving dual antithrombotic treatment (therapy changed from two antiplatelet agents to only one after the first 3–6 months). It is interesting to note that bleeding reduction is less dramatic in patients with major bleeding history. The EWOLUTION study reported that after 2 years, patients with HAS-BLED scores <3 showed relative reductions of 50% (1.8% vs. expected 3.6%) compared to relative reductions of 41% in patients with HAS-BLED scores >3 (4.2% vs. expected 7.1%), and these figures were even lower in patients with a major bleeding history (30%) [14]. In our study, in patients with GIB history, major bleeding events were 6.1 per 100 patient-years (HAS-BLED score 3.8 ± 1.1), compared to 2.7 per 100 patient-years in patients with no previous GIB history (HAS-BLED score 3.4 ± 1.2; *p* = 0.029).

5.2. The Importance of Age

Age is a risk factor in the prediction of both stroke and bleeding as a whole [7]. Elderly patients receiving treatment with OAC present a high bleeding risk that ranges from 9% to 13%, and for that reason they are not well represented in NOAC randomized trials [15,16]. It is still debated whether age has more influence on major bleedings than on thromboembolic events, as several studies support opposite claims in this respect [17–19]. Thus, it was observed that even in patients who were able to take OAC in the ENGAGE AF-TIMI 48 study, age had a greater influence on major bleeding than on thromboembolic risk [17].

It is crucial to clarify if age has more impact on major bleeding risk or on thromboembolic events in NVAF patients undergoing left atrial appendage closure (LAAC) and with a history of frequent bleeding events. In our study, patients ≥75 years had higher HAS-BLED scores (3.5 ± 1.1) than patients <75 years (3.3 ± 1.2; $p = 0.004$), and bleeding events were 9 per 100 patient-years (26.7% increase) versus 3.7 per 100 patient-years in the younger group (40.3% decrease).

The question as to whether age is the main factor or a secondary factor responsible for the accumulation in the percentage of patients with bleeding history was clarified by the multivariate analysis, which showed that age and bleeding history were independent predictors of subsequent bleeding events, especially a history of GIB.

There are no specific studies on the importance of age in bleeding events in LAAC patients, although there are two published LAAC series from the Multicentre and EWOLUTION registries [4,20].

The study published by Freixa and colleagues, based on the Multicentre Registry with the AMPLATZER Cardiac Plug, compared two populations of patients under or over 75 years old [4] and found no differences in major bleeding events (1.7% vs. 2.6%; $p = 0.54$) during a mean follow-up of 16.8 months. In addition, in the series of Freixa and collaborators, the percentage of patients <75 or ≥75 years with a previous history of major bleeding was similar between the two groups (48.4% vs. 47.7%; $p = 0.83$), whereas in our study, the percentage was significantly different between the two groups and even higher in patients ≥75 years (39.9% vs. 53.3%; $p = 0.001$) [4,5].

Cruz-González and colleagues published a sub-analysis of the EWOLUTION Registry of patients undergoing LAAC, comparing patients <85 and ≥85 years old. Although the differences between younger and older patients were not statistically significant (due to a limited sample size), after a follow-up of 24 months the group aged >85 years presented higher rates of major or severe non-procedural bleeding events than the younger group (5.1 per 100 patient-years vs. 2.6 per 100 patient-years, or 7.5 vs. 4.3 respectively, if procedural severe bleedings were included) [20].

5.3. Post-Implantation Treatment is an Important Variable

Most of the patients included in our study underwent dual antiplatelet treatment (DAPT) for 3 months, and after that, treatment was reduced to only one antiplatelet agent (APT), which is the usual procedure in current studies. It is clear that post-interventional treatment is an important variable to take into account, but in all studies, with the exception of randomized series, patients present a high percentage of bleeding events of different natures and origins. This makes it difficult to standardize treatment guidelines, and doctors must make decisions based on the specific risk associated with each patient [14]. The analysis of this variable can be confusing as data from the Amulet Registry showed that patients that were not taking antiplatelet agents developed more bleeding events than the group that was medicated, reflecting the current trend to treat patients with lower bleeding risk instead of patients with a very high bleeding risk [2]. The EWOLUTION study showed that patients treated with DAPT presented more major bleeding events after 105 days than those who discontinued this treatment (3.5% vs. 1.1%) [14].

Our study has the limitations of any registry since it is not a randomized trial. However, patients cannot be randomized for ethical reasons. Nevertheless, our data reflect a very exhaustive collection of events in a highly complex population, and their comparison with expected outcomes according to the risk scores has been widely validated. Despite the difficulty of reaching a consensus regarding appropriate post-interventional antiplatelet treatment (generally DAPT for 3 months), our analyses took into consideration the duration of antiplatelet treatment when comparing patients with or without bleeds.

6. Conclusions

In our Iberian Registry II, 46% of patients referred for LAAC had previous major bleedings, mostly of gastrointestinal origin. A history of severe GIB is an independent predictor of new severe bleeding events during follow-up. The percentage of patients aged ≥75 years may also significantly influence the incidence of major bleeding events beyond that expected using the HAS-BLED score, especially due to the high frequency of GIB, as age appears to have greater influence on major bleeding than on thromboembolic risk in these patients. Despite this, after the first year, bleeding events fell significantly, although they continued to be higher than in the group aged <75 years, in whom fewer bleeding complications were observed than expected from the HAS-BLED score. Efficacy in thromboembolic events remains very high, regardless of age, even from the first year.

6.1. What is Known about the Topic?

-   LAAC is an effective therapeutic option for atrial fibrillation patients with a contraindication for the use of anticoagulants.
-   However, these patients present a high bleeding risk even in the absence of antiplatelet treatment.
-   Age influences the emergence of complications during follow-up of LAAC patients.

6.2. What does this Study add?

-   This study shows that age has a greater influence on the occurrence of major bleedings than on thromboembolic events.
-   Our analysis also shows that GIB history is the main predictive factor of major bleeding events during the first year of follow-up after LAAC.
-   Differences in the rates of major bleeding events reported in different series of LAAC patients may be due to the number of patients ≥ 75 years and the percentage of patients with GIB history included in those series.

Author Contributions: J.R.L.-M.: conceptualization, methodology, validation, investigation, writing—original draft preparation, writing—review and editing, visualization, supervision, J.M.N.-A.: methodology, validation, data curation, supervision, project administration, E.I.D.O., L.S., R.R.-S., D.A.-A., M.C., H.G.-G., J.A.F.-D., X.F., I.C.-G., R.M., A.Í.-R., F.A.-M.: methodology, validation, investigation, writing—review and editing, visualization, supervision. All authors have read and agreed to the published version of the manuscript.

Acknowledgments: Reyes González-Fernández, Ginés Martínez-Cáceres, Roman Arnold, Ignacio J. Amat-Santos, Javier Goicolea Ruigómez, Rocio Gonzalez-Ferreiro, Javier Rodríguez Collado, Guillermo Galeote García, Rodrigo Estevez Loureiro, Guillermo Bastos Fernández, Antonio de Miguel Castro, and Fernando Rivero Crespo: have contributed as collaborators of Iberian Registry II in: methodology and investigation.

Abbreviations

LAAC	left atrial appendage closure
GIB	gastrointestinal bleeding
OAC	oral anticoagulants
NOAC	new oral anticoagulants
NVAF	non-valvular atrial fibrillation

References

1. Sharma, D.; Reddy, V.Y.; Sandri, M.; Schulz, P.; Majunke, N.; Hala, P.; Wiebe, J.; Mraz, T.; Miller, M.A.; Neuzil, P.; et al. Left Atrial Appendage Closure in Patients With Contraindications to Oral Anticoagulation. *J. Am. Coll. Cardiol.* **2016**, *67*, 2190–2192. [CrossRef] [PubMed]

2. Landmesser, U.; Tondo, C.; Camm, J.; Diener, H.C.; Paul, V.; Schmidt, B.; Settergren, M.; Teiger, E.; Nielsen-Kudsk, J.E.; Hildick-Smith, D. Left atrial appendage occlusion with the AMPLATZER Amulet device: One-year follow-up from the prospective global Amulet observational registry. *EuroIntervention* **2018**, *14*, e590–e597. [CrossRef] [PubMed]

3. Phillips, K.P.; Santoso, T.; Sanders, P.; Alison, J.; Chan, J.L.K.; Pak, H.N.; Chandavimol, M.; Stein, K.M.; Gordon, N.; Razali, O.B. Left atrial appendage closure with WATCHMAN in Asian patients: 2 year outcomes from the WASP registry. *Int. J. Cardiol Heart Vasc.* **2019**, *23*, 100358. [CrossRef] [PubMed]

4. Freixa, X.; Gafoor, S.; Regueiro, A.; Cruz-Gonzalez, I.; Shakir, S.; Omran, H.; Berti, S.; Santoro, G.; Kefer, J.; Landmesser, U.; et al. Comparison of Efficacy and Safety of Left Atrial Appendage Occlusion in Patients Aged <75 to >/= 75 Years. *Am. J. Cardiol.* **2016**, *117*, 84–90. [CrossRef] [PubMed]

5. Lopez-Minguez, J.R.; Nogales-Asensio, J.M.; Infante De Oliveira, E.; De Gama Ribeiro, V.; Ruiz-Salmeron, R.; Arzamendi-Aizpurua, D.; Costa, M.; Gutierrez-Garcia, H.; Fernandez-Diaz, J.A.; Martin-Yuste, V.; et al. Long-term Event Reduction After Left Atrial Appendage Closure. Results of the Iberian Registry II. *Rev. Esp. Cardiol.* **2019**, *72*, 449–455. [CrossRef] [PubMed]

6. Friberg, L.; Rosenqvist, M.; Lip, G.Y. Evaluation of risk stratification schemes for ischaemic stroke and bleeding in 182 678 patients with atrial fibrillation: The Swedish Atrial Fibrillation cohort study. *Eur. Heart J.* **2012**, *33*, 1500–1510. [CrossRef] [PubMed]

7. Lip, G.Y.; Frison, L.; Halperin, J.L.; Lane, D.A. Comparative validation of a novel risk score for predicting bleeding risk in anticoagulated patients with atrial fibrillation: The HAS-BLED (Hypertension, Abnormal Renal/Liver Function, Stroke, Bleeding History or Predisposition, Labile INR, Elderly, Drugs/Alcohol Concomitantly) score. *J. Am. Coll. Cardiol.* **2011**, *57*, 173–180. [CrossRef] [PubMed]

8. Kappetein, A.P.; Head, S.J.; Genereux, P.; Piazza, N.; van Mieghem, N.M.; Blackstone, E.H.; Brott, T.G.; Cohen, D.J.; Cutlip, D.E.; van Es, G.A.; et al. Updated standardized endpoint definitions for transcatheter aortic valve implantation: The Valve Academic Research Consortium-2 consensus document. *EuroIntervention* **2012**, *8*, 782–795. [CrossRef] [PubMed]

9. Lopez Minguez, J.R.; Asensio, J.M.; Gragera, J.E.; Costa, M.; Gonzalez, I.C.; de Carlos, F.G.; Diaz, J.A.; Martin Yuste, V.; Gonzalez, R.M.; Dominguez-Franco, A.; et al. Two-year clinical outcome from the Iberian registry patients after left atrial appendage closure. *Heart* **2015**, *101*, 877–883. [CrossRef] [PubMed]

10. Ruff, C.T.; Giugliano, R.P.; Braunwald, E.; Hoffman, E.B.; Deenadayalu, N.; Ezekowitz, M.D.; Camm, A.J.; Weitz, J.I.; Lewis, B.S.; Parkhomenko, A.; et al. Comparison of the efficacy and safety of new oral anticoagulants with warfarin in patients with atrial fibrillation: A meta-analysis of randomised trials. *Lancet* **2014**, *383*, 955–962. [CrossRef]

11. Boersma, L.V.; Ince, H.; Kische, S.; Pokushalov, E.; Schmitz, T.; Schmidt, B.; Gori, T.; Meincke, F.; Protopopov, A.V.; Betts, T.; et al. Efficacy and safety of left atrial appendage closure with WATCHMAN in patients with or without contraindication to oral anticoagulation: 1-Year follow-up outcome data of the EWOLUTION trial. *Heart Rhythm* **2017**, *14*, 1302–1308. [CrossRef] [PubMed]

12. Tzikas, A.; Shakir, S.; Gafoor, S.; Omran, H.; Berti, S.; Santoro, G.; Kefer, J.; Landmesser, U.; Nielsen-Kudsk, J.E.; Cruz-Gonzalez, I.; et al. Left atrial appendage occlusion for stroke prevention in atrial fibrillation: Multicentre experience with the AMPLATZER Cardiac Plug. *EuroIntervention* **2016**, *11*, 1170–1179. [CrossRef] [PubMed]

13. Berti, S.; Santoro, G.; Brscic, E.; Montorfano, M.; Vignali, L.; Danna, P.; Tondo, C.; D'Amico, G.; Stabile, A.; Sacca, S.; et al. Left atrial appendage closure using AMPLATZER devices: A large, multicenter, Italian registry. *Int. J. Cardiol.* **2017**, *248*, 103–107. [CrossRef] [PubMed]

14. Boersma, L.V.; Ince, H.; Kische, S.; Pokushalov, E.; Schmitz, T.; Schmidt, B.; Gori, T.; Meincke, F.; Protopopov, A.V.; Betts, T.; et al. Evaluating Real-World Clinical Outcomes in Atrial Fibrillation Patients Receiving the WATCHMAN Left Atrial Appendage Closure Technology. *Circ. Arrhythm Electrophysiol.* **2019**, *12*, e006841. [CrossRef] [PubMed]

15.   Hylek, E.M.; Evans-Molina, C.; Shea, C.; Henault, L.E.; Regan, S. Major hemorrhage and tolerability of warfarin in the first year of therapy among elderly patients with atrial fibrillation. *Circulation* **2007**, *115*, 2689–2696. [CrossRef] [PubMed]
16.   Kwon, C.H.; Kim, M.; Kim, J.; Nam, G.B.; Choi, K.J.; Kim, Y.H. Real-world comparison of non-vitamin K antagonist oral anticoagulants and warfarin in Asian octogenarian patients with atrial fibrillation. *J. Geriatr. Cardiol.* **2016**, *13*, 566–572. [CrossRef] [PubMed]
17.   Kato, E.T.; Giugliano, R.P.; Ruff, C.T.; Koretsune, Y.; Yamashita, T.; Kiss, R.G.; Nordio, F.; Murphy, S.A.; Kimura, T.; Jin, J.; et al. Efficacy and Safety of Edoxaban in Elderly Patients With Atrial Fibrillation in the ENGAGE AF-TIMI 48 Trial. *J. Am. Heart Assoc.* **2016**, *5*, e003432. [CrossRef] [PubMed]
18.   Lauw, M.N.; Eikelboom, J.W.; Coppens, M.; Wallentin, L.; Yusuf, S.; Ezekowitz, M.; Oldgren, J.; Nakamya, J.; Wang, J.; Connolly, S.J. Effects of dabigatran according to age in atrial fibrillation. *Heart* **2017**, *103*, 1015–1023. [CrossRef] [PubMed]
19.   Patti, G.; Lucerna, M.; Pecen, L.; Siller-Matula, J.M.; Cavallari, I.; Kirchhof, P.; De Caterina, R. Thromboembolic Risk, Bleeding Outcomes and Effect of Different Antithrombotic Strategies in Very Elderly Patients With Atrial Fibrillation: A Sub-Analysis From the PREFER in AF (PREvention oF Thromboembolic Events-European Registry in Atrial Fibrillation). *J. Am. Heart Assoc.* **2017**, *6*. [CrossRef] [PubMed]
20.   Cruz-Gonzalez, I.; Ince, H.; Kische, S.; Schmitz, T.; Schmidt, B.; Gori, T.; Foley, D.; De Potter, T.; Tschishow, W.; Vireca, E.; et al. Left atrial appendage occlusion in patients older than 85 years. Safety and efficacy in the EWOLUTION registry. *Rev. Esp. Cardiol.* **2019**. [CrossRef] [PubMed]

4

Utilization of Percutaneous Mechanical Circulatory Support Devices in Cardiogenic Shock Complicating Acute Myocardial Infarction and High-Risk Percutaneous Coronary Interventions

Rabea Asleh and Jon R. Resar *

Division of Cardiology, Department of Medicine, Johns Hopkins University School of Medicine, Baltimore, MD 21205, USA
* Correspondence: jresar@jhmi.edu;

Abstract: Given the tremendous progress in interventional cardiology over the last decade, a growing number of older patients, who have more comorbidities and more complex coronary artery disease, are being considered for technically challenging and high-risk percutaneous coronary interventions (PCI). The success of performing such complex PCI is increasingly dependent on the availability and improvement of mechanical circulatory support (MCS) devices, which aim to provide hemodynamic support and left ventricular (LV) unloading to enable safe and successful coronary revascularization. MCS as an adjunct to high-risk PCI may, therefore, be an important component for improvement in clinical outcomes. MCS devices in this setting can be used for two main clinical conditions: patients who present with cardiogenic shock complicating acute myocardial infarction (AMI) and those undergoing technically complex and high-risk PCI without having overt cardiogenic shock. The current article reviews the advancement in the use of various devices in both AMI complicated by cardiogenic shock and complex high-risk PCI, highlights the available hemodynamic and clinical data associated with the use of MCS devices, and presents suggestive management strategies focusing on appropriate patient selection and optimal timing and support to potentially increase the clinical benefit from utilizing these devices during PCI in this high-risk group of patients.

Keywords: mechanical circulatory support; percutaneous coronary intervention; cardiogenic shock; acute myocardial infarction; outcome; patient selection

1. Introduction

Recent advances in percutaneous coronary intervention (PCI) technologies, including mechanical circulatory support (MCS) devices, have facilitated treatment of high-risk patients with complex coronary artery disease (CAD) and low left ventricular (LV) systolic function as well as patients with acute myocardial infarction (AMI) complicated by cardiogenic shock. These high-risk patients would otherwise be poor candidates for coronary artery bypass grafting (CABG) due to high surgical morbidity and mortality risks, and the ability to provide adequate hemodynamic support using MCS devices would potentially enable safer PCI and improve outcomes as compared to unprotected PCI strategy, surgical revascularization, or medical therapy alone [1]. However, despite the preemptive improvement in hemodynamics with the use of MCS devices [2], randomized trials using intraaortic balloon pump (IABP) or Impella 2.5 devices have not demonstrated significant reduction in mortality during high-risk and complex PCI as compared to unprotected PCI [3,4]. A clinical benefit from the use of MCS in the setting of cardiogenic shock complicating AMI has also not yet been conclusively demonstrated [5,6]. Besides possible methodological flaws in these trials, other important factors might have contributed to the lack of benefit seen in these studies and should be taken into consideration, such as inadequate hemodynamic support, inappropriate patient selection, and deferred or inappropriate timing of device insertion during the course of cardiogenic shock and also in relation to PCI.

In light of the development of new generation MCS devices with greater hemodynamic support and lower device-associated complications combined with careful planning and optimal timing of device utilization, a growing body of data is suggestive of improvement in procedural success and clinical outcomes [7,8], and thus opens the door for future research in this field to examine the benefit of optimal MCS use in the setting of high risk PCI among a highly selective group of patients. Herein, we provide the most updated data available on MCS in two different situations involving high risk patients undergoing PCI: (1) high risk patients without cardiogenic shock undergoing complex PCI, and (2) patients with AMI complicated by cardiogenic shock.

2. High-Risk Percutaneous Coronary Interventions

Over the last few decades, there has been a tremendous progression in coronary interventional techniques that enables performance of PCI in complex coronary lesions (heavily calcified and type C) that would previously not have been amenable to intervention. This includes improved guide catheters and wires, mother-child guide catheters, low-profile balloons, coronary atherectomy devices, dedicated chronic total occlusion devices and algorithms, and superior stent designs that enhance deliverability to achieve complete multivessel revascularization including those involving chronic totally occluded coronary vessels. However, each aspect of PCI, beginning from guide catheter engagement and ending with balloon inflation and stent deployment, is associated with potential risk of vascular damage and impairment of myocardial perfusion. For instance, patients at advanced age, with increased comorbidities, and underlying left ventricular dysfunction, may pose a clinical challenge, as complex PCI among these patients may incur a substantial risk that overweighs any benefit achieved from revascularization [4]. On the other hand, utilization of PCI even in older adults with AMI and cardiogenic shock has been shown to be associated with substantial reduction in mortality in a recent contemporary analysis involving older adults ≥75 years of age [9]. Although clinical judgment is important, one should not, therefore, exclude patients from PCI solely based on advanced age in the absence of clear contraindications.

Among high-risk patients with active ischemia, the need and the type of revascularization should be discussed by Heart Team in an individual base. The recommendation with respect to the type of revascularization (PCI versus CABG) should be generally guided by important criteria including the predicted surgical mortality (based on the Society of Thoracic Surgeons (STS) score), the anatomical complexity of CAD (based on the SYNTAX (Synergy between Percutaneous Coronary Intervention with Taxus and Cardiac Surgery) score), and the anticipated completeness of revascularization. The risks of periprocedural complications should be weighed up against the anticipated improvement in quality of life and long-term freedom from death, MI, and repeat vascularization for electing whether conservative therapy, PCI, or CABG is the recommended strategy. According to the current ESC guidelines [10], when suitable coronary anatomy for both procedures and low predicted surgical mortality exist, patients with three-vessel disease and diabetes in particular achieve greater benefit from CABG than PCI regardless of the SYNTAX score, while in patients without diabetes CABG is favored over PCI only when SYNTAX score is intermediate or high (>22). In the presence of significant left main CAD, CABG is preferred for patients with SYNTAX score >22 irrespective of the diabetic state. However, in the presence of complex CAD anatomy (i.e., unprotected left main CAD or three-vessel disease) and high surgical mortality (i.e., previous cardiac surgery, severe comorbidities, and frailty) precluding CABG, high-risk PCI with MCS protection may be suggested as an alternative strategy for achieving complete revascularization safely in this high-risk group of patients. Although high-risk PCI has not been well defined, it can be generally categorized into three major groups based on patient characteristics, lesion characteristics, and clinical presentation [2,11] (Table 1). Patient characteristics include increased age, comorbidities (such as diabetes mellitus, chronic kidney disease, and chronic obstructive lung disease), reduced left ventricular systolic function, and prior myocardial infarction [12–14]. Lesion characteristics include anatomical and procedural variables that determine the complexity of PCI from the technical perspectives and the potential risk of complications. These include PCI of unprotected left main stenosis, bifurcation disease, heavily calcified lesions, saphenous vein grafts, and chronic total occlusions [15,16]. Finally, the clinical characteristics, among which acute coronary syndrome presentation and heart failure symptoms are important elements to take into consideration when assessing PCI risk [17]. An example of a high-risk PCI that can be facilitated by MCS is in an elderly patient with comorbidities who presents acutely with reduced LV systolic function and has a heavily calcified left main bifurcation or three-vessel coronary artery disease.

Table 1. High-Risk Percutaneous Coronary Intervention Characteristics.

Patient Characteristics
Increased age
Comorbidities (diabetes mellitus, chronic lung disease, prior myocardial infarction, peripheral arterial disease, frailty)
Severe LV systolic dysfunction (EF < 20–30%)
Severe renal function impairment (eGFR < 30 mL/min/1.73 m^2).
Lesion Characteristics
Severe three-vessel coronary artery disease
Unprotected left main stenosis
Bifurcation disease or ostial stenosis
High SYNTAX score or type C lesions
Chronic total occlusions
Saphenous vein graft disease
Heavily calcified lesions requiring coronary atherectomy
Clinical Presentation
Acute coronary syndrome
Heart failure symptoms (dyspnea, orthopnea, PND, exercise intolerance, peripheral edema)
Arrhythmias (atrial fibrillation with RVR, ventricular tachycardia)
Elevated LV end-diastolic pressure
Severe mitral regurgitation (or other valvular disease)

Abbreviations: EF, ejection fraction; eGFR, estimated glomerular filtration rate; LV, left ventricular; PND, paroxysmal nocturnal dyspnea; RVR, rapid ventricular response; SYNTAX, Synergy between Percutaneous Coronary Intervention with Taxus and Cardiac Surgery.

As high-risk PCI is associated with increased risk of myocardial ischemia and hemodynamic compromise that may lead to circulatory collapse, the purpose of MCS is to diminish myocardial oxygen consumption and provide adequate cardiac output and myocardial perfusion during the procedure. Use of appropriate MCS devices allows adequate time to safely perform complex PCI with optimal results in these high-risk patients who would not otherwise tolerate complete revascularization [18].

It is critical, therefore, that MCS device insertion in this setting is performed prior to PCI as this enables confident proceeding with revascularization without the risk of circulatory collapse that may subsequently require emergent bailout MCS implementation. Although several patient- and lesion-specific variables are well-recognized predictors of adverse outcomes after PCI, a risk score to assess the need for MCS during PCI has not yet been developed and warrants further research. Despite the lack of a risk calculator, most interventional cardiologists would now consider the use of MCS devices in patients with severely reduced LV systolic function and complex coronary artery disease involving a large territory (such as sole-remaining vessel, unprotected left main, or three-vessel disease) [11].

3. Cardiogenic Shock Complicating Acute Myocardial Infarction

Cardiogenic shock is defined as the combination of sustained systemic tissue hypoperfusion and decreased cardiac output despite adequate circulatory volume and LV filling pressure. Specific clinical and hemodynamic criteria that define cardiogenic shock include systolic blood pressure of <90 mmHg for >30 min, cardiac index <2.2 L/min/m^2 with hemodynamic support or <1.8 L/min/m^2 without support, pulmonary capillary wedge pressure (PCWP) >15 mmHg, and evidence of end-organ damage (such as urinary output <30 mL/h, high lactate levels, or cool extremities) [19,20]. Cardiogenic shock can develop because of various pathologies that affect the heart with AMI involved in the majority of cases. It occurs in 6–10% of patients with AMI and remains a leading cause of death with in-hospital mortality exceeding 50% despite the implementation of guideline-directed medical therapy and early myocardial reperfusion by primary PCI [21,22]. Consequently, patients with cardiogenic shock complicating MI represent a high-risk group of patients with compromised cardiac function and hemodynamics who are more susceptible to circulatory collapse during PCI [23]. Indeed, even though a substantial improvement in PCI techniques and pharmacology has occurred over time, this has not translated to further improvement in outcomes beyond what is achieved with prompt revascularization in the setting of cardiogenic shock [5,6]. Therefore, utilization of percutaneous MCS devices to augment cardiac output and decrease LV filling pressures by LV unloading may act as a successful adjunct to PCI as a bridge to myocardial recovery in these critically ill patients [24].

4. Hemodynamic Effects of Percutaneous Mechanical Circulatory Support Devices

The hemodynamic condition in steady state as well as in various cardiac abnormalities is illustrated by the pressure-volume loop, which provides fundamental information to the understanding of the underlying hemodynamic imbalance and the anticipated effect with the use of each type of the available MCS devices (Figure 1) [11,18]. Pressure-volume loops not only provides a platform for explaining ventricular mechanics, such as contractile and relaxation properties, stroke volume, and cardiac work, but provides a platform for understanding the determinants of myocardial oxygen consumption represented mainly by LV work [11,18,25,26]. Each one of these hemodynamic variables can be compromised based on the clinical presentation. In AMI, for example, patients may mainly present with decreased myocardial contractility and stroke volume in addition to increased myocardial oxygen demand and diminished coronary blood flow (Figure 1B). In cardiogenic shock, LV contractility and stroke volume are severely reduced, while LV end-diastolic volume (LVEDV) and pressure (LVEDP) as well as myocardial oxygen demand are considerably increased (Figure 1C). In the setting of mechanical support, the change in the volume-pressure loops is dependent on the type of the MCS device and the amount of support [18,27,28]. IABP provides modest hemodynamic support demonstrated by modest reduction in both LV systolic and diastolic pressures with afterload reduction and increase in stroke volume (Figure 1D). Percutaneous LV assist devices (including Impella and TandemHeart) result in remarkable reduction in LV systolic and diastolic pressures, LV volumes, and stroke volume resulting in significant decrease in LV work. Unlike the other forms of support, continuous pumping of blood directly from the LV by Impella is not dependent on blood ejection through the aortic valve and LV unloading can, therefore, be augmented by increasing the flow rate, thus resulting in further reduction in LV filling pressures and in myocardial oxygen demand (Figure 1E). Venoarterial extracorporeal membrane oxygenation (VA-ECMO) has the capacity to assume responsibility for the entire cardiac output providing biventricular support in combination with full gas exchange. Strictly on a hemodynamic basis and without an LV venting strategy, use of VA-ECMO results in increased LV systolic and diastolic pressures and reduced stroke volume, with a final flow-dependent increase in afterload and LVEDP (Figure 1F). Therefore, LV venting assisted by Impella or IABP may be ultimately required to mitigate LV loading and decrease left-sided filling pressures and myocardial oxygen demand, especially when the aortic valve remains persistently closed during ECMO support indicating a maximal LV loading condition.

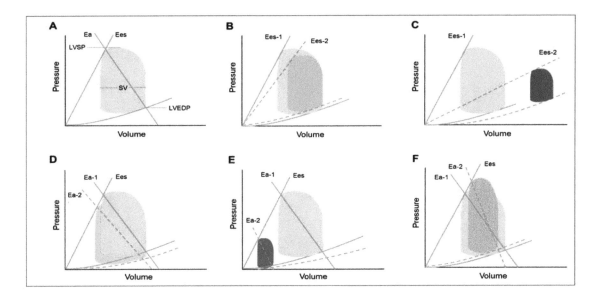

Figure 1. (**A**) Normal pressure-volume (PV) loop. Effective arterial elastance (Ea) is the slope of the line extending from the left ventricular (LV) end-diastolic pressure-volume point through the end-systolic pressure-volume point of the loop. Ea is determined by the total peripheral resistance and heart rate and gives an estimate of the LV afterload. End-systolic elastance (Ees) is the slope of the line extending from the volume-axis intercept V_0 through the end-systolic pressure-volume point of the loop and represents the ventricular contractility. The width of the PV loop represents stroke volume (SV), which can be extracted by calculating the difference between the end-diastolic and end-systolic volumes. (**B**) PV loop in the setting of acute myocardial infarction (AMI) showing decreased contractility (Ees) and SV in addition to increased LV end-diastolic pressure (LVEDP). (**C**) PV loop of patients with cardiogenic shock showing severe reduction in contractility (Ees) and SV in addition to markedly increased LVEDP and LV end-diastolic volume (LVEDV). (**D**) Illustration of PV loop change after intraaortic balloon (IABP) counterpulsation showing mildly reduced LVEDP and LV end systolic pressure (LVESP) resulting in modest afterload (Ea) reduction and increase in SV. (**E**) PV loop with percutaneous LV assist device support (Impella or TandemHeart) showing marked reduction in LVEDP, LVESP, and SV, with a net effect of substantial afterload, preload, and LV workload reduction. (**F**) LV loop with veno-arterial extracorporeal membrane oxygenation (VA-ECMO) without LV venting increases LVEDP and LVESP, while reduces stroke volume and an ultimate increase in afterload (Ea) and LV loading.

5. Available Percutaneous Mechanical Circulatory Support Devices

Several percutaneous MCS devices are currently available to assist interventional cardiologists during high-risk PCIs both for patients undergoing a complex PCI and for those requiring PCI in the setting of cardiogenic sock complicating AMI. Types of available percutaneous MCS devices and comparisons of their characteristics and hemodynamic impact are presented in Table 2 [29,30]. Generally, the goal of MCS devices is to improve cardiac power (defined as the product of mean arterial blood pressure and cardiac output), which has been demonstrated to be a strong predictor of outcomes in patients with cardiogenic shock [31,32]. Therefore, each device has its unique impact on cardiovascular hemodynamics, but an ideal MCS device should ultimately provide circulatory support to achieve adequate systemic tissue perfusion, by increasing mean arterial pressure, while concurrently decreasing myocardial oxygen demand, by reducing both LV volume (preload) and pressure (afterload).

Table 2. Comparison of Technical and Clinical Features of Contemporary Percutaneous Mechanical Circulatory Support Devices.

Features	IABP	Impella 2.5	Impella CP	iVAC 2L	TandemHeart	VA-ECMO
Inflow/outflow	Aorta	LV→aorta	LV→aorta	LV→aorta	LA→aorta	RA→aorta
Mechanism of action	Pneumatic	Axial flow	Axial flow	Pulsatile flow	Centrifugal flow	Centrifugal flow
Insertion approach	Pc (FA)	Pc (FA)	Pc (FA)	Pc (FA)	Pc (FA/FV)	Pc (FA/FV)
Sheath size	7–8 F	13 F	14 F	17 F	Venous: 21 F Arterial: 12–19 F	Venous: 17–21 F Arterial: 16–19 F
Flow (L/min)	0.3–0.5	Max 2.5	3.7–4.0	Max 2.8 40 mL/beat	Max 4.0	Max 7.0
Pump speed (RPM)	N/A	Max 51,000	Max 51,000	40 mL/beat	Max 7500	Max 5000
Duration of support	2–5 days	6 h–10 days	6 h–10 days	6 h–10 days	UP to 14 days	7–10 days
LV function dependency	+	–	–	–	–	–
Synchrony with the cardiac cycle	+	–	–	+	–	–
LV unloading	+	++	+++	+	+++	–
Afterload	↓	→	→	→	↑	↑↑
MAP	↑	↑↑	↑↑	↑↑	↑↑	↑↑
Cardiac index	↑	↑↑	↑↑↑	↑↑	↑↑↑	↑↑↑
PCWP	↓	→	↓↓	→	↓↓	↕
LVEDP	↓	↓↓	↓↓	↓↓	↓↓↓	↕
Coronary perfusion	↑	↑	↑	↑	↓↔	↕
Myocardial oxygen demand	↓	↓↓	↓↓	↓↓	↓↔	↕
Anticoagulation	+	+	+	+	+	+
Implant complexity	+	++	++	++	+++	++
Management complexity	+	++	++	++	+++	+++
Complications	Limb ischemia, bleeding	Hemolysis, limb ischemia, bleeding	Hemolysis, limb ischemia, bleeding	Hemolysis, limb ischemia, bleeding	Limb ischemia, bleeding, hemolysis	Bleeding, limb ischemia, hemolysis
Contraindications	Moderate-to-severe AR, severe PAD	Severe AS/AR, mechanical AoV, LV thrombus, CI to AC	Severe AS/AR, mechanical AoV, LV thrombus, CI to AC	Severe AS/AR, mechanical AoV, LV thrombus, CI to AC	Moderate-to-severe AR, severe PAD, CI to AC, LA thrombus	Moderate-to-severe AR, severe PAD, CI to AC
CE-certification	+	+	+	+	+	+
FDA approval	+	+	+	–	+	+

Abbreviations: AC, anticoagulation; AoV, aortic valve; AR, aortic regurgitation; AS, aortic stenosis; CI, contraindication; FA, femoral artery; FDA, US Food and Drug Administration; FV, femoral vein; LV, left ventricle; LVEDP, left ventricular end-diastolic pressure; IABP, intraaortic balloon pump; MAP, mean arterial pressure; Max, maximum; PAD, peripheral arterial disease; Pc, percutaneous; PCWP, pulmonary capillary wedge pressure; PS, peripheral surgical; RA, right atrium; RPM, rotations per minute; VA-ECMO, venoarterial extracorporeal membrane oxygenation.

5.1. Intraaortic Balloon Bump

Since its introduction in the 1960s, IABP remains the most widely used device for temporary support in hemodynamically unstable patients due to its greater availability and ease of insertion as compared to other temporary devices [33]. It is typically inserted via femoral arterial access, though axillary or subclavian approaches are also feasible and have the advantage of enabling ambulation among stabilized patients. IABP support is driven by electrocardiogram (ECG)-guided balloon inflation with helium (due to its low viscosity that facilitates easy transfer in and out of the balloon in addition to its rapid absorption in blood in case of balloon rupture) at the onset of diastole and deflation at the onset of LV systole. This diastolic pressure augmentation results in increased coronary perfusion, decreased afterload, decreased cardiac work, and decreased myocardial oxygen demand. Despite these favorable effects, the increase in cardiac output is usually minimal and it may not, therefore, provide adequate support to improve end-organ perfusion in patients with severe cardiogenic shock. Moreover, optimal support is dependent on the underlying heart work and also on other factors, such as a stable electrical rhythm, optimal balloon position and sizing, and the timing of balloon inflation in diastole and deflation in systole [34].

The complications associated with IABP use are mainly vascular, including limb ischemia, vascular injury, and stroke [35]. Although it rarely occurs, trauma to the aorta or ostia of the visceral arteries can result in life-threatening complications, including acute renal failure, bowel ischemia, and atheroembolic events. Other complications include bleeding, infection, and thrombocytopenia. Anticoagulation therapy (usually with heparin) is generally recommended for patients supported with an IABP to prevent ischemic complications though no definitive evidence exists to support this approach and some centers do not use anticoagulation with 1:1 pumping, particularly in patients at high bleeding risk. IABP is contraindicated in patients with severe peripheral arterial or aortic disease and in those with moderate or severe aortic valve regurgitation. With the emergence of newer short term support strategies that provide greater hemodynamic support and ventricular unloading, the role of IABP support in the setting of cardiogenic shock or high risk PCI will continue to decline as experience grows with more promising short-term MCS therapies. According to the current European Society of Cardiology (ESC) guidelines, IABP is not indicated for patients with cardiogenic shock complicating AMI (Class III) [10], and a recent study has found that IABP is considered one of the medical reversals in clinical practice as this widespread therapeutic strategy bolstered by retrospective studies and previous guidelines was strongly challenged by subsequent large prospective and randomized studies showing no clinical benefit of its utilization in this clinical setting [36].

5.2. Impella Devices

The Impella pumps are continuous nonpulsatile microaxial flow devices that are deployed into the LV across the aortic valve and unload the LV by pumping blood from the LV cavity to the ascending aorta. The Impella 2.5 and CP pumps (Abiomed Inc, Danvers, MA, USA) can be placed percutaneously and provide maximal flow rates of 2.5 and 3.0–4.0 L/min, respectively, while the Impella 5.0 and Impella LD (Abiomed Inc, Danvers, MA, USA) devices are larger LV assist axial-flow pumps that require surgical cutdown and provide up to 5.0 L/min of cardiac output [14,37,38]. Similarly, the right-sided Impella RP is designed for right ventricular (RV) hemodynamic support by propelling blood from the inferior vena cava and right atrium (RA) to the pulmonary arteries and can also be deployed percutaneously. The percutaneous Impella devices for LV support are inserted most commonly through the femoral artery and then advanced in a retrograde fashion to the LV with a flexible pigtail loop that stabilizes the pump in the LV chamber and protects from LV perforation. Impella insertion requires large-bore arterial cannulation (13-F for Impella 2.5 and 14-F for Impella CP) and therefore, it is essential to ensure adequate femoral and iliac arterial diameters to enable device delivery via a femoral approach. Alternatively, though less commonly used, axillary or subclavian arterial accesses can be used to deliver these pumps percutaneously. For high-risk PCI, the device is usually removed at the end of the procedure. However, in patients with persistent cardiogenic shock despite revascularization, Impella should be retained for further hemodynamic support, a condition that may pose some challenges and thus requires careful assessment and management in the cardiac care unit. Optimal device functioning is crucial and largely depends on appropriate positioning in the LV cavity, as device migration can lead to low flow, ventricular arrhythmias, and hemolysis [39]. In such cases, bedside transthoracic echocardiography-guided device repositioning is usually successful without the need for fluoroscopy [11].

Unlike IABP, Impella (as other percutaneous ventricular assist devices) functions independently of the remaining LV function and does not require synchronization with the cardiac cycle. Therefore, Impella devices are more helpful than IABP in patients with severely depressed LV function who present with significant arrhythmias. Impella results in effective LV unloading thus resulting in decreased LV filling pressures (LVEDP) and myocardial oxygen consumption, while improving cardiac output, mean arterial pressure, and coronary perfusion [40]. All the hemodynamic parameters, including cardiac output, are more markedly improved with Impella use compared with an IABP. Additionally, the more powerful Impella CP and 5.0 devices provide greater hemodynamic support than Impella 2.5 and thereby are more beneficial in patients with profound cardiogenic shock requiring greater hemodynamic support [30].

Despite the improvement in hemodynamic parameters, device-related complications are not rare and can be clinically meaningful, thereby contradicting the potential hemodynamic benefits that can be achieved with the use of Impella devices in some cases. As with any mechanical support device, common complications associated with Impella include vascular trauma, limb ischemia, and bleeding requiring blood transfusion. Moreover, hemolysis is frequently encountered during Impella support due to mechanical erythrocyte shearing, but usually improves after repositioning the device. Based on the Impella EUROSHOCK Registry [39], utilization of Impella 2.5 in the setting of acute cardiogenic shock was found to be associated bleeding at the vascular access site requiring blood transfusion in 24% of cases and hemolysis requiring blood transfusion in 7.5% of cases after a mean Impella support duration of approximately 48 h. Impella may also worsen right-to-left shunting and hypoxemia among patients with a preexisting ventricular or atrial septal defect. As device technology continues to improve and the Impella-associated complications continue to decrease, the use of Impella devices has been steadily increasing over the last several years [41]. This is also owing to its relative ease of deployment and more efficient hemodynamic support compared with other MCS devices.

Impella should not be used in patients with a mechanical aortic valve or LV thrombus as well as in those with severe peripheral arterial disease or who cannot tolerate systemic anticoagulation therapy. Although severe aortic stenosis and regurgitation are considered relative contraindication, the use of Impella in this setting has been shown to be feasible and may be considered in selected high-risk patients with severe aortic stenosis and cardiogenic shock or those with severe LV dysfunction and CAD who require high-risk PCI and/or balloon aortic valvuloplasty as well as in selected patients who develop hemodynamic collapse during transcatheter aortic valve replacement (TAVR) [42].

5.3. TandemHeart

The TandemHeart (CardiacAssist) system is an extracorporeal, centrifugal, continuous flow pump, which is available on the market for left, right, and biventricular failure. For LV support, TandemHeart device is percutaneously inserted to pump blood extracorporeally from the left atrium through a transseptal cannula back into the femoral/iliac artery through an arterial cannula using a centrifugal pump that provides 3 to 5 L/min of continuous flow at 3000 to 7500 rpm, respectively [11,37]. The transseptal inflow cannula is a 21-F and contains a large end-hole and 14 side holes that enable effective blood aspiration from the left atrium while the arterial outflow cannula ranges in size between 15-F and 19-F according to the flow rate via the iliofemoral arterial system [43]. The pump is also FDA-approved and available in market for an oxygenator to be added to the circuit thereby allowing for blood oxygenation with simultaneous LV unloading. As with Impella support, anticoagulation (typically with unfractionated heparin) is required with a recommended activated clotting time (ACT) goal of about 250–300 s prior to device activation.

By propelling blood from the left atrium directly to the arterial system, TandemHeart results in a significantly reduced LV preload, filling pressures, and myocardial oxygen demand, while cardiac output and mean arterial pressures are improved. However, because LV output through the aortic valve competes with the retrograde flow from the device, LV afterload increases as the device support is augmented, which may ultimately result in aortic valve closure requiring LV venting [44,45].

Similar to other percutaneous MCS devices, TandemHeart use may infrequently cause limb ischemia and vascular injury [37]. Additionally, as transseptal puncture is needed to insert a large caliber venous cannula, expertise with this technique is crucial for TandemHeart application in clinical practice, which may limit its widespread use, particularly among inexperienced interventional cardiologists not regularly performing transseptal punctures in their practice. Although rare, unique complications related to the transseptal puncture required for MCS with TandemHeart may occur and include cardiac tamponade, hemolysis, and thrombus or air embolism. Finally, device migration with dislodgement of the left atrial cannula to the RA during patient transport or leg movement may cause significant right-to-left shunt, resulting in severe hypoxemia and hemodynamic collapse. Severe peripheral arterial disease, left atrial thrombus, and profound coagulopathy are considered contraindications for TandemHeart use. Moreover, limited experience exists regarding the use of this device among patients with moderate to severe aortic regurgitation or those with ventricular septal defect [46].

5.4. Venoarterial Extracorporeal Membrane Oxygenation (VA-ECMO)

Based on the Extracorporeal Life Support Organization (ELSO) registry data, the number of ECMO devices and the number of centers utilizing ECMO are markedly increasing [47,48]. VA-ECMO provides both circulatory and oxygenation support, and therefore it is ideally used in patients with biventricular failure who develop cardiogenic shock and impaired oxygenation requiring cardiopulmonary resuscitation at the time PCI is initiated [49]. This is unlike venovenous ECMO (VV-ECMO), which is reserved for patients with respiratory failure but without significant cardiac dysfunction. When percutaneously inserted, VA-ECMO bypasses both the right and left side of the heart by draining deoxygenated blood from a central vein or RA with an 18-F to 21-F venous cannula and pumping oxygenated blood, after passing via an extracorporeal membrane oxygenator, into the iliofemoral arterial circulation (14-F to 19-F arterial cannula). The VA-ECMO system provides cardiac flow between 3 and 7 L/min depending on cannula sizes and can potentially be maintained for several days to weeks among patients with persistent cardiogenic shock as a bridge to recovery, permanent LV assist device implantation, or heart transplantation. Due to the substantial hemodynamic support provided by VA-ECMO, the hemodynamic and metabolic derangement resulted from cardiogenic shock is generally corrected within hours of device activation. Unfractionated heparin is typically used during ECMO support but other anticoagulants, such as bivalirudin, particularly in patients with heparin-induced thrombocytopenia who are unable to receive heparin, have been increasingly used as alternatives. The extent of anticoagulation during ECMO support is largely dependent on the type of membrane oxygenator and ranges from 180–250 s [50].

VA-ECMO support results in a remarkable increase in cardiac output and mean arterial pressure. However, its use is limited by retrograde blood flow leading to LV afterload mismatch, inadequate LV decompression, and high myocardial oxygen demand. The concurrent use of IABP or Impella can add further support by direct unloading of the LV and reducing ventricular wall stress [51,52]. Recently, a novel electrocardiogram (ECG)-synchronized, pulsatile VA-ECMO system, labeled i-cor (Xenios AG), has been introduced. The i-cor system consists of an ECG-triggered diagonal pump, which has a feature of diastolic augmentation and a capacity of providing a support up to 8 L/min. The main difference of the i-cor pump is the ability to generate a physiological pulse and to manage rotational timing to synchronize the pulse with the cardiac cycle of the native heart in order to provide adequate and physiologic circulatory support. By decreasing extracorporeal blood flow during systole and increasing flow during diastole, i-cor assist device flow decreases afterload and LV end-diastolic pressure and improves LV function and coronary flow compared with standard continuous VA-ECMO flow [53–55]. The first-in-man study, involving 15 patients with cardiogenic shock (71% due to AMI), showed that the i-cor pump was safe and applicable in clinical practice and implicated a hemodynamic benefit [56]. A multicenter study designed to test the safety and feasibility of this innovative pulsatile cardiac-synchronous MCS system in a larger population (the "SynCor" trial) is still ongoing.

One of the recent advancements in the percutaneous extracorporeal life support (ECLS) technology is the development of the Lifebridge B2T "bridge to therapy" system (Zoll Medical GmbH, Köln, Germany), which is a miniaturized and portable heart-lung support system similar in design to standard ECMO systems with an ability to provide cardiovascular stabilization and sufficient end-organ perfusion immediately after circulatory arrest. The Lifebridge system enables rapid application within 5 min due to its automated set-up and portable design in addition to less cumbersome transportation of the patient than standard ECMO equipment due to its smaller size and suitcase configuration. Other technical features include a battery life of 2 h, an overall weight of 18 kg (39.6 lb.), and a maximal blood flow of 6 L/min. Real-world clinical data of the German Lifebridge Registry involving 444 patients from 60 tertiary cardiovascular centers has been recently published [57] showing that this transportable automated ECLS system was safely applicable for hemodynamic stabilization with acceptable complications. However, mortality rates remained extremely high in these critically ill patients with immediate survival rates of 36% and 16% at 30-days after device implementation, especially in those with high lactate levels on admission.

Adverse events related to VA-ECMO include bleeding (with excessive anticoagulation), thromboembolic events in the circuit or systemically (if anticoagulation is inadequate), cannula-induced vascular injuries, infection, stroke (ischemic or hemorrhagic), hemolysis, and limb ischemia [58]. To reduce the risk of limb ischemia, a second antegrade arterial sheath can be inserted into the superficial femoral artery and when fed by the main arterial cannula can provide secured antegrade perfusion to the limb. Contraindications to peripheral VA-ECMO include patients with severe chronic organ dysfunction (renal failure, cirrhosis, or emphysema), prolonged cardiopulmonary resuscitation without adequate tissue perfusion, severe peripheral arterial disease, and patients unable to receive anticoagulation [11].

5.5. Other Percutaneous Mechanical Support Devices

Percutaneous LV MCS pumps under investigation include the pulsatile iVAC 2L (PulseCath BV, Arnhem, The Netherlands), which has been recently evaluated prospectively in a pilot study of 14 patients undergoing high-risk PCI demonstrating 100% angiographic success [59]. The Aortix (Procyrion, Houston, TX, USA) and Reitan (Cardiobridge, Hechingen, Germany) devices are other investigational devices that are deployed in the descending aorta similar to the IABP.

Apart from LV support, RV failure refractory to medical therapy is increasingly becoming a clinical challenge, thereby prompting the development of devices to specifically provide RV support. Large inferior AMI may cause predominant RV failure with cardiogenic shock with or without severe LV dysfunction. When cardiogenic shock is persistent despite maximal medical therapy, the options for MCS in this setting include VA-ECMO, surgical implantation of RVAD or total artificial heart (TAH), and heart transplantation [60]. The recent development of Impella RP launched an evolving field of percutaneous mechanical therapies for refractory RV failure. Impella RP is an intracardiac microaxial pump designed predominantly for management of primary RV failure, particularly in the setting of AMI, and can be inserted through the femoral vein to eject blood from the inferior vena cava directly to the pulmonary artery. The safety and reliability of the RP Impella has been established in the prospective RECOVER RIGHT study for severe isolated RV dysfunction [61]. Like LV Impella devices, complications that may occur with RP Impella support include bleeding, thrombosis, hemolysis, or infection.

6. Clinical Benefit of Percutaneous MCS Devices for PCI

The most recent clinical practice guidelines regarding the use of percutaneous MCS for PCI and management of ACS recommend consideration of the use of these devices in the setting of high-risk PCI and AMI complicated by cardiogenic shock [11]. However, despite accumulating evidence of hemodynamic improvement using various MCS devices, a convincing clinical benefit based on randomized controlled trials has not yet been demonstrated among this population. Because this is an extremely high-risk group of patients, improving clinical outcomes can be challenging and further research is still necessary to examine the optimal device features, the timing of support, and the appropriate patient for achieving maximal clinical benefit from these devices during PCI. The salient findings of contemporary studies examining the effect of MCS devices on outcomes in cardiogenic shock complicating AMI and high-risk PCI are summarized in Tables 3 and 4, respectively.

6.1. Intraaortic Balloon Bump

In the setting of PCI with cardiogenic shock complicating AMI, a previous retrospective study has suggested a potential benefit with early IABP support placed prior to PCI showing decreased rates of in-hospital mortality and cardiac adverse events compared with IABP placed only following PCI [62]. In a meta-analysis by Sjauw et al. [63], no mortality benefit or improvement in LV ejection fraction were found with utilizing IABP among patients undergoing PCI for ST-elevation myocardial infarction (STEMI), while higher stroke and bleeding rates were observed in the IABP group. Furthermore, among patients with cardiogenic shock undergoing PCI, there was a 6% increase in 30-day mortality [63]. Not only were randomized studies analyzed but cohort studies were also included in this meta-analysis; therefore, it could be subject to selection bias as sicker patients with more profound cardiogenic shock were more likely to be supported with IABP. In the SHOCK trial [64], IABP was not been shown to reduce mortality or major adverse events in patients with cardiogenic shock or high-risk PCI except in patients with STEMI. Subsequently, the IABP-SHOCK II trial [5], a prospective randomized controlled trial designed to study the effect of IABP involving 600 patients with AMI and cardiogenic shock undergoing early revascularization, showed no improvement in survival with IABP at 30 days [5] and subsequently at 1 year [65] and 6 years [66] post AMI. Moreover, there were no significant differences in any of the secondary clinical and laboratory (including lactate and creatinine) endpoints, and there were no significant differences in subgroup analyses. Based on the current guidelines, IABP is largely recommended in patients with mechanical complications post AMI or during transport of unstable patients from PCI centers without to centers with on-site cardiac surgery [12,67].

Among patients undergoing PCI without evident cardiogenic shock, IABP use was tested in the CRISP-AMI (Counterpulsation to Reduce Infarct Size Pre-PCI Acute Myocardial Infarction) trial [68]; a 30-center randomized controlled trial involving 337 patients with anterior STEMI, which found that routine IABP placement immediately prior to PCI had no significant effect on the infarct size as assessed by magnetic resonance imaging 3 to 5 days post PCI or on survival rates after 6 months of follow-up. Similarly, in a nonrandomized study using the National Cardiovascular Data Registry database, IABP utilization in high-risk PCI was not associated with lower mortality, and wide regional variations in the use of IABP was noted among the different centers [69]. Finally, the BCIS-1 trial [3], a prospective randomized controlled trial involving 301 patients randomized to routine IABP versus provisional IABP support for high-risk PCI, found no significant differences in mortality between the two groups. However, a long-term follow-up of more than four years showed a 34% relative reduction in all-cause mortality risk with routine IABP in patients with severe ischemic cardiomyopathy undergoing high-risk PCI, which might be attributed to lower incidence of procedural hypotension with preplanned IABP insertion [70].

Given these conflicting results and the controversy surrounding its benefit, the use of IABP in the setting of STEMI complicated with cardiogenic shock is decreasing and its routine use has been recently downgraded to class III (harm) by the ESC [10] and to class IIa (should be considered) by the American Heart Association (AHA)/American College of Cardiology (ACC) [71] guidelines. Furthermore, due to the introduction of new devices, such as Impella, and the continuous advancement in MCS technology, which provides superior hemodynamic support and potentially more favorable outcomes, the future role of IABP in management of cardiogenic shock and ventricular unloading may continue to decline.

6.2. Impella Devices

There are currently limited available data to establish a significant clinical benefit of Impella use in patients with cardiogenic shock undergoing PCI. Impella devices provide greater hemodynamic support with a more pronounced cardiac output augmentation and LV unloading than IABP. In 2008, the ISAR-SHOCK (Impella LP 2.5 versus IABP in Cardiogenic SHOCK) trial [72] was the first randomized clinical study to assess the safety and efficacy of Impella 2.5 in the setting of AMI complicated by cardiogenic shock as compared to IABP. Twenty-five patients were randomized to the Impella 2.5 LP device or IABP, and the primary endpoint was a change in cardiac index after 30 min of support. All patients received PCI of the infarct-related artery and remained in shock. Patients supported with an Impella had greater increase in cardiac index and mean arterial blood pressure after 30 min of support. However, there was no difference in mortality or in the rates of bleeding or limb ischemia between the two groups [72]. Subsequently, the safety and efficacy of Impella 2.5 LP was examined in the EUROSHOCK multicenter registry [39] involving 120 patients with severe cardiogenic shock refractory to conventional therapy, among which cardiopulmonary resuscitation was performed in more than 40%, showing high overall in-hospital mortality rates reaching 64% without survival benefit in the group treated with an Impella. Similarly, the IMPRESS in Severe SHOCK (IMPella versus IABP Reduces mortality in STEMI patients treated with primary PCI in Severe cardiogenic SHOCK) trial [6] enrolled 48 mechanically ventilated patients with severe cardiogenic shock after AMI who were randomized 1:1 to Impella CP or IABP and followed for all-cause mortality at 30 days and 6 months post AMI. Importantly, 44 (92%) patients had cardiac arrest prior to randomization with interquartile time till return of spontaneous circulation ranging from 15 to 52 min and a considerable proportion of patients (46%) died due to anoxic brain damage. The overall mortality in the study was 50% and there were no significant differences between the two arms (50% versus 46% at 30 days and 50% versus 50% at 6 months in the IABP and Impella CP groups, respectively), thus reflecting a very high risk cohort presenting with late-stage cardiogenic shock [6,73]. The only study reporting a mortality benefit of Impella in the setting of cardiogenic shock complicating AMI was by Karatolios et al. [74], who conducted a retrospective, single-center study including 90 patients suffering from AMI and cardiogenic shock treated with Impella (n = 27) or medical treatment alone (n = 63). Patients in the Impella group were sicker, evidenced by higher lactate levels, longer low cardiac output duration, and lower LV ejection fraction than those treated medically. When 20 patients of each group were matched, patients supported with Impella had decreased rates of in-hospital (35% versus 80%; $p = 0.01$) and 6-month (40% versus 80%; $p = 0.02$) mortality [74]. More recently, using IABP-SHOCK II trial inclusion and exclusion criteria, a retrospective analysis of 237 patients with AMI and cardiogenic shock treated with Impella 2.5 (~30% of patients) or Impella CP (~70% of patients) were propensity matched to the same number of patients from the IABP-SHOCK II trial [75]. There was no significant difference in 30-day all-cause mortality. Moreover, severe or life-threatening bleedings as well as peripheral vascular complications occurred more often in the Impella group. Limiting the analysis to IABP-treated patients as the control group showed comparable results with no evidence of favorable outcomes with Impella use [75]. Finally, a meta-analysis including 588 patients from the main aforementioned studies, the use of MCS with Impella in the setting of AMI and cardiogenic shock was not associated with improved short-time survival but there were higher rates of complications when compared with IABP and medical treatment [76]. It is important to recognize, however, that the vast majority of patients included in these studies were in profound cardiogenic shock and after cardiac arrest. As the use of Impella in patients with less severe shock or pre-shock conditions was not the focus of these studies, its effect on outcomes cannot, therefore, be addressed based on the current data and further studies are still warranted in these settings.

The effectiveness and safety of Impella support for planned high-risk coronary interventions have been investigated in small studies showing encouraging results. In the AMC MAC1 study [77], 19 consecutive high-risk and poor surgical candidates with moderate-to-severe LV dysfunction (ejection fraction < 40%) underwent PCI of an unprotected left main or the last remaining vessel with Impella 2.5 support showing 100% procedural success and no important device-related adverse events, thereby demonstrating safety and feasibility of utilizing Impella devices for high-risk PCI. This has also been confirmed in the PROTECT I trial [78], a prospective and multicenter study, which showed that Impella 2.5 system is safe, easy to implant, and provides excellent hemodynamic support for a mean duration of 1.7 h (range: 0.4–2.5 h) during high-risk PCI. The real-world use of the Impella 2.5 in complex high-risk PCI showed an angiographic revascularization success of 99% in the overall cohort and in 90% of patients with multivessel revascularization. Survival rates were 91% and 81% at 6 months and 12 months, respectively, despite including inoperable patients with a high prevalence of LV dysfunction, New York Heart Association (NYHA) class III and IV heart failure, and chronic renal dysfunction [14].

The largest prospective randomized clinical study to examine the effect of hemodynamic support with Impella in patients undergoing high-risk PCI was the PROTECT II trial [4]. In this multi-center study, 452 patients with complex three-vessel disease or unprotected left main CAD and severely depressed LV function were assigned to IABP or Impella 2.5 during non-emergent high-risk PCI. The composite primary endpoint of 30-day incidence of 11 major adverse events was similar between the Impella and IABP groups (35.1% for Impella 2.5 versus 40.1% for IABP, $p = 0.227$ in the intention-to-treat population, and 34.3% versus 42.2%, $p = 0.092$ in the per-protocol population). Impella did provide greater hemodynamic support and at 90-day follow-up there was a trend towards a decreased incidence of adverse events with Impella in the intention-to-treat population (40.6% versus 49.3%, $p = 0.066$) and significantly decreased events in the per-protocol population (40.0% versus 51.0%, $p = 0.023$) [4]. A subsequent analysis of the outcomes using a prognostic ally important definition of AMI based on new Q-waves or >8× increase in creatinine kinase-MB, demonstrated that that Impella resulted in improved event-free survival after 90 days of follow-up, supporting a late benefit that could be attributed to more stable procedural hemodynamics that facilitate the performance of more complete revascularization and complex PCI procedures, such as rotational atherectomy and bifurcation coronary disease intervention, more safely [79]. A more recent consecutive real-world cohort of high-risk PCI patients, new generation MCS devices (including Impella CP, Heartmate PHP, and PulseCath iVAC2L) have demonstrated a significant reduction in the composite endpoint of serious peri-procedural adverse events, including cardiac arrest and 30-day mortality despite worse LV function and higher Synergy between Percutaneous Coronary Intervention with TAXUS and Cardiac Surgery (SYNTAX)-I score observed in patients protected with MCS [8]. Interestingly, patients under age of 75, with a SYNTAX-I score > 32, and with an LV ejection fraction < 30% derived most potential benefit from MCS utilization during PCI. These promising findings indicate that the more powerful LV support obtained using new generation MCS devices may be necessary for improving clinical outcomes, which has not been evidently seen using the IABP or Impella 2.5 devices.

6.3. TandemHeart

Small studies have shown a significant improvement in hemodynamics with TandemHeart use, but were underpowered to show improvement in survival. In an observational study by Kar et al. [43], TandemHeart placement in patients with severe cardiogenic shock refractory to conventional inotropic or IABP therapy was associated with improvement in cardiac index (increased from 0.5 to 3 L/min/m^2), PCWP (decreased from 31 to 17 mmHg), and mixed venous oxygen saturation (increased from 49 to 69%), as well as improvement in kidney function (urine output increased from 70 to 1200 mL/day and creatinine decreased from 1.5 to 1.2 mg/dL) and lactic acid level (decreased from 11 to 1.5 mg/dL). However, overall mortality (40.2% at 30 days and 45.3% at 6 months) and bleeding complications remained high [43]. In a small randomized study involving patients in cardiogenic shock after AMI, with intended PCI to the infarcted artery, who were assigned to either IABP (n = 20) or TandemHeart (n = 21), hemodynamic and metabolic parameters was more effectively reversed by TandemHeart than by IABP treatment. However, adverse events, such as severe bleeding and limb ischemia, were encountered more frequently after TandemHeart support, and 30-day mortality was similar [80]. Similarly, a small randomized trial of patients presenting within 24 h of the development of cardiogenic shock and assigned to IABP or TandemHeart showed superior hemodynamic parameters with TandemHeart, even in patients failing IABP, but no significant differences in in-hospital mortality or severe adverse events when compared with IABP alone [81].

Data on the use of TandemHeart in high-risk PCI is limited to observational studies. A study from the Mayo Clinic summarized data on 54 consecutive patients undergoing high-risk PCI using a TandemHeart device for support, demonstrating feasibility and safety of this device to allow performance of high-risk and complex intervention [82]. All patients were deemed high risk for surgery and underwent complex PCI, with a Society of Thoracic Surgery (STS) mortality risk score of 13%, a median SYNTAX score of 33, and the majority of patients underwent left main and multivessel PCI. Procedural success was achieved in 97% of cases, with hemodynamic improvement during the procedure, and 6-month survival was 87%. However, major vascular complications occurred in 13% of cases [82]. Additional small series of patients undergoing TandemHeart-assisted high-risk PCI have shown comparable results. A meta-analysis of usefulness of percutaneous MCS devices, including eight cohort studies with 205 patients supported by TandemHeart and 12 studies with 1346 patients supported with Impella 2.5 during high-risk PCI, found 30-day mortality rates of 8% and major bleeding rates of 3.6% with TandemHeart compared with 3.5% and 7.1% with Impella 2.5, respectively. Overall periprocedural outcomes were comparable between the two groups [83].

6.4. Venoarterial Extracorporeal Membrane Oxygenation (VA-ECMO)

While ECMO provides excellent cardiopulmonary support with a relative ease of implementation, its use in the setting of AMI and shock is limited by the need for specialized perfusion expertise and nursing as well as the possibility for increased LV stroke work and myocardial oxygen demand, which can precipitate further myocardial ischemia. Additionally, there is need for large bore cannulas and aggressive antithrombotic therapy which increase the risk of bleeding. A recent single-center study [84] reported a 67% survival to discharge rate among 18 consecutive patients who received femoral VA-ECMO in the cardiac catheterization lab for severe shock due to ACS. The average length of ECMO support was 3.2 days and 17 (94%) patients required at least one blood transfusion with higher bleeding rates observed among those treated with glycoprotein IIb/IIIa inhibitors [84]. In another small retrospective study [85], a total of 15 patients undergoing VA-ECMO placement for AMI with refractory cardiogenic shock were analyzed. One-third of patients presented with out-of-hospital resuscitation and 60% had IABP placed for LV venting. The survival rate after 30 days was 47% and vascular complications occurred in 53% of patients. There is a growing utilization of VA-ECMO in patients suffering from cardiac arrest requiring prolonged cardiopulmonary resuscitation (CPR) showing acceptable survival rate and outcome [86]. A meta-analysis including 1866 patients treated with VA-ECMO for cardiogenic shock or cardiac arrest showed an approximate overall survival of 30% and significant associated morbidity with the performance of this intervention [58]. These data suggest that use of VA-ECMO should be individualized based on risk-benefit analysis derived from vascular anatomy and comorbidities to maximize clinical benefit. Finally, LV unloading during VA-ECMO treatment for cardiogenic shock appears beneficial either with predominant use of IABP [51] or Impella [87] demonstrating significant improvement in survival with the two unloading tools.

7. Recommendations for MCS Use During PCI

A suggested algorithmic approach to MCS use during PCI for cardiogenic shock complicating AMI and high-risk PCI without cardiogenic shock is depicted in Figure 2. Interventional cardiologists are challenged with a growing number of patients in need of coronary revascularization but who are hemodynamically unstable or deemed poor surgical candidates and too high risk for PCI. The use of percutaneous MCS devices has been proven to be feasible and safe in clinical conditions previously considered for conservative therapy only. However, data on survival benefit as a result of utilizing these percutaneous devices is still lacking. It is not therefore surprising that there has been a modest adoption of these devices in the current practice, reflecting the equivocal results from the current evidence base in addition to the uncertainty as to which patients MCS will add a real benefit. Optimal timing of device insertion is also an important variable. In light of the currently available data, it is reasonable that utilization of MCS devices in clinical practice should be advocated in an individualized manner based on a detailed review of the risks and benefits rather than as a standard of care for every complex procedure. The recommendations on the use of a specific MCS device are based on the anticipated hemodynamic effects and risks as well as clinical outcome data. Based on the recent SCAI/ACC/HFSA/STS Clinical Expert Consensus Statement published in 2015 [11], percutaneous MCS may be considered in carefully selected patients with severe cardiogenic shock complicating AMI unresponsive to pharmacologic support as a bridge to recovery following PCI or definitive therapy. The evidence is stronger in the setting of mechanical complications post MI, such as ischemic mitral regurgitation when hemodynamic derangement is usually acute and more substantial and the benefit from these devices is more pronounced. There is an increasing indication for temporary MCS use during and after primary PCI for patients presenting with large AMI causing severe LV dysfunction, and RV mechanical support with Impella RP can be considered for RV infarction complicated by cardiogenic shock. Early insertion of MCS devices is essential to attenuate the sequelae that may result from persistent cardiac ischemia and systemic hypoperfusion. The type of MCS device is dependent on multiple factors including the amount of hemodynamic support needed and the ultimate goal of support as well as technical characteristics that should be taken into consideration, such as the ease or deployment, and availability of these devices. IABP is more often used due to the ease of insertion and availability although the benefit of its utility is questionable in patients with AMI and cardiogenic shock. Impella 2.5 or CP provide more powerful hemodynamic support and can be inserted as rapidly as an IABP in experienced centers and are thus considered more favorable devices in appropriate patients. Finally, TandemHeart, VA-ECMO, or Impella 5 (which requires surgical cutdown for delivery) should be reserved for patients who continue to deteriorate despite such support. In patients who present with biventricular or cardiopulmonary failure, VA-ECMO is recommended as the first choice. For isolated RV failure with cardiogenic shock, Impella RP is an available percutaneous MCS option that may be considered in such cases [28].

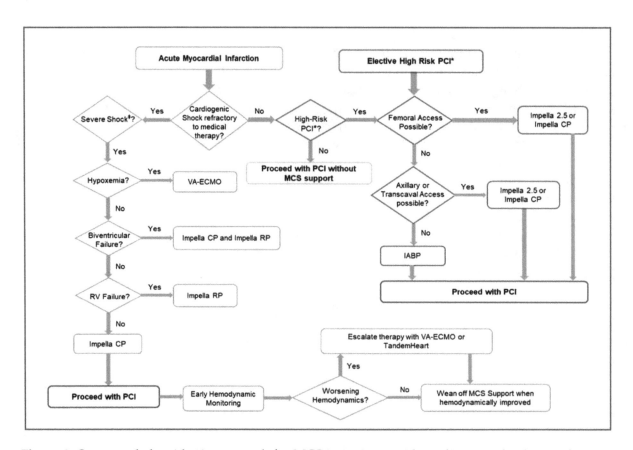

Figure 2. Suggested algorithmic approach for MCS in patients with cardiogenic shock complicating AMI and high-risk PCI. MCS, mechanical circulatory support; AMI, acute myocardial infarction; PCI, percutaneous coronary intervention. IABP, intraaortic balloon bump; VA-ECMO, venoarterial extracorporeal membrane oxygenation. * High-risk PCI is defined as presented in Table 1 and mainly include comorbidities, severe LV dysfunction (EF < 35%), and complex coronary artery disease involving a large territory, such as unprotected left main, sole-remaining vessel, or three-vessel disease. ‡ Severe cardiogenic shock is defined as markedly abnormal hemodynamic parameters (systolic blood pressure < 90 mmHg, heart rate > 120 beats per minute, cardiac index < 1.5 L/min/m², pulmonary capillary wedge pressure/left ventricular end-diastolic pressure > 30 mmHg), metabolic (lactate > 4 mg/dL), and clinical (confusion, cool extremities, on ≥2 vasopressors/inotropes) parameters.

For prophylactic percutaneous MCS use in the setting of high-risk PCI, great emphasis should be on identifying the patient's anatomic, hemodynamic, and procedural features that indicate adjunctive MCS support may be necessary and also determine the optimal device to utilize [2]. The current recommendation is to consider using MCS devices in patients with severe LV dysfunction (EF < 35%) or recent presentation with decompensated heart failure in the setting of complex coronary artery disease involving a large territory, such as unprotected left main, sole-remaining vessel, or three-vessel disease. Generally, patients with anticipated noncomplex PCI may be considered for IABP as the first-line MCS option with Impella as back up support, whereas those with anticipated technically challenging or prolonged procedure (rotational atherectomy or bifunctional stenting) may be considered for Impella, TandemHeart, or VA-ECMO depending on vascular anatomy, RV function, expertise, and availability [2,88]. The more severe the clinical and anatomic circumstances, the greater the potential benefit of MCS use [11]. MCS support should be initiated before the start of the PCI and in most cases can be removed immediately after the intervention. In cases with hemodynamic derangement after PCI, prolonged MCS support should be considered until hemodynamic improvement. Continuous hemodynamic monitoring with pulmonary arterial catheter in encouraged as early as possible to tailor therapy and help with determining the amount and duration of MCS support needed. Finally, the use of MCS devices in the emergent setting has been suggested to be cost-effective compared with surgical ECMO or ventricular assist device support [89], as well as in the elective setting when compared with IABP [90].

8. Future Directions

The majority of studies involving the new MCS devices for cardiogenic shock and high risk PCI have demonstrated superior hemodynamic improvement as compared to IABP but these studies were largely underpowered to find mortality benefit and therefore should be regarded as feasibility trials and a basis for larger clinical trials in the future. The DanGer Shock study [91] is an ongoing prospective randomized multicenter study with planned enrollment of 360 patients with AMI complicated by cardiogenic shock randomized 1:1 immediately after shock diagnosis to either Impella CP prior to PCI or current guideline-driven therapy. Patients with coma after out of hospital cardiac arrest are excluded. The primary endpoint is all-cause mortality at 180 days. The DanGer trial will be the first adequately powered randomized controlled trial to examine whether MCS with Impella CP improves survival among patients with cardiogenic shock complicating AMI and will therefore provide fundamental knowledge on the use of transvalvular LV unloading in this setting [91].

Despite the lack of current evidence, we believe that advanced MCS devices may improve clinical outcomes, including survival, in a selected group of patients and in specific circumstances. Future studies should largely focus on three major considerations when examining the clinical benefit of MCS. First, the optimal MCS device design and amount of support needed to achieve hemodynamic as well as metabolic improvement is unclear. For instance, in the IMPRESS in Severe Shock trial, one third of the patients died due to refractory cardiogenic shock and lactate levels remained high in many patients while being on Impella CP support, suggesting that the actual level of support was not sufficient [6,73]. Second, appropriate patient selection is a key factor that should be emphasized in future studies. Because utilization is currently determined based on subjective criteria, many patients may survive without MCS while others with irreversible anoxic brain injury from prolonged shock may not survive even with adequate hemodynamic support. Additionally, patients with shock and multiorgan dysfunction are at significantly higher risk of bleeding due to increased inflammation and coagulopathy which may progress to disseminated intravascular coagulation. Therefore, studies focusing on identifying patients are higher risk of device-associated complications among whom the harm of these complications may outweigh the benefit is clinically meaningful for mitigating device complications. For example, lactate has been shown to be an important biomarker for risk stratification in the setting of cardiogenic shock. Among patients undergoing extracorporeal cardiopulmonary resuscitation due to cardiac arrest, lactate clearance was the sole predictor of neurological outcome as assessed by the Glasgow Outcome Scale (GOS) [92] and in patients with refractory cardiogenic shock requiring VA-ECMO support, lactate levels and lactate clearance during ECMO therapy were predictive markers for 30-day mortality [93]. In patients with cardiac arrest, lactate levels prior to ECMO initiation was significantly associated with increased risk of all-cause mortality at 90 days. Interestingly, lactate was found to be more predictive of outcome than duration of cardiopulmonary resuscitation or absence of return of spontaneous circulation [94]. These findings suggest that early metabolic assessment by measuring plasma lactate levels may be an important prognostic marker for risk stratification when considering MCS in patients with cardiogenic shock. One study has shown that high body mass index (BMI) was an additional predictor of 30-day mortality in patients with AMI and cardiogenic shock supported by VA-ECMO [95]. However, the influence of BMI on outcomes among patients supported by other MCS devices is unclear.

Third, the timing of MCS device insertion in relation to primary PCI among patients with AMI and cardiogenic shock can be critical to achieve survival benefit and future studies should focus on determining the optimal timing of MCS, which remains elusive. Recent studies have shown in an animal model that mechanical support with LV unloading reduces infarct size and favorably mediates key biological pathways associated with inflammation and maladaptive cardiac remodeling when mechanical support is initiated prior to coronary reperfusion compared with early reperfusion without support [96–99]. In a prospective safety and feasibility first-in-human study known as the Door to Unloading With Impella CP System in Acute Myocardial Infarction to Reduce Infarct Size (DTU), LV unloading with the Impella CP with a 30-min delay prior to reperfusion in patient with STEMI is feasible with similar rates of adverse cardiovascular events and 30-day mean infarct size and without prohibitive safety signals [100]. These data suggest that LV unloading prior to PCI initiation in the setting of myocardial ischemia may be pivotal to achieve significant benefit from MCS devices but clinical evidence from randomized control trials is still awaiting. In support of this hypothesis, in the setting of AMI and cardiogenic shock, data from the catheter-based ventricular assist device registry have shown that early MCS implantation (either the Impella 2.5 or Impella CP) before PCI, prior to escalating doses of inotropes or vasopressors and within 75 min from shock onset, was independently associated with improved survival compared with later MCS support [24]. Similarly, data from a quality improvement registry including over 15,000 patients with AMI complicated by cardiogenic shock and supported with Impella have shown wide variation in outcomes across centers with higher survival rates seen when Impella was used as first support strategy, when invasive hemodynamic monitoring was used, and at higher institutional Impella implantation volume [101]. A meta-analysis of 3 available studies on the use of early Impella in patients with AMI and cardiogenic shock found that early initiation of Impella decreased in-hospital or 30-day mortality by 48% compared with late initiation of Impella [102].

Based on these promising retrospective data, and after the FDA's approval of Impella for cardiogenic shock complicating AMI, investigators have organized the construct of a multicenter national shock protocol now referred to as the "National Cardiogenic Shock Initiative" (NCSI) emphasizing invasive hemodynamic monitoring and rapid initiation of percutaneous MCS support. The analysis of the first 171 patients enrolled in NCSI was recently published [7] and included patients presenting with AMI and cardiogenic shock using the same inclusion and exclusion criteria from the "SHOCK" trial (with an additional exclusion criteria of IABP use prior to MCS). The majority of patients were supported with Impella CP (92%) prior to PCI (74%) with an average door to support of 85 min in STEMI cases. Moreover, right heart catheterization with hemodynamic monitoring was performed in 92% of cases. The use of a protocol-based approach showed improved survival compared with previously reported studies [7]. Despite the limitations of being an observational single arm study, these findings highlight the importance of early MCS prior to PCI for achieving the most benefit from MCS. Future studies are still warranted to confirm these promising findings. Finally, it is necessary to derive efficient risk scores for identifying patients at high risk of developing cardiogenic shock following AMI as this may aid in risk stratification and potential prophylactic utilization of MCS during PCI to mitigate subsequent hemodynamic derangement in this high-risk population [103].

Another field of future research is the percutaneous LV unloading strategy using Impella in combination with VA-ECMO (ECMELLA) to improve outcomes in patients with refractory cardiogenic shock [87,104]. In an all-comers retrospective study, percutaneous LV unloading with Impella on top of VA-ECMO showed improved outcomes, including higher 30-day survival, as compared to predicted outcomes by established risk scores [87]. In addition to the ECMELLA approach, previous studies have also suggested that a combination of VA-ECMO plus IABP is safe and associated with improved in-hospital survival in cardiogenic shock patients [105]. However, given the retrospective nature of these studies, prospective and randomized studies are still warranted to further investigate this therapeutic strategy.

Table 3. Main Clinical Studies of Percutaneous MCS devices in AMI with Cardiogenic Shock.

First Author/Study (Ref. #)	N	Study Type	Study Arms	Definition	Primary Endpoint	Salient Findings
			IABP			
IABP-SHOCK-II [5,65,66]	600	RCT	IABP versus no IABP	AMI with cardiogenic shock (SBP < 90 mmHg for >30 min or need for vasoactive agents, pulmonary congestion, impaired organ perfusion)	30-day, 1-year, 6-year all-cause mortality	No difference in survival at 30 days [5], 1 year [65], and 6 years [66]. No differences recurrent MI, stroke, ischemic comp, severe bleeding, or sepsis.
TACTICs [106]	57	RCT	Fibrinolytic therapy with IABP versus without IABP	AMI with sustained hypotension and heart failure with signs of hypoperfusion	6-month all-cause Mortality	No survival benefit except for patients with Killip III/IV supported with IABP.
Waksman et al. [107]	45	Prospective, nonrandomized	Fibrinolytic therapy with IABP versus without IABP	AMI complicated by cardiogenic shock	In-hospital and 1-year all-cause mortality	In-hospital and 1-year survival improved with IABP after early revascularization with fibrinolytic therapy.
NRMI [108]	23,180	Observational	Fibrinolytic or PCI with IABP versus no IABP	AMI with cardiogenic shock at initial presentation or during hospitalization	In-hospital all-cause mortality	IABP was associated with decreased in-hospital mortality in patients received fibrinolysis but not PCI.
Hariss et al. [62]	48	Observational	IABP prior to PCI versus late IABP	AMI complicated by cardiogenic shock	In-hospital all-cause mortality	Early IABP was associated with decreased in-hospital mortality compared with late IABP.
Sjauw et al. [63]	1009 (RCTs) 10,529 (cohort studies)	Meta-analysis (7 RCTs, 9 cohort studies)	IABP versus no IABP	AMI complicated by cardiogenic shock	30-day all-cause mortality	No survival benefit or improvement in LV ejection fraction with IABP.

Table 3. *Cont.*

First Author/Study (Ref. #)	N	Study Type	Study Arms	Definition	Primary Endpoint	Salient Findings
Impella						
ISAR-SHOCK [72]	25	RCT	Impella 2.5 versus IABP	AMI complicated by cardiogenic shock	Change in the CI at 30 min post implantation	Superior hemodynamics with Impella. Mortality was similar between the two groups.
EUROSHOCK [39]	120	Observational	Impella 2.5	AMI complicated by cardiogenic shock	30-day all-cause mortality	30-day mortality was high at 64% despite improvement in hemodynamic and metabolic parameters with Impella.
IMPRESS in Severe Shock [6]	48	RCT	Impella CP versus IABP	AMI with severe shock (SBP < 90 mmHg or the need for vasoactive agents, and all required mechanical ventilation)	30-day all-cause mortality	Mortality occurred in 50% of patients with no significant survival benefit with Impella.
Karatolios et al. [74]	90	Observational	Impella versus medical therapy	AMI with post-cardiac arrest cardiogenic shock	In-hospital all-cause mortality	Impella group had better survival at discharge and after 6 months despite being a sicker group.
Schrage et al. [75]	237	Observational	Impella 2.5 (~30%), Impella CP (~70%) versus IABP (matched from IABP-SHOCK trial)	AMI with cardiogenic shock (SBP < 90 mmHg for >30 min or need for vasoactive agents, pulmonary congestion, impaired organ perfusion)	30-day all-cause mortality	Impella was not associated with lower 30-day mortality. Severe bleedings and peripheral vascular complications were more common with Impella use.
Wernly et al. [76]	588	Meta-analysis (4 studies)	Impella versus IABP or medical therapy alone	AMI with cardiogenic shock	30-day all-cause mortality	No improvement in short-term survival with Impella. Higher risk of major bleeding and peripheral ischemic events with Impella.

Table 3. *Cont.*

First Author/Study (Ref. #)	N	Study Type	Study Arms	Definition	Primary Endpoint	Salient Findings
Cheng et al. [109]	100	Meta-analysis (3 RCTs; 1 for Impella versus IABP and 2 for TandemHeart versus IABP))	Impella or TandemHeart versus IABP	AMI with cardiogenic shock	30-day all-cause mortality	No significant differences in 30-day mortality. Improved hemodynamics with Impella and TandemHeart. Higher rates of bleeding with TandemHeart and of hemolysis with Impella.
Alushi et al. [110]	116	Observational	Impella 2.5 (~30%), Impella CP (~70%) versus IABP	AMI with cardiogenic shock	30-day all-cause mortality	No significant differences in 30-day mortality. Impella significantly reduced the inotropic score, lactate levels, and improved LVEF compared with IABP. Higher rates of bleeding with Impella.
TandemHeart						
Kar et al. [43]	117	Observational	TandemHeart	Severe cardiogenic shock despite vasopressor and IABP support	30-day all-cause mortality	30-day mortality: 40%. Improvement in hemodynamics refractory to vasopressors and IABP.
Thiele et al. [80]	41	RCT	TandemHeart versus IABP	AMI with cardiogenic shock (CI < 2.1 L/min/m^2, lactate > 2)	Change in cardiac index	Hemodynamic and metabolic parameters were reversed more effectively by TandemHeart. 30-day mortality was similar. Bleeding and ischemic events were more common with TandemHeart.
Burkhoff et al. [81]	42	RCT	TandemHeart versus IABP	Severe cardiogenic shock (most had AMI and failed IABP)	30-day all-cause mortality	Similar mortality rates and adverse events at 30 days. Superior hemodynamics with TandemHeart.

Table 3. *Cont.*

First Author/Study (Ref. #)	N	Study Type	Study Arms	Definition	Primary Endpoint	Salient Findings
			VA-ECMO			
Esper et al. [84]	18	Observational	VA-ECMO	Severe cardiogenic shock due to ACS	Survival to hospital discharge	Survival rates at discharge: 67%. High bleeding rates (94% required blood transfusion).
Negi et al. [85]	15	Observational	VA-ECMO	AMI with severe cardiogenic shock (60% had STEMI and IABP support)	Survival to hospital discharge	Survival rates at discharge: 47%. Vascular complications: 53%.
Nichol et al. [111]	1494 (84 studies)	Systematic review	VA-ECMO	Cardiogenic shock or cardiac arrest	Survival to hospital discharge	Survival to hospital discharge: 50%.
Sheu et al. [112]	Group 1: 115 Group 2: 219	Observational	Group 1: profound shock without ECMO versus group 2: profound shock with ECMO	AMI and profound cardiogenic shock (SBP <75 mmHg despite IABP and vasopressor support)	30-day survival	ECMO group had higher survival rates: 60.9% versus 28% in non-ECMO group.
Takayama et al. [113]	90	Observational	VA-ECMO	Refractory cardiac shock (AMI in 49%)	Survival to hospital discharge	Survival to hospital discharge: 49%. Bleeding and stroke rates: 26%; and LV distension and pulmonary edema: 18%.

Abbreviations: ACS, acute coronary syndrome; AMI, acute myocardial infarction; CI, cardiac index; IABP, intraaortic balloon pump; IMPRESS in Severe SHOCK, IMPella versus IABP Reduces mortality in STEMI patients treated with primary PCI in Severe cardiogenic SHOCK; ISAR-SHOCK, Impella LP 2.5 versus IABP in Cardiogenic SHOCK; LVEF, left ventricular ejection fraction; MCS, mechanical circulatory support; NRMI, National Registry of Myocardial Infarction; PCI, percutaneous coronary intervention; RCT, randomized controlled study; SBP, systolic blood pressure; STEMI, ST-elevation myocardial infarction; VA-ECMO, venoarterial extracorporeal membrane oxygenation.

Table 4. Main Clinical Studies of Percutaneous MCS devices in High-Risk PCI.

First Author/Study (Ref. #)	N	Study Type	Study Arms	Definition	Primary Endpoint	Salient Findings
IABP						
BCIS-1 [3]	301	RCT	Elective IABP versus no IABP before PCI	High-risk PCI without cardiogenic shock, LVEF < 30%, severe CAD (jeopardy score > 8)	MACE: Composite of death, AMI, stroke, revascularization at hospital discharge	No reduction in MACE. No difference in survival rates at 6 months. Decreased major procedural complications with planned IABP (mainly hypotension).
Extended BCIS-1 [70]	301	RCT	Elective IABP versus no IABP before PCI	High-risk PCI without cardiogenic shock, LVEF < 30%, severe CAD (jeopardy score > 8)	Long-term All-cause mortality	Elective IABP use was associated with a 34% relative reduction in all-cause mortality at 4 years post PCI.
CRISP-AMI [68]	337	RCT	Elective IABP prior to PCI until at least 12 h post versus no IABP	Acute anterior MI without cardiogenic shock	Infarct size measured by cardiac MRI at 3–5 days post PCI	No reduction in infarct size with IABP use. Survival at 6 months and procedural complications were similar between groups.
NCDR [69]	181,599	Observational	Elective IABP versus no IABP before PCI	LVEF < 30%, severe CAD, including patients with cardiogenic shock	In-hospital mortality	IABP use varied significantly across hospitals. No association with differences in in-hospital mortality.

Table 4. *Cont.*

First Author/Study (Ref. #)	N	Study Type	Study Arms	Definition	Primary Endpoint	Salient Findings
				Impella		
Henriques et al. [77]	19	Observational	Impella 2.5	High-risk PCI (elderly, most with prior MI, poor surgical candidates, LVEF < 40%)	Safety and feasibility of Impella use	A 100% procedural success and no important device-related adverse events.
PROTECT I [78]	20	Prospective, nonrandomized	Impella 2.5	High-risk PCI (LVEF < 35%, UPLM disease or last patent vessel)	Safety and feasibility of Impella use	Impella is safe, easy to implant, and provides excellent hemodynamic support during high-risk PCI.
USPella [14]	175	Observational	Impella 2.5	High-risk PCI (severe three-vessel disease or UPLM, mean SYNTAX score 36, low LVEF)	MACE at 30 days	MACE: 8%. 30-day, 6-month, and 12-month survival: 96%, 91%, and 88%, respectively.
PROTECT II [4]	452	RCT	Impella 2.5 versus IABP	High-risk PCI (LVEF < 35%, UPLM, three-vessel or last patent vessel disease)	MACE (a composite of 11 adverse events) at 30 days	30-day MACE was similar between groups (ITT) and trend for lower MACE with Impella (PP). 90-day MACE was similar (ITT) and significantly lower with Impella (PP).
Ameelot et al. [8]	198	Observational	Impella CP, heartmate PHP, or PulseCath iVAC2L versus unprotected PCI	Prophylactic high-risk PCI	A composite of procedure-related adverse events	Lower rates of periprocedural adverse events with Impella devices. 30-day survival was significantly higher with Impella versus unsupported PCI.

Table 4. *Cont.*

First Author/Study (Ref. #)	N	Study Type	Study Arms	Definition	Primary Endpoint	Salient Findings
TandemHeart						
Alli et al. [82]	54	Observational	TandemHeart	Prophylactic high-risk PCI (STS score 13%, SYNTAX score 33, three-vessel and UPLM disease)	6-month survival	6-month survival: 87%. Major vascular complications: 13%.
Briasoulis et al. [83]	205	Meta-analysis (8 cohort studies)	TandemHeart	Prophylactic high-risk PCI	30-day all-cause mortality	30-day mortality: 8%. Major bleeding rates: 3.6%.
VA-ECMO						
Teirstein et al. [114]	389 (prophylactic support) 180 (standby support)	Observational	VA-ECMO	High-risk PCI (LVEF < 25%, culprit lesion supplying > 50% of the myocardium)	PCI success rates and major complications rates	Comparable results in the prophylactic compared with the standby VA-ECMO support groups. Patients with extremely low LVEF may benefit more from prophylactic support.
Schreiber et al. [115]	149	Observational	VA-ECMO versus IABP	High-risk PCI (low LVEF and multivessel PCI)	MACE: Composite of MI, stroke, death, CABG	No difference in MACE between VA-ECMO and IABP groups. Higher multivessel PCI success rates with VA-ECMO.

Abbreviations: AMI, acute myocardial infarction; BCIS-1, the Balloon pump-assisted Coronary Intervention Study; CRISP-AMI, the Counterpulsation to Reduce Infarct Size Pre-PCI Acute Myocardial Infarction; CABG, coronary artery bypass grafting; IABP, intraaortic balloon pump; ITT, intention to treat analysis; LVEF, left ventricular ejection fraction; MACE, major adverse cardiac events; MCS, mechanical circulatory support; MI, myocardial infarction; NCDR, National Cardiovascular Data Registry; PCI, percutaneous coronary intervention; PP, per protocol analysis; RCT, randomized controled study; SYNTAX, Synergy between Percutaneous Coronary Intervention with TAXUS and Cardiac Surgery; UPLM, unprotected left main; VA-ECMO, venoarterial extracorporeal membrane oxygenation.

9. Conclusions

The use of MCS devices is expanding and several MCS devices are currently available and can provide varying magnitude of hemodynamic support during high-risk and complex PCIs. Small randomized controlled trials have provided conflicting results regarding survival benefit using these devices despite substantial hemodynamic and metabolic benefit. However, given the high morbidity and mortality burden among patients undergoing high-risk and complex PCI, detailed hemodynamic assessment and careful patient selection is mandatory to achieve incremental benefit over early revascularization and pharmacologic therapy with utilizing these devices. Furthermore, the optimal timing and magnitude of hemodynamic support during PCI as well as prevention of device-related complications are all important considerations in future research in this field. Until adequate data supporting MCS use in a broader patient population is available, MCS devices during PCI should be individualized based on multiple factors with a recommended use in patients with the greatest potential benefit and a relatively low risk of device-related complications.

Author Contributions: Conceptualization, R.A. and J.R.R.; methodology, R.A. and J.R.R.; formal analysis, R.A. and J.R.R.; data curation, R.A. and J.R.R.; writing—original draft preparation, R.A. and J.R.R.; writing—review and editing, R.A. and J.R.R.

References

1.   Waldo, S.W.; Secemsky, E.A.; O'Brien, C.; Kennedy, K.F.; Pomerantsev, E.; Sundt, T.M., 3rd; McNulty, E.J.; Scirica, B.M.; Yeh, R.W. Surgical ineligibility and mortality among patients with unprotected left main or multivessel coronary artery disease undergoing percutaneous coronary intervention. *Circulation* **2014**, *130*, 2295–2301. [CrossRef] [PubMed]

2.   Atkinson, T.M.; Ohman, E.M.; O'Neill, W.W.; Rab, T.; Cigarroa, J.E. A practical approach to mechanical circulatory support in patients undergoing percutaneous coronary intervention an interventional perspective. *JACC Cardiovasc. Interv.* **2016**, *9*, 871–883. [CrossRef] [PubMed]

3.   Perera, D.; Stables, R.; Thomas, M.; Booth, J.; Pitt, M.; Blackman, D.; de Belder, A.; Redwood, S. BCSI-1 Investigators. Elective intra-aortic balloon counterpulsation during high-risk percutaneous coronary intervention: A randomized controlled trial. *JAMA* **2010**, *304*, 867–874. [CrossRef] [PubMed]

4.   O'Neill, W.W.; Kleiman, N.S.; Moses, J.; Henriques, J.P.; Dixon, S.; Massaro, J.; Palacios, I.; Maini, B.; Mulukutla, S.; Dzavík, V. A prospective, randomized clinical trial of hemodynamic support with impella 2.5 versus intra-aortic balloon pump in patients undergoing high-risk percutaneous coronary intervention: The PROTECT II study. *Circulation* **2012**, *126*, 1717–1727. [CrossRef] [PubMed]

5.   Thiele, H.; Zeymer, U.; Neumann, F.J.; Ferenc, M.; Olbrich, H.G.; Hausleiter, J.; Richardt, G.; Hennersdorf, M.; Empen, K.; Fuernau, G. Intraaortic balloon support for myocardial infarction with cardiogenic shock. *N. Engl. J. Med.* **2012**, *367*, 1287–1296. [CrossRef] [PubMed]

6.   Ouweneel, D.M.; Eriksen, E.; Sjauw, K.D.; van Dongen, I.M.; Hirsch, A.; Packer, E.J.; Vis, M.M.; Wykrzykowska, J.J.; Koch, K.T.; Baan, J.; et al. Percutaneous mechanical circulatory support versus intra-aortic balloon pump in cardiogenic shock after acute myocardial infarction. *J. Am. Coll. Cardiol.* **2017**, *69*, 278–287. [CrossRef] [PubMed]

7.   Basir, M.B.; Kapur, N.K.; Patel, K.; Salam, M.A.; Schreiber, T.; Kaki, A.; Hanson, I.; Almany, S.; Timmis, S.; Dixon, S.; et al. Improved outcomes associated with the use of shock protocols: Updates from the national cardiogenic shock initiative. *Catheter Cardiovasc. Interv.* **2019**, *93*, 1173–1183. [CrossRef] [PubMed]

8.   Ameloot, K.; Bastos, M.B.; Daemen, J.; Schreuder, J.; Boersma, E.; Zijlstra, F.; Van Mieghem, N.M. New generation mechanical circulatory support during high-risk PCI: A cross sectional analysis. *EuroIntervention* **2019**. [CrossRef]

9.   Damluji, A.A.; Bandeen-Roche, K.; Berkower, C.; Boyd, C.M.; Al-Damluji, M.S.; Cohen, M.G.; Forman, D.E.; Chaudhary, R.; Gerstenblith, G.; Walston, J.D.; et al. Percutaneous coronary intervention in older patients

with ST-segment elevation myocardial infarction and cardiogenic shock. *J. Am. Coll. Cardiol.* **2019**, *73*, 1890–1900. [CrossRef] [PubMed]

10. Ibanez, B.; James, S.; Agewall, S.; Antunes, M.J.; Bucciarelli-Ducci, C.; Bueno, H.; Caforio, A.L.P.; Crea, F.; Goudevenos, J.A.; Halvorsen, S.; et al. 2017 ESC Guidelines for the management of acute myocardial infarction in patients presenting with ST-segment elevation. *Eur. Heart J.* **2018**, *39*, 119–177. [CrossRef] [PubMed]

11. Rihal, C.S.; Naidu, S.S.; Givertz, M.M.; Szeto, W.Y.; Burke, J.A.; Kapur, N.K.; Kern, M.; Garratt, K.N.; Goldstein, J.A.; Dimas, V.; et al. 2015 SCAI/ACC/HFSA/STS clinical expert consensus statement on the use of percutaneous mechanical circulatory support devices in cardiovascular care. *J. Am. Coll. Cardiol.* **2015**, *65*, e7–e26. [CrossRef] [PubMed]

12. Levine, G.N.; Bates, E.R.; Blankenship, J.C.; Bailey, S.R.; Bittl, J.A.; Cercek, B.; Chambers, C.E.; Ellis, S.G.; Guyton, R.A.; Hollenberg, S.M.; et al. 2011 ACCF/AHA/SCAI guideline for percutaneous coronary intervention. *J. Am. Coll. Cardiol.* **2011**, *124*, e574–e651. [CrossRef]

13. Wallace, T.W.; Berger, J.S.; Wang, A.; Velazquez, E.J.; Brown, DL. Impact of left ventricular dysfunction on hospital mortality among patients undergoing elective percutaneous coronary intervention. *Am. J. Cardiol.* **2009**. [CrossRef] [PubMed]

14. Maini, B.; Naidu, S.S.; Mulukutla, S.; Kleiman, N.; Schreiber, T.; Wohns, D.; Dixon, S.; Rihal, C.; Dave, R.; O'Nell, W. Real-world use of the Impella 2.5 circulatory support system in complex high-risk percutaneous coronary intervention: The USpella registry. *Catheter Cardiovasc. Interv.* **2012**, *80*, 717–725. [CrossRef] [PubMed]

15. Krone, R.J.; Shaw, R.E.; Klein, L.W.; Block, P.C.; Anderson, H.V.; Weintraub, W.S.; Brindis, R.G.; McKay, C.R.; ACC-National Cardiovascular Data Registry. Evaluation of the American College of Cardiology/American Heart Association and the Society for Coronary Angiography and Interventions lesion classification system in the current "stent era" of coronary interventions (from the ACC-National Cardiovascular. *Am. J. Cardiol.* **2003**, *92*, 389–394. [CrossRef]

16. Sakakura, K.; Ako, J.; Wada, H.; Kubo, N.; Momomura, S.I. ACC/AHA classification of coronary lesions reflects medical resource use in current percutaneous coronary interventions. *Catheter Cardiovasc. Interv.* **2012**. [CrossRef] [PubMed]

17. Brennan, J.M.; Curtis, J.P.; Dai, D.; Fitzgerald, S.; Khandelwal, A.K.; Spertus, J.A.; Rao, S.V.; Singh, M.; Shaw, R.E.; Ho, K.K.; et al. Enhanced mortality risk prediction with a focus on high-risk percutaneous coronary intervention: Results from 1,208,137 procedures in the NCDR (national cardiovascular data registry). *JACC Cardiovasc. Interv.* **2013**, *6*, 790–799. [CrossRef] [PubMed]

18. Burkhoff, D.; Sayer, G.; Doshi, D.; Uriel, N. Hemodynamics of mechanical circulatory support. *J. Am. Coll. Cardiol.* **2015**. [CrossRef]

19. Van Diepen, S.; Katz, J.N.; Albert, N.M.; Henry, T.D.; Jacobs, A.K.; Kapur, N.K.; Kilic, A.; Menon, V.; Ohman, E.M.; Sweitzer, N.K.; et al. Contemporary management of cardiogenic shock: A scientific statement from the american heart association. *Circulation* **2017**, *136*, e232–e268. [CrossRef]

20. Reynolds, H.R.; Hochman, J.S. Cardiogenic shock current concepts and improving outcomes. *Circulation* **2008**. [CrossRef]

21. Miller, L. Cardiogenic shock in acute myocardial infarction the era of mechanical support. *J. Am. Coll. Cardiol.* **2016**. [CrossRef]

22. Masoudi, F.A.; Ponirakis, A.; de Lemos, J.A.; Jollis, J.G.; Kremers, M.; Messenger, J.C.; Moore, J.W.M.; Moussa, I.; Oetgen, W.J.; Varosy, P.D.; et al. Trends in U.S. cardiovascular care: 2016 report from 4 ACC national cardiovascular data registries. *J. Am. Coll. Cardiol.* **2017**, *69*, 1427–1450. [CrossRef] [PubMed]

23. Babaev, A.; Frederick, P.D.; Pasta, D.J.; Every, N.; Sichrovsky, T.; Hochman, J.S. Trends in management and outcomes of patients with acute myocardial infarction complicated by cardiogenic shock. *J. Am. Med. Assoc.* **2005**. [CrossRef] [PubMed]

24. Basir, M.B.; Schreiber, T.L.; Grines, C.L.; Dixon, S.R.; Moses, J.W.; Maini, B.J.; Khandelwal, A.K.; Ohman, E.M.; O'Nell, W.W. Effect of early initiation of mechanical circulatory support on survival in cardiogenic shock. *Am. J. Cardiol.* **2017**, *119*, 845–851. [CrossRef] [PubMed]

25. Remmelink, M.; Sjauw, K.D.; Henriques, J.P.S.; Vis, M.M.; van der Schaaf, R.J.; Koch, K.T.; Tijssen, J.G.; de Wintr, R.J.; Piek, J.J.; Baan, J., Jr. Acute left ventricular dynamic effects of primary percutaneous coronary intervention. From occlusion to reperfusion. *J. Am. Coll. Cardiol.* **2009**, *53*, 1498–1502. [CrossRef] [PubMed]

26. Borlaug, B.A.; Kass, D.A. Invasive hemodynamic assessment in heart failure. *Cardiol. Clin.* **2011**. [CrossRef] [PubMed]

27. Uriel, N.; Sayer, G.; Annamalai, S.; Kapur, N.K.; Burkhoff, D. Mechanical unloading in heart failure. *J. Am. Coll. Cardiol.* **2018**. [CrossRef] [PubMed]

28. Rab, T.; O'Neill, W. Mechanical circulatory support for patients with cardiogenic shock. *Trends Cardiovasc. Med.* **2018**. [CrossRef]

29. Thiele, H.; Ohman, E.M.; Desch, S.; Eitel, I.; De Waha, S. Management of cardiogenic shock. *Eur. Heart J.* **2015**. [CrossRef]

30. Csepe, T.A.; Kilic, A. Advancements in mechanical circulatory support for patients in acute and chronic heart failure. *J. Thorac. Dis.* **2017**. [CrossRef]

31. Tan, L.B. Cardiac pumping capability and prognosis in heart failure. *Lancet* **1986**. [CrossRef]

32. Lang, C.C.; Karlin, P.; Haythe, J.; Levy, W.; Lim, T.K.; Mancini, D.M. Peak cardiac power, measured non-invasively, is a powerful predictor of mortality in chronic heart failure. *Circulation* **2007**, *22*, 33–38.

33. WEBER, KT. Intra-aortic balloon pumping. *Ann. Intern. Med.* **2013**. [CrossRef]

34. Papaioannou, T.G.; Stefanadis, C. Basic principles of the intraaortic balloon pump and mechanisms affecting its performance. *ASAIO J.* **2005**. [CrossRef]

35. Rastan, A.J.; Tillmann, E.; Subramanian, S.; Lehmkuhl, L.; Funkat, A.K.; Leontyev, S.; Doenst, T.; Walther, T.; Gutberlet, M.; Mohr, F.W. Visceral arterial compromise during intra-aortic balloon counterpulsation therapy. *Circulation* **2010**. [CrossRef]

36. Herrera-Perez, D.; Haslam, A.; Crain, T.; Gill, J.; Livingston, C.; Kaestner, V.; Hayes, M.; Morgan, D.; Cifu, A.S.; Prasad, V. A comprehensive review of randomized clinical trials in three medical journals reveals 396 medical reversals. *Elife* **2019**. [CrossRef] [PubMed]

37. Basra, S.S.; Loyalka, P.; Kar, B. Current status of percutaneous ventricular assist devices for cardiogenic shock. *Curr. Opin. Cardiol.* **2011**. [CrossRef] [PubMed]

38. Möbius-Winkler, S.; Fritzenwanger, M.; Pfeifer, R.; Schulze, P.C. Percutaneous support of the failing left and right ventricle—Recommendations for the use of mechanical device therapy. *Heart Fail. Rev.* **2018**. [CrossRef]

39. Lauten, A.; Engström, A.E.; Jung, C.; Empen, K.; Erne, P.; Cook, S.; Windecker, S.; Bergmann, M.W.; Klingenberg, R.; Lüscher, T.F.; et al. Percutaneous left-ventricular support with the impella-2.5-assist device in acute cardiogenic shock results of the impella-EUROSHOCK-registry. *Circ. Hear Fail.* **2013**, *6*, 23–30. [CrossRef] [PubMed]

40. Remmelink, M.; Sjauw, K.D.; Henriques, J.P.; De Winter, R.J.; Vis, M.M.; Koch, K.T.; Paulus, W.J.; De Mol, B.A.; Tijssen, J.G.; Piek, J.J.; et al. Effects of mechanical left ventricular unloading by impella on left ventricular dynamics in high-risk and primary percutaneous coronary intervention patients. *Catheter Cardiovasc. Interv.* **2010**. [CrossRef]

41. Doshi, R.; Patel, K.; Decter, D.; Gupta, R.; Meraj, P. Trends in the utilisation and in-hospital mortality associated with short-term mechanical circulatory support for heart failure with reduced ejection fraction. *Hear Lung Circ.* **2019**. [CrossRef] [PubMed]

42. Martinez, C.A.; Singh, V.; Londoño, J.C.; Cohen, M.G.; Alfonso, C.E.; O'Neill, W.W.; Heldman, A.W. Percutaneous retrograde left ventricular assist support for patients with aortic stenosis and left ventricular dysfunction. *J. Am. Coll. Cardiol.* **2011**, *80*, 1201–1209. [CrossRef] [PubMed]

43. Kar, B.; Gregoric, I.D.; Basra, S.S.; Idelchik, G.M.; Loyalka, P. The percutaneous ventricular assist device in severe refractory cardiogenic shock. *J. Am. Coll. Cardiol.* **2010**. [CrossRef] [PubMed]

44. Burkhoff, D.; Naidu, S.S. The science behind percutaneous hemodynamic support: A review and comparison of support strategies. *Catheter Cardiovasc. Interv.* **2012**. [CrossRef] [PubMed]

45. Kono, S.; Nishimura, K.; Nishina, T.; Komeda, M.; Akamatsu, T. Auto-synchronized systolic unloading during left ventricular assist with centrifugal pump. *ASAIO J.* **1999**. [CrossRef]

46. Pham, D.T.; Al-Quthami, A.; Kapur, N.K. Percutaneous left ventricular support in cardiogenic shock and severe aortic regurgitation. *Catheter Cardiovasc. Interv.* **2013**. [CrossRef]

47. Ouweneel, D.M.; Schotborgh, J.V.; Limpens, J.; Sjauw, K.D.; Engström, A.E.; Lagrand, W.K.; Cherpanath, T.G.V.; Driessen, A.H.G.; De Mol, B.A.J.M.; Henriques, J.P.S. Extracorporeal life support during cardiac arrest and cardiogenic shock: A systematic review and meta-analysis. *Intensive Care Med.* **2016**. [CrossRef]

48. Thiagarajan, R.R.; Barbaro, R.P.; Rycus, P.T.; McMullan, D.M.; Conrad, S.A.; Fortenberry, J.D.; Paden, M.L. Extracorporeal life support organization registry international report 2016. *ASAIO J.* **2017**. [CrossRef]

49. Aghili, N.; Kang, S.; Kapur, N.K. The fundamentals of extra-corporeal membrane oxygenation. *Minerva Cardioangiol.* **2015**, *63*, 75–85.

50. MacLaren, G.; Combes, A.; Bartlett, R.H. Contemporary extracorporeal membrane oxygenation for adult respiratory failure: Life support in the new era. *Intensive Care Med.* **2012**. [CrossRef]

51. Russo, J.J.; Aleksova, N.; Pitcher, I.; Couture, E.; Parlow, S.; Faraz, M.; Visintini, S.; Simard, T.; Di Santo, P.; Mathew, R.; et al. Left ventricular unloading during extracorporeal membrane oxygenation in patients with cardiogenic shock. *J. Am. Coll. Cardiol.* **2019**. [CrossRef]

52. Koeckert, M.S.; Jorde, U.P.; Naka, Y.; Moses, J.W.; Takayama, H. Impella LP 2.5 for left ventricular unloading during venoarterial extracorporeal membrane oxygenation support. *J. Cardiol. Surg.* **2011**. [CrossRef]

53. Ostadal, P.; Mlcek, M.; Gorhan, H.; Simundic, I.; Strunina, S.; Hrachovina, M.; Krüger, A.; Vondrakova, D.; Janotka, M.; Hala, P.; et al. Electrocardiogram-synchronized pulsatile extracorporeal life support preserves left ventricular function and coronary flow in a porcine model of cardiogenic shock. *PLoS ONE* **2018**. [CrossRef]

54. Wang, S.; Izer, J.M.; Clark, J.B.; Patel, S.; Pauliks, L.; Kunselman, A.R.; Leach, D.; Cooper, T.K.; Wilson, R.P.; Ündar, A. In vivo hemodynamic performance evaluation of novel electrocardiogram-synchronized pulsatile and nonpulsatile extracorporeal life support systems in an adult swine model. *Artif. Organs* **2015**. [CrossRef]

55. Wolfe, R.; Strother, A.; Wang, S.; Kunselman, A.R.; Ündar, A. Impact of pulsatility and flow rates on hemodynamic energy transmission in an adult extracorporeal life support system. *Artif. Organs* **2015**. [CrossRef]

56. Pöss, J.; Kriechbaum, S.; Ewen, S.; Graf, J.; Hager, I.; Hennersdorf, M.; Petros, S.; Link, A.; Bohm, M.; Thiele, H.; et al. First-in-man analysis of the i-cor assist device in patients with cardiogenic shock. *Eur. Heart J. Acute Cardiovasc. Care* **2015**. [CrossRef]

57. Masyuk, M.; Abel, P.; Hug, M.; Wernly, B.; Haneya, A.; Sack, S.; Sideris, K.; Langwieser, N.; Graf, T.; Fuernau, G.; et al. Real-world clinical experience with the percutaneous extracorporeal life support system: Results from the German Lifebridge® Registry. *Clin. Res. Cardiol.* **2019**. [CrossRef]

58. Cheng, R.; Hachamovitch, R.; Kittleson, M.; Patel, J.; Arabia, F.; Moriguchi, J.; Esmailian, F.; Azarbal, B. Complications of extracorporeal membrane oxygenation for treatment of cardiogenic shock and cardiac arrest: A meta-analysis of 1,866 adult patients. *Ann. Thorac. Surg.* **2014**. [CrossRef]

59. Uil, C.D.; Daemen, J.; Lenzen, M.; Maugenest, A.-M.; Joziasse, L.; Van Geuns, R.; Van Mieghem, N. Pulsatile iVAC 2L circulatory support in high-risk percutaneous coronary intervention. *EuroIntervention* **2017**. [CrossRef]

60. McLaughlin, V.V.; Archer, S.L.; Badesch, D.B.; Barst, R.J.; Farber, H.W.; Lindner, J.R.; Mathier, M.A.; McGoon, M.D.; Park, M.H.; Rosenson, R.S.; et al. ACCF/AHA 2009 expert consensus document on pulmonary hypertension. A report of the American College of Cardiology Foundation task force on expert consensus documents and the American Heart Association Developed in Collaboration with the American College of Chest Physicians; American Thoracic Society, Inc.; and the Pulmonary Hypertension Association. *J. Am. Coll. Cardiol.* **2009**. [CrossRef]

61. Anderson, M.B.; Goldstein, J.; Milano, C.; Morris, L.D.; Kormos, R.L.; Bhama, J.; Kapur, N.K.; Bansal, A.; Garcia, J.; Baker, J.N.; et al. Benefits of a novel percutaneous ventricular assist device for right heart failure: The prospective RECOVER RIGHT study of the Impella RP device. *J. Heart Lung Transplant.* **2015**. [CrossRef]

62. Harris, S.; Tepper, D.; Ip, R. Comparison of hospital mortality with intra-aortic balloon counterpulsation insertion before vs after primary percutaneous coronary intervention for cardiogenic shock complicating acute myocardial infarction. *Congest. Heart Fail.* **2010**. [CrossRef]

63. Sjauw, K.D.; Engström, A.E.; Vis, M.M.; van der Schaaf, R.J.; Baan, J., Jr.; Koch, K.T.; de Winter, R.J.; Piek, J.J.; Tijssen, J.G.; Henriques, J.P. A systematic review and meta-analysis of intra-aortic balloon pump therapy in ST-elevation myocardial infarction: Should we change the guidelines? *Eur. Heart J.* **2009**. [CrossRef]

64. Hochman, J.S.; Sleeper, L.A.; Webb, J.G.; Sanborn, T.A.; White, H.D.; Talley, J.D.; Buller, C.E.; Jacobs, A.K.; Slater, J.N.; Col, J.; et al. Early revascularization in acute myocardial infarction complicated by cardiogenic shock. SHOCK Investigators. Should we emergently revascularize occluded coronaries for cardiogenic shock. *N. Engl. J. Med.* **1999**. [CrossRef]

65. Thiele, H.; Zeymer, U.; Neumann, F.-J.; Ferenc, M.; Olbrich, H.-G.; Hausleiter, J.; De Waha, A.; Richardt, G.; Hennersdorf, M.; Empen, K.; et al. Intra-aortic balloon counterpulsation in acute myocardial infarction complicated by cardiogenic shock (IABP-SHOCK II): Final 12 month results of a randomised, open-label trial. *Lancet* **2013**. [CrossRef]

66. Thiele, H.; Zeymer, U.; Thelemann, N.; Neumann, F.J.; Hausleiter, J.; Abdel-Wahab, M.; Meyer-Saraei, R.; Fuernau, G.; Eitel, I.; Hambrecht, R.; et al. Intraaortic balloon pump in cardiogenic shock complicating acute myocardial infarction: Long-term 6-year outcome of the randomized IABP-SHOCK II trial. *Circulation* **2018**. [CrossRef]

67. Dehmer, G.J.; Blankenship, J.C.; Cilingiroglu, M.; Dwyer, J.G.; Feldman, D.N.; Gardner, T.J.; Grines, C.L.; Singh, M. SCAI/ACC/AHA Expert consensus document: 2014 update on percutaneous coronary intervention without on-site surgical backup. *Catheter Cardiovasc. Interv.* **2014**. [CrossRef]

68. Patel, M.R.; Smalling, R.W.; Thiele, H.; Barnhart, H.X.; Zhou, Y.; Chandra, P.; Chew, D.; Choen, M.; French, J.; Perera, D.; et al. Intra-aortic balloon counterpulsation and infarct size in patients with acute anterior myocardial infarction without shock: The CRISP AMI randomized trial. *JAMA-J. Am. Med. Assoc.* **2011**. [CrossRef]

69. Curtis, J.P.; Rathore, S.S.; Wang, Y.; Chen, J.; Nallamothu, B.K.; Krumholz, H.M. Use and effectiveness of intra-Aortic balloon pumps among patients undergoing high risk percutaneous coronary intervention: Insights from the national cardiovascular data registry. *Circ. Cardiovasc. Qual. Outcomes* **2012**. [CrossRef]

70. Perera, D.; Stables, R.; Clayton, T.; De Silva, K.; Lumley, M.; Clack, L.; Thomas, M.; Redwood, S.; BCSI-1 Investigators. Long-term mortality data from the balloon pump–assisted coronary intervention study (BCIS-1). *Circulation* **2012**. [CrossRef]

71. O'Gara, P.T.; Kushner, F.G.; Ascheim, D.D.; E Casey, D.; Chung, M.K.; A De Lemos, J.; Ettinger, S.M.; Fang, J.C.; Fesmire, F.M.; A Franklin, B.; et al. 2013 ACCF/AHA guideline for the management of st-elevation myocardial infarction: Executive summary: A report of the American college of cardiology foundation/american heart association task force on practice guidelines. *J. Am. Coll. Cardiol.* **2013**. [CrossRef]

72. Seyfarth, M.; Sibbing, D.; Bauer, I.; Fröhlich, G.; Bott-Flügel, L.; Byrne, R.; Dirschinger, J.; Kastrati, A.; Schömig, A. A Randomized clinical trial to evaluate the safety and efficacy of a percutaneous left ventricular assist device versus intra-aortic balloon pumping for treatment of cardiogenic shock caused by myocardial infarction. *J. Am. Coll. Cardiol.* **2008**. [CrossRef]

73. Zeymer, U.; Thiele, H. Mechanical support for cardiogenic shock: Lost in translation? *J. Am. Coll. Cardiol.* **2017**. [CrossRef]

74. Karatolios, K.; Chatzis, G.; Markus, B.; Luesebrink, U.; Ahrens, H.; Dersch, W.; Betz, S.; Ploeger, B.; Boesl, E.; O'Neill, W.; et al. Impella support compared to medical treatment for post-cardiac arrest shock after out of hospital cardiac arrest. *Resuscitation* **2018**. [CrossRef]

75. Schrage, B.; Ibrahim, K.; Loehn, T.; Werner, N.; Sinning, J.-M.; Pappalardo, F.; Pieri, M.; Skurk, C.; Lauten, A.; Landmesser, U.; et al. Impella support for acute myocardial infarction complicated by cardiogenic shock. *Circulation* **2019**. [CrossRef]

76. Wernly, B.; Seelmaier, C.; Leistner, D.; Stähli, B.E.; Pretsch, I.; Lichtenauer, M.; Jung, C.; Hoppe, U.C.; Landmesser, U.; Thiele, H.; et al. Mechanical circulatory support with Impella versus intra-aortic balloon pump or medical treatment in cardiogenic shock—A critical appraisal of current data. *Clin. Res. Cardiol.* **2019**. [CrossRef]

77. Henriques, J.P.; Remmelink, M.; Baan, J.; Van Der Schaaf, R.J.; Vis, M.M.; Koch, K.T.; Scholten, E.W.; De Mol, B.A.; Tijssen, J.G.; Piek, J.J.; et al. Safety and feasibility of elective high-risk percutaneous coronary intervention procedures with left ventricular support of the impella recover LP 2.5. *Am. J. Cardiol.* **2006**. [CrossRef]

78. Dixon, S.R.; Henriques, J.P.; Mauri, L.; Sjauw, K.; Civitello, A.; Kar, B.; Loyalka, P.; Resnic, F.S.; Teirstein, P.; Makkar, R.; et al. A prospective feasibility trial investigating the use of the impella 2.5 system in patients undergoing high-risk percutaneous coronary intervention (The PROTECT I Trial). Initial U.S. Experience. *JACC Cardiovasc. Interv.* **2009**. [CrossRef]

79. Dangas, G.D.; Kini, A.S.; Sharma, S.K.; Henriques, J.P.; Claessen, B.E.; Dixon, S.R.; Massaro, J.M.; Palacios, I.; Popma, J.J.; Ohman, E.M.; et al. Impact of hemodynamic support with impella 2.5 versus intra-aortic balloon pump on prognostically important clinical outcomes in patients undergoing high-risk percutaneous coronary intervention (from the PROTECT II randomized trial). *Am. J. Cardiol.* **2014.** [CrossRef]

80. Thiele, H.; Sick, P.; Boudriot, E.; Diederich, K.-W.; Hambrecht, R.; Niebauer, J.; Schuler, G. Randomized comparison of intra-aortic balloon support with a percutaneous left ventricular assist device in patients with revascularized acute myocardial infarction complicated by cardiogenic shock. *Eur. Heart J.* **2005.** [CrossRef]

81. Burkhoff, D.; Cohen, H.; Brunckhorst, C.; O'Neill, W.W. A randomized multicenter clinical study to evaluate the safety and efficacy of the TandemHeart percutaneous ventricular assist device versus conventional therapy with intraaortic balloon pumping for treatment of cardiogenic shock. *Am. Heart J.* **2006.** [CrossRef]

82. Alli, O.O.; Singh, I.M.; Holmes, D.R.; Pulido, J.N.; Park, S.J.; Rihal, C.S. Percutaneous left ventricular assist device with TandemHeart for high-risk percutaneous coronary intervention: The Mayo Clinic experience. *Catheter Cardiovasc. Interv.* **2012.** [CrossRef]

83. Briasoulis, A.; Telila, T.; Palla, M.; Mercado, N.; Kondur, A.; Grines, C.; Schreiber, T. Meta-analysis of usefulness of percutaneous left ventricular assist devices for high-risk percutaneous coronary interventions. *Am. J. Cardiol.* **2016.** [CrossRef]

84. Bermudez, C.; Kormos, R.; Subramaniam, K.; Mulukutla, S.; Sappington, P.; Waters, J.; Khandhar, S.J.; Esper, S.A.; Dueweke, E.J. Extracorporeal Membrane oxygenation support in acute coronary syndromes complicated by cardiogenic shock. *Catheter Cardiovasc. Interv.* **2015.** [CrossRef]

85. Negi, S.I.; Sokolovic, M.; Koifman, E.; Kiramijyan, S.; Torguson, R.; Lindsay, J.; Ben-Dor, I.; Suddath, W.; Pichard, A.; Satler, L.; et al. Contemporary use of veno-arterial extracorporeal membrane oxygenation for refractory cardiogenic shock in acute coronary syndrome. *J. Invasive Cardiol.* **2016,** *28,* 52–57.

86. Chen, Y.-S.; Chao, A.; Yu, H.-Y.; Ko, W.-J.; Wu, I.-H.; Chen, R.J.-C.; Huang, S.-C.; Lin, F.-Y.; Wang, S.-S. Analysis and results of prolonged resuscitation in cardiac arrest patients rescued by extracorporeal membrane oxygenation. *J. Am. Coll. Cardiol.* **2003.** [CrossRef]

87. Schrage, B.; Burkhoff, D.; Rübsamen, N.; Becher, P.M.; Schwarzl, M.; Bernhardt, A.; Grahn, H.; Lubos, E.; Söffker, G.; Clemmensen, P.; et al. Unloading of the left ventricle during venoarterial extracorporeal membrane oxygenation therapy in cardiogenic shock. *JACC Heart Fail.* **2018.** [CrossRef]

88. Myat, A.; Patel, N.; Tehrani, S.; Banning, A.P.; Redwood, S.R.; Bhatt, D.L. Percutaneous circulatory assist devices for high-risk coronary intervention. *JACC Cardiovasc. Interv.* **2015.** [CrossRef]

89. Maini, B.; Gregory, D.; Scotti, D.J.; Buyantseva, L. Percutaneous cardiac assist devices compared with surgical hemodynamic support alternatives: Cost-effectiveness in the emergent setting. *Catheter Cardiovasc. Interv.* **2014.** [CrossRef]

90. Roos, J.B.; Doshi, S.N.; Konorza, T.; Palacios, I.; Schreiber, T.; Borisenko, O.V.; Henriques, J.P.S. The cost-effectiveness of a new percutaneous ventricular assist device for high-risk PCI patients: mid-stage evaluation from the European perspective. *J. Med. Econ.* **2013.** [CrossRef]

91. Udesen, N.J.; Møller, J.E.; Lindholm, M.G.; Eiskjær, H.; Schäfer, A.; Werner, N.; Holmvang, L.; Terkelsen, C.J.; Jensen, L.O.; Junker, A.; et al. Rationale and design of DanGer shock: Danish-German cardiogenic shock trial. *Am. Heart J.* **2019.** [CrossRef]

92. Jung, C.; Bueter, S.; Wernly, B.; Masyuk, M.; Saeed, D.; Albert, A.; Fuernau, G.; Kelm, M.; Westenfeld, R. Lactate clearance predicts good neurological outcomes in cardiac arrest patients treated with extracorporeal cardiopulmonary resuscitation. *J. Clin. Med.* **2019.** [CrossRef]

93. Slottosch, I.; Liakopoulos, O.; Kuhn, E.; Scherner, M.; Deppe, A.-C.; Sabashnikov, A.; Mader, N.; Choi, Y.-H.; Wippermann, J.; Wahlers, T. Lactate and lactate clearance as valuable tool to evaluate ECMO therapy in cardiogenic shock. *J. Crit. Care* **2017.** [CrossRef]

94. Fux, T.; Holm, M.; Corbascio, M.; van der Linden, J. cardiac arrest prior to venoarterial extracorporeal membrane oxygenation. *Crit. Care Med.* **2019.** [CrossRef]

95. Lee, W.-C.; Fang, C.-Y.; Chen, H.-C.; Chen, C.-J.; Yang, C.-H.; Hang, C.-L.; Yip, H.-K.; Fang, H.-Y.; Wu, C.-J. Associations with 30-day survival following extracorporeal membrane oxygenation in patients with acute ST segment elevation myocardial infarction and profound cardiogenic shock. *Heart Lung J. Acute Crit. Care* **2016.** [CrossRef]

96. Kapur, N.K.; Paruchuri, V.; Urbano-Morales, J.A.; Mackey, E.E.; Daly, G.H.; Qiao, X.; Pandian, N.; Perides, G.; Karas, R.H. Mechanically unloading the left ventricle before coronary reperfusion reduces left ventricular wall stress and myocardial infarct size. *Circulation* **2013**. [CrossRef]

97. Esposito, M.L.; Zhang, Y.; Qiao, X.; Reyelt, L.; Paruchuri, V.; Schnitzler, G.R.; Morine, K.J.; Annamalai, S.K.; Bogins, C.; Natov, P.S.; et al. Left ventricular unloading before reperfusion promotes functional recovery after acute myocardial infarction. *J. Am. Coll. Cardiol.* **2018**. [CrossRef]

98. Meyns, B.; Stolinski, J.; Leunens, V.; Verbeken, E.; Flameng, W. Left ventricular support by catheter-mounted axial flow pump reduces infarct size. *J. Am. Coll. Cardiol.* **2003**, *41*, 1087–1095. [CrossRef]

99. Kapur, N.K.; Qiao, X.; Paruchuri, V.; Morine, K.J.; Syed, W.; Dow, S.; Shah, N.; Pandian, N.; Karas, R.H. Mechanical pre-conditioning with acute circulatory support before reperfusion limits infarct size in acute myocardial infarction. *JACC Heart Fail.* **2015**. [CrossRef]

100. Kapur, N.K.; Alkhouli, M.A.; DeMartini, T.J.; Faraz, H.; George, Z.H.; Goodwin, M.J.; Hernandez-Montfort, J.A.; Iyer, V.S.; Josephy, N.; Kalra, S.; et al. Unloading the left ventricle before reperfusion in patients with anterior st-segment-elevation myocardial infarction: A pilot study using the impella CP. *Circulation* **2019**. [CrossRef]

101. O'Neill, W.W.; Grines, C.; Schreiber, T.; Moses, J.; Maini, B.; Dixon, S.R.; Ohman, E.M.; O'Neill, W.W. Analysis of outcomes for 15,259 US patients with acute myocardial infarction cardiogenic shock (AMICS) supported with the Impella device. *Am. Heart J.* **2018**. [CrossRef]

102. Flaherty, M.P.; Khan, A.R.; O'Neill, W.W. Early initiation of impella in acute myocardial infarction complicated by cardiogenic shock improves survival: A meta-analysis. *JACC Cardiovasc. Interv.* **2017**. [CrossRef]

103. Auffret, V.; Cottin, Y.; Leurent, G.; Gilard, M.; Beer, J.-C.; Zabalawi, A.; Chagué, F.; Filippi, E.; Brunet, D.; Hacot, J.-P.; et al. Predicting the development of in-hospital cardiogenic shock in patients with ST-segment elevation myocardial infarction treated by primary percutaneous coronary intervention: The ORBI risk score. *Eur. Heart J.* **2018**. [CrossRef]

104. Schrage, B.; Westermann, D. Reply: Does VA-ECMO plus impella work in refractory cardiogenic shock? *JACC Heatr Fail.* **2019**. [CrossRef]

105. Li, Y.; Yan, S.; Gao, S.; Liu, M.; Lou, S.; Liu, G.; Ji, B.; Gao, B. Effect of an intra-aortic balloon pump with venoarterial extracorporeal membrane oxygenation on mortality of patients with cardiogenic shock: A systematic review and meta-analysis. *Eur. J. Cardio-Thoracic Surg.* **2019**. [CrossRef]

106. Ohman, E.M.; Nanas, J.; Stomel, R.J.; Leesar, M.A.; Nielsen, D.W.T.; O'Dea, D.; Rogers, F.J.; Harber, D.; Hudson, M.P.; Fraulo, E.; et al. Thrombolysis and counterpulsation to improve survival in myocardial infarction complicated by hypotension and suspected cardiogenic shock or heart failure: Results of the TACTICS trial. *J. Thromb. Thrombolysis* **2005**. [CrossRef]

107. Waksman, R.; Weiss, A.T.; Gotsman, M.S.; Hasin, Y. Intra-aortic balloon counterpulsation improves survival in cardiogenic shock complicating acute myocardial infarction. *Eur. Heart J.* **1993**. [CrossRef]

108. Barron, H.V.; Every, N.R.; Parsons, L.S.; Angeja, B.; Goldberg, R.J.; Gore, J.M.; Chou, T.M. The use of intra-aortic balloon counterpulsation in patients with cardiogenic shock complicating acute myocardial infarction: Data from the national registry of myocardial infarction 2. *Am. Heart J.* **2001**. [CrossRef]

109. Cheng, J.M.; Uil, C.A.D.; Hoeks, S.E.; Van Der Ent, M.; Jewbali, L.S.; Van Domburg, R.T.; Serruys, P.W. Percutaneous left ventricular assist devices vs. intra-aortic balloon pump counterpulsation for treatment of cardiogenic shock: A meta-analysis of controlled trials. *Eur. Heart J.* **2009**. [CrossRef]

110. Alushi, B.; Douedari, A.; Froehlich, G.; Knie, W.; Leistner, D.; Staehli, B.; Mochmann, H.-C.; Pieske, B.; Landmesser, U.; Krackhardt, F.; et al. P2481Impella assist device or intraaortic balloon pump for treatment of cardiogenic shock due to acute coronary syndrome. *Eur. Heart J.* **2018**. [CrossRef]

111. Nichol, G.; Karmy-Jones, R.; Salerno, C.; Cantore, L.; Becker, L. Systematic review of percutaneous cardiopulmonary bypass for cardiac arrest or cardiogenic shock states. *Resuscitation* **2006**. [CrossRef]

112. Sheu, J.-J.; Tsai, T.-H.; Lee, F.-Y.; Fang, H.-Y.; Sun, C.-K.; Leu, S.; Yang, C.-H.; Chen, S.-M.; Hang, C.-L.; Hsieh, Y.-K.; et al. Early extracorporeal membrane oxygenator-assisted primary percutaneous coronary intervention improved 30-day clinical outcomes in patients with ST-segment elevation myocardial infarction complicated with profound cardiogenic shock. *Crit. Care Med.* **2010**. [CrossRef]

113. Takayama, H.; Truby, L.; Koekort, M.; Uriel, N.; Colombo, P.; Mancini, D.M.; Jorde, U.P.; Naka, Y. Clinical outcome of mechanical circulatory support for refractory cardiogenic shock in the current era. *J. Heart Lung Transplant* **2013**. [CrossRef]

114. Teirstein, P.S.; Vogel, R.A.; Dorros, G.; Stertzer, S.H.; Vandormael, M.; Smith, S.C.; Overlie, P.A.; O'Neill, W.W. Prophylactic versus standby cardiopulmonary support for high risk percutaneous transluminal coronary angioplasty. *J. Am. Coll. Cardiol.* **1993**. [CrossRef]

115. Schreiber, T.L.; Kodali, U.R.; O'Neill, W.W.; Gangadharan, V.; Puchrowicz-Ochocki, S.B.; Grines, C.L. Comparison of acute results of prophylactic intraaortic balloon pumping with cardiopulmonary support for percutaneous transluminal coronary angioplasty (PTCA). *Catheter Cardiovasc. Diagn.* **1998**. [CrossRef]

5

Transcatheter Aortic Valve Replacement with Self-Expandable ACURATE neo as Compared to Balloon-Expandable SAPIEN 3 in Patients with Severe Aortic Stenosis

Mirosław Gozdek [1,2], Kamil Zieliński [2,3], Michał Pasierski [2,4], Matteo Matteucci [5,6],
Dario Fina [5,7], Federica Jiritano [5,8], Paolo Meani [5,9], Giuseppe Maria Raffa [10],
Pietro Giorgio Malvindi [11], Michele Pilato [10], Domenico Paparella [12,13], Artur Słomka [2,14],
Jacek Kubica [1], Dariusz Jagielak [15], Roberto Lorusso [5], Piotr Suwalski [4] and
Mariusz Kowalewski [2,4,5,*] on behalf of Thoracic Research Centre

[1] Department of Cardiology and Internal Medicine, Nicolaus Copernicus University, Collegium Medicum, 85067 Bydgoszcz, Poland; gozdekm@wp.pl (M.G.); kubicajw@gmail.com (J.K.)
[2] Thoracic Research Centre, Nicolaus Copernicus University, Collegium Medicum in Bydgoszcz, Innovative Medical Forum, 85067 Bydgoszcz, Poland; kamilziel@gmail.com (K.Z.); michalpasierski@gmail.com (M.P.); artur.slomka@cm.umk.pl (A.S.)
[3] Department of Cardiology, Warsaw Medical University, 02091 Warsaw, Poland
[4] Clinical Department of Cardiac Surgery, Central Clinical Hospital of the Ministry of Interior and Administration, Centre of Postgraduate Medical Education, 02607 Warsa, Poland; suwalski.piotr@gmail.com
[5] Department of Cardio-Thoracic Surgery, Heart and Vascular Centre, Maastricht University Medical Centre, 6229 HX Maastricht, The Netherlands; teo.matte@libero.it (M.M.); dario.fina88@gmail.com (D.F.); fede.j@hotmail.it (F.J.); paolo.meani@ospedaleniguarda.it (P.M.); roberto.lorussobs@gmail.com (R.L.)
[6] Department of Cardiac Surgery, Circolo Hospital, University of Insubria, 21100 Varese, Italy
[7] Department of Cardiology, IRCCS Policlinico San Donato, University of Milan, 20097 Milan, Italy
[8] Department of Cardiac Surgery, University Magna Graecia of Catanzaro, 88100 Catanzaro, Italy
[9] Department of Intensive Care Unit, Maastricht University Medical Centre (MUMC+), 6229 HX Maastricht, The Netherlands
[10] Department for the Treatment and Study of Cardiothoracic Diseases and Cardiothoracic Transplantation, IRCCS-ISMETT (Instituto Mediterraneo per i Trapianti e Terapie ad alta specializzazione), 90127 Palermo, Italy; giuseppe.raffa78@gmail.com (G.M.R.); mpilato@ISMETT.edu (M.P.)
[11] Wessex Cardiothoracic Centre, University Hospital Southampton, Southampton SO16 6YD, UK; pg.malvindi@hotmail.com
[12] GVM Care & Research, Department of Cardiovascular Surgery, Santa Maria Hospital, 70124 Bari, Italy; domenico.paparella@uniba.it
[13] Department of Emergency and Organ Transplant, University of Bari Aldo Moro, 70121 Bari, Italy
[14] Chair and Department of Pathophysiology, Nicolaus Copernicus University, Collegium Medicum, 85067 Bydgoszcz, Poland
[15] Department of Cardiac Surgery, Gdańsk Medical University, 80210 Gdańsk, Poland; kardchir@gumed.edu.pl
*   Correspondence: kowalewskimariusz@gazeta.pl;

Abstract: Frequent occurrence of paravalvular leak (PVL) after transcatheter aortic valve replacement (TAVR) was the main concern with earlier-generation devices. Current meta-analysis compared outcomes of TAVR with next-generation devices: ACURATE neo and SAPIEN 3. In random-effects meta-analysis, the pooled incidence rates of procedural, clinical and functional outcomes according to VARC-2 definitions were assessed. One randomized controlled trial and five observational studies including 2818 patients (ACURATE neo $n = 1256$ vs. SAPIEN 3 $n = 1562$) met inclusion criteria. ACURATE neo was associated with a 3.7-fold increase of moderate-to-severe PVL (RR (risk ratio): 3.70 (2.04–6.70); $P < 0.0001$), which was indirectly related to higher observed 30-day mortality with

ACURATE valve (RR: 1.77 (1.03–3.04); $P = 0.04$). Major vascular complications, acute kidney injury, periprocedural myocardial infarction, stroke and serious bleeding events were similar between devices. ACURATE neo demonstrated lower transvalvular pressure gradients both at discharge ($P < 0.00001$) and at 30 days ($P < 0.00001$), along with lower risk of patient–prosthesis mismatch (RR: 0.29 (0.10–0.87); $P = 0.03$) and pacemaker implantation (RR: 0.64 (0.50–0.81); $P = 0.0002$), but no differences were observed regarding composite endpoints early safety and device success. In conclusion, ACURATE neo, as compared with SAPIEN 3, was associated with higher rates of moderate-to-severe PVL, which were indirectly linked with increased observed 30-day all-cause mortality.

Keywords: meta-analysis; ACURATE neo; SAPIEN 3; transcatheter aortic valve replacement

---

1. Introduction

Since first its mention by Cribier in 2002 [1], transcatheter aortic valve replacement (TAVR) has been complementary method to surgical aortic valve replacement (SAVR) in inoperable or high-risk patients with severe symptomatic aortic stenosis. Similar [2] or even lower [3] one-year mortality rate of TAVR, as compared to SAVR, was shown in selected groups of patients. Hence, TAVR is now considered to be an alternative treatment option and is recommended not only in inoperable, high or increased risk surgical patients [2–5] but also in intermediate and lower risk individuals [6–10]. Commercially available earlier-generation transcatheter valves, despite providing good clinical outcomes, were not free from shortcomings; indeed, high rates of conduction abnormalities, permanent pacemaker implantation (PPI) or vascular complications remained important issues to be addressed. More importantly, though, higher incidence of paravalvular leak (PVL), in turn associated with increased late mortality and higher rate of other adverse clinical incidents, as compared to SAVR [11–13], often outweigh the benefits of transcatheter approach.

To minimize these shortcomings, technological innovations were developed in next-generation valves including the following: balloon-expandable SAPIEN 3 (Edwards Lifesciences, Irvine, CA, USA) and self-expandable ACURATE neo (Boston Scientific Corporation, Marlborough, MA, USA). Since direct comparisons of these two devices are few and one recent randomized controlled trial (RCT) [14] did not demonstrate non-inferiority of the ACURATE neo device as compared to SAPIEN 3 as opposed to previous observational studies [15–21] that, however, pointed to comparable or superior results with ACURATE, the debate is ongoing.

The objective of the present investigation was to evaluate and compare short-term results of TAVR with ACURATE neo and SAPIEN 3 in patients presenting with symptomatic severe native aortic valve stenosis.

2. Experimental Section

2.1. Data Sources and Search Strategy

The systematic review and meta-analysis were performed in accordance to MOOSE statement and PRISMA guidelines [22,23]. The MOOSE checklist is available as Table A1. We searched PubMed, ClinicalKey, the Web of Science and Google Scholar all until October 2019. Search terms were as follows: "ACURATE neo" (or "ACCURATE neo"), "Symetic ACURATE", "Boston ACURATE" and/or "SAPIEN 3", "SAPIEN III" and "transcatheter valve" or "aortic". The literature was limited to peer-reviewed articles published in English. References of original articles were reviewed manually and cross-checked.

2.2. Selection Criteria and Quality Assessment

Studies were included if having met all of the following criteria: (1) human study; (2) study or study arms comparing directly strategy of transcatheter aortic valve replacement with ACURATE neo and SAPIEN 3; (3) RCT or propensity score matched observational study. Studies were excluded if they fell into the following categories: (1) in-vitro study; (2) single arm; (3) adjustment not PS or methods not reported; (4) outcomes of interest not reported; and (5) sub-studies or overlapping populations. No restrictions regarding number of patients included or characteristic of the population were imposed. Two reviewers (M.G. and K.Z.) selected the studies for the inclusion, extracted studies and patients' characteristics of interest and relevant outcomes. Two authors (M.G. and K.Z.) independently assessed the trials' eligibility and risk of bias. Any divergences were resolved by consensus.

Quality of RCTs was appraised by using the components recommended by the Cochrane Collaboration [24]; observational studies were, instead, appraised with ROBINS-I (Risk of Bias in Nonrandomised Studies-of Interventions), a tool used for assessment of the bias (the selection of the study groups; the comparability of the groups; and the ascertainment of either the exposure or outcome of interest) in cohort studies included in a systematic review and/or meta-analysis [25].

2.3. Endpoints Selection

Endpoints were established according to the Valve Academic Research Consortium-2 (VARC-2) definitions [26]. Procedural outcomes of interest were predilatation and postdilatation, procedural times and contrast volume. Clinical endpoints assessed included the following: PPI, major vascular complications (MVC), serious bleeding (life-threatening and/or major), acute kidney injury (AKI), stroke, myocardial infarction and 30-day mortality. Functional outcomes were as follows: mean transvalvular gradients, prosthesis-patient mismatch (PPM), and mild and moderate-to-severe paravalvular leak (PVL). Composite endpoints were as per VARC-2: device success (defined as absence of procedural death, correct position of 1 valve in the proper location, mean gradient < 20 mm Hg or peak velocity < 3 m/s, absence of moderate-to-severe PVL and absence of PPM) and early safety (composite of all-cause death, any stroke, life-threatening or disabling bleeding, major vascular complications, coronary artery obstruction requiring intervention, acute kidney injury (stage 2 or higher), rehospitalization for valve-related symptoms or congestive heart failure, valve-related dysfunction requiring repeat procedure, and valve-related dysfunction determined by echocardiography (mean aortic valve gradient ≥ 20 mm Hg and either effective orifice area ≤ 0.9–1.1 cm^2 (depending on body surface area) or Doppler velocity index < 0.35; or moderate or severe prosthetic PVL).

2.4. Statistical Analysis

Data were analyzed according to intention-to-treat principle, wherever applicable. Risks ratios (RR) and 95% confidence intervals (95% CI) served as primary index statistics for dichotomous outcomes. For continuous outcomes, mean difference (MD) and corresponding 95% CI were calculated by using a random effects model. To overcome the low statistical power of Cochran Q test, the statistical inconsistency test $I^2 = [(Qdf)/Q] \times 100\%$, where Q is the chi-square statistic and df is its degrees of freedom, was used to assess heterogeneity [27]. It examines the percentage of inter-study variation, with values ranging from 0% to 100%. An I^2 value of 25% indicates low heterogeneity, 50% are suggestive of moderate heterogeneity and 70% of high heterogeneity. Because of high degree of heterogeneity anticipated among predominantly nonrandomized trials, an inverse variance (DerSimonian–Laird) random-effects model was applied as a more conservative approach for observational data accounting for between- and within-study variability. Whenever a single study reported median values and interquartile ranges instead of mean and standard deviation (SD), the latter were approximated as described by Wan and colleagues [28]. In case there were "0 events" reported in both arms, calculations were repeated, as a sensitivity analysis, using risk difference (RD) and respective 95% CI. Additionally, we performed a set of meta-regression analyses to address potential relationships between 30-day all-cause mortality and other endpoints and baseline characteristics assessed. For the analyses of clinical endpoints, RCTs and PS-matched studies were analyzed separately. Review Manager 5.3 (The Nordic Cochrane Centre, Copenhagen, Denmark) was used for statistical computations. *P*-values ≤ 0.05 were considered statistically significant and reported as two-sided, without adjustment for multiple comparisons.

3. Results

3.1. Study Selection and Bias

Study selection process and reasons for exclusion of some studies are described in Figure 1.

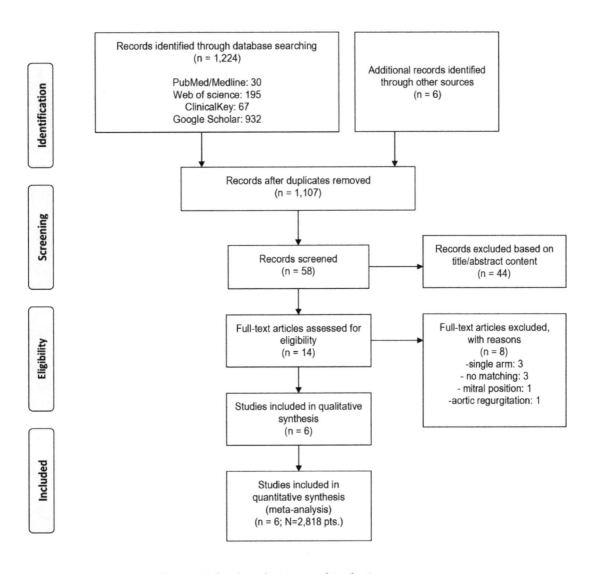

Figure 1. Study selection and inclusion process.

Systematic search of the online databases allowed collection of 58 potentially eligible records that were retrieved for scrutiny. Of those, 52 were further excluded because they were not pertinent to the design of the meta-analysis or did not meet the explicit inclusion criteria. One RCT [14] and five observational studies [15–19] enrolling the total of 2818 patients were eventually included in the analysis. Potential sources of the studies' bias were analyzed with the use of components recommended by the Cochrane Collaboration and ROBINS-I tool, and the results are enclosed as Table A2. Overall, the studies reported moderate risk of bias. Most commonly, biases arose from participants selection for the study by designated heart teams and subjective distribution of the participants within the study arms. All but one study [14] lacked a core lab assessment of PVL and central adjudication of clinical events.

Patients were divided into two groups: those treated with ACURATE neo transcatheter valve ($n = 1256$) and SAPIEN 3 transcatheter valve ($n = 1562$). Summary of the valve characteristics is available as Table 1.

Table 1. Valve characteristics and features.

ACURATE neo (Boston Scientific Corporation)	SAPIEN 3 (Edwards Lifesciences)
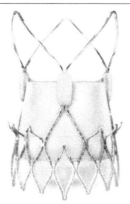	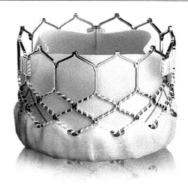
Supra-annular	Intra-annular
Porcine pericardial leaflet tissue	Bovine pericardial leaflet tissue
Self-expanding, deployment in a top-down mechanism of nitinol frame.	Balloon-expandable cobalt-chromium frame

Transfemoral sheath size (valve size)

18-French for all devices: Small (23 mm), Medium (25 mm), Large (27 mm).	Ready for ultra-low profile: 14 F (20, 23, 26 mm); 16 F (29 mm), 18 F (20, 23, 26 mm), 21 F (29 mm)

Special features

-Upper and lower crown; -Three stabilization arches; -Outer and inner pericardial skirt.	-Outer sealing and inner skirt at the inflow

Studies' characteristics, as well as definitions or diagnostic criteria for assessed clinical endpoints, are reported in Table 2. Table A3 lists selection criteria for the procedure and valve, as well as inclusion and exclusion criteria within particular studies. Patients' baseline characteristics and detailed procedural characteristics are available as Tables A4 and A5. All studies reported data on 30-day clinical outcomes; three reported Kaplan–Meier estimates of survival at longer-term follow-ups [15,16,18].

Table 2. Baseline characteristics of included studies.

Study	Barth S et al. 2019 [15]		Costa et al. 2019 [16]		Husser O et al. 2017 [17]		Lanz J et al. 2019 [14]		Mauri V et al. 2017 [18]		Schaefer A et al. 2017 [19]	
	ACURATE neo	SAPIEN 3	ACURATE neo	SAPIEN 3	ACURATE neo	SAPIEN 3	ACURATE neo	SAPIEN 3	ACURATE neo	SAPIEN 3	ACURATE neo	SAPIEN 3
Study period	2012–2016		09.2014–02.2018		01.2014–01.2016		02.2017–02.2019		02.2014–08.2016		2012–2016	
Design	MC, RCS, PM		SC, RCS, PM		MC, RCS, PM		MC, RCT		MC, RCS, PM		SC, RCS, PM	
Number of pts.	329	329	48	48	311	622	372	367	92	92	104	104
Age	81.0 ± 5.0	81.0 ± 6.0	82.3 ± 3.8	83.3 ± 2.3	81.0 ± 6.0	81.0 ± 6.0	82.6 ± 4.3	83.0 ± 3.9	82.8 ± 6.5	81.9 ± 5.3	81.7 ± 5.5	81.2 ± 6.2
Female (%)	NR	NR	70.8	68.8	60.8	55.3	59.0	55.0	92.4	92.4	69.2	65.4
BMI (kg/m^2)	28.7 ± 5.5	28.4 ± 5.8	27.8 ± 4.6	27.1 ± 3.9	27.0 ± 5.0	27.0 ± 5.0	27.3 ± 4.4	27.9 ± 4.7	27.3 ± 5.5	26.0 ± 4.7	27.1 ± 5.1	26.8 ± 5.0
STS-PROM (%)	NR		4.0 ± 3.3	3.8 ± 1.7	NR		3.7 ± 1.8	3.7 ± 1.9	NR		5.8 ± 3.8	5.4 ± 3.6
Logistic EuroSCORE (%)	18.8 ± 14.7	19.1 ± 13.6	NR	NR	18.0 ± 10.0	18.0 ± 12.0	NR	NR	16.2 ± 8.8	16.6 ± 8.8	15.9 ± 9.3	13.7 ± 9.0
NYHA III/IV (%)	79.0	78.1	NR		256	489	77.0	73.0	NR		86.5	88.5
EF (%)	53.0 ± 13.0	54.0 ± 15.0	54.5 ± 9.7	56.1 ± 9.7	NR	NR	56.4 ± 11.1	57.1 ± 10.7	59.0 ± 8.0	59.0 ± 10.0	NR	NR
EF <35% (%)	9.4	10.3	NR		5.8	5.5	NR		NR		26.0*	22.1[1]
Mean aortic gradient (mmHg)	44.0 ± 15.0	45.0 ± 14.0	51.3 ± 14.5	51.3 ± 17.2	45.0 ± 15.0	44.0 ± 16.0	42.9 ± 17.2	41.5 ± 15.1	46.0 ± 16.0	47.0 ± 16.0	35.9 ± 16.6	37.6 ± 16.7
Aortic annulus diameter (mm)	21.0 ± 2.0	21.0 ± 3.0	NR		NR		23.6 ± 1.6	23.7 ± 1.6	NR		24.5 ± 2.5	25.3 ± 2.6
Access site (%)	TF 74.5, TA 25.5	TF 75.7, TA 24.3	TF 100.0	TF 100.0	TF 100.0	TF 100.0	TF 99.0, TA <1.0	TF 100.0	TF 100.0	TF 100.0	TF 100.0	TF 100.0
VARC-2 outcomes definitions	yes		Yes		yes		yes		yes		yes	
Follow-up (months)	10.8 ± 9.7	12.2 ± 9.9	12		1		1		12.7 ± 2.6		1	

[1] <44% EF; RCT, randomized control trial; SC, single center; MC, multi center; RCS, retrospective cases series; PM, propensity matching; NYHA, New York Heart Association; STS-PROM, Society of Thoracic Surgeons Predicted Risk of Mortality; EuroSCORE, European System for Cardiac Operative Risk Evaluation; VARC, Valve Academic Research Consortium; EF, ejection fraction; TF, trans femoral; TA, trans apical; NR, not reported. In bold are highlighted the variables that differed significantly between study groups.

3.2. Patients Characteristic

Groups treated with ACURATE neo and SAPIEN 3 did not differ regarding patients' age ($P = 0.363$), body mass index ($P = 0.708$), NYHA III/IV status ($P = 0.115$) or left ventricle ejection fraction ($P = 0.178$). No difference was found in the baseline logistic EuroSCORE as well ($P = 0.749$). SAPIEN 3 group included significantly fewer female individuals, 59.7% vs. 64.1%, respectively ($P = 0.037$). Aortic valve baseline echo-parameters, i.e., mean trans-aortic gradient were comparable: 43.4 ± 15.8 vs. 43.6 ± 15.5 mmHg ($P = 0.861$) in ACURATE neo and SAPIEN 3, respectively (Figure 2), although the aortic annulus plane area were on average 4 mm^2 smaller in the ACURATE neo recipients 439.7 ± 62.4 vs. 446.7 ± 76.3; $P = 0.037$ as compared to SAPIEN 3. Transfemoral access was mostly widely employed during TAVR procedure; in five studies, it was used exclusively [14,16–19]. Barth et al. [15] included both transfemoral and transapical access in 75.7% vs. 24.3% and 74.5% vs. 25.5% for ACURATE neo and SAPIEN 3, respectively. For the transapical approach, ACUARATE TA device was used.

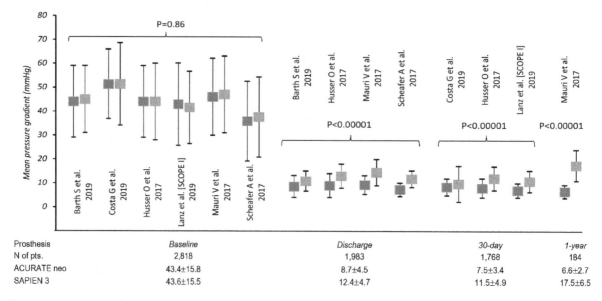

Prosthesis	Baseline	Discharge	30-day	1-year
N of pts.	2,818	1,983	1,768	184
ACURATE neo	43.4±15.8	8.7±4.5	7.5±3.4	6.6±2.7
SAPIEN 3	43.6±15.5	12.4±4.7	11.5±4.9	17.5±6.5

Figure 2. Analysis of mean transaortic gradients before and after transcatheter aortic valve replacement (TAVR).

3.3. Procedural Outcomes

Five studies [14,15,17–19] and 2722 patients contributed to the analysis of procedural outcomes between two devices. Both predilatation and postdilatation were more common with ACURATE neo valve; predilatation was necessary in 1124/1271 (88.4%) of cases as compared to 801/1514 (52.9%); RR 2.05, 95% CI, (1.44, 2.94) $P < 0.0001$; $I^2 = 97\%$); postdilatation: RR 3.10, 95% CI, (2.01, 4.77) $P < 0.00001$; $I^2 = 88\%$) with respective rates of 45.3% vs. 17.2% for ACURATE neo and SAPIEN 3, respectively. Figure 1 and A2. The procedures performed with ACURATE neo required significantly greater amount of contrast: 130.3 ± 56.1 mL vs. 109.7 ± 50.3 mL (MD 18.22 95% CI, (10.04, 26.40) mL; $P < 0.0001$). Figure 3). Four studies [14,15,17,19] including 1116 ACURATE neo and 1411 SAPIEN 3 cases provided data on procedure duration, which on average 3 minutes longer in the former: 60.1 ± 28.6 min. vs. 56.5.9 ± 26.0 min. (MD 3.06, 95% CI, (−0.66, 6.76) min) without reaching statistical significance (Figure 4). Use of >1 valve was necessary in 35 cases (26 ACURATE neo vs. nine SAPIEN 3; RR 3.24, 95% CI, (1.47, 7.13) $P = 0.004$; $I^2 = 0\%$). Incidence of cardiac tamponade was reported in three studies [14,15,18] with respective event rates of 1.0% vs. 0.7% for ACURATE neo and SAPIEN 3 valves: RR 1.17, 95% CI, (0.52, 2.63) $P = 0.70$; $I^2 = 0\%$. Early procedural complications included the following: coronary obstruction in three ACURATE neo patients and total of eight annular ruptures, 20 conversions to surgery and 20 valve malpositionings without differences between two devices.

3.4. Clinical Outcomes

Six studies [14–19] enrolling 2818 patients contributed data for the analysis of early safety as defined by VARC-2; with the corresponding rates of 13.9% (174/1256) and 12.6% (197/1562) for ACURATE neo and SAPIEN 3 valves, respectively, there were no statistical differences between two devices (RR 1.15, 95% CI, (0.94, 1.40) $P = 0.16$; $I^2 = 0\%$) and pooled estimates of RCT and PS-matched studies in subgroup analysis ($P_{interaction} = 0.47$) (Figure 3a). In the pooled analysis of device success (five studies included (2634 patients.)), there were no differences between two types of valve in the pooled analysis: RR 1.01, 95% CI, (0.92, 1.10) $P = 0.89$; $I^2 = 89\%$). Analyzed separately, there were strong between-subgroup differences between RCT and pooled estimate from PS-matched studies: RR 1.44, 95% CI, (1.24, 1.66); $P < 0.00001$; $I^2 = NA$ and RR 0.95, 95% CI, (0.91, 0.99); $P = 0.01$; $I^2 = 47\%$ with $P_{interaction} < 0.00001$ (Figure 3b).

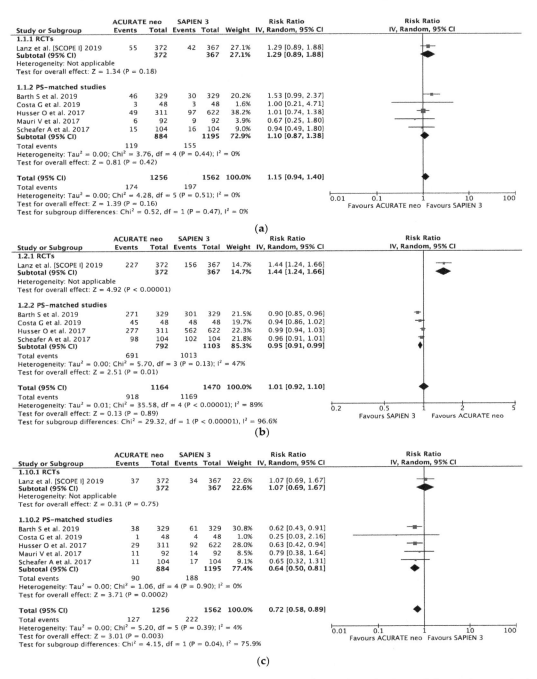

Figure 3. Individual and summary risk ratios with corresponding 95% confidence intervals for the comparison of ACURATE neo vs. SAPIEN 3 in the analysis of clinical outcomes: (**a**) early safety, (**b**)·device success and (**c**) permanent pacemaker implantation.

There were no differences between ACURATE neo and SAPIEN 3 valves in terms of risk of major vascular complications (RR 1.21, 95% CI, (0.89, 1,65); P = 0.23; I^2 = 6%; Figure 5), acute kidney injury (RR 1.28, 95% CI, (0.71, 2,31); P = 0.42; I^2 = 15%; Figure 6), periprocedural myocardial infarction (RR 1.76, 95% CI, (0.36, 8.47); P = 0.428 I^2 = 0%; Figures 7 and 8), stroke (RR 0.95, 95% CI, (0.57, 1.57); P = 0.84 I^2 = 0%; Figures 9 and 10), and serious bleeding events (RR 1.23, 95% CI, (0.95, 1.61); P = 0.12; I^2 = 0%; Figure 11).

Based on the data from six studies (2818 pts.), PPI was required nearly 30% less often after ACURATE neo implantation as compared to SAPIEN 3 (RR 0.72, 95% CI, (0.58, 0.89); P = 0.003; I^2 = 75.9%) with corresponding frequency of 10.1% vs. 14.2%, respectively (Figure 3c). Importantly, the estimates derived from SCOPE I differed from the pooled estimates ($P_{interaction}$ = 0.04) with higher rates of PPI observed in SAPIEN 3 arm in PS-matched studies (9.3% vs. 15.8%) Table 6 lists the VARC-2 derived quality criteria for PPI appraisal

3.5. Functional Outcomes

With five studies [14–16,18,19] and 1885 patients included, mild PVL occurred less frequently in SAPIEN 3 recipients, 28.0% (263 of 940), compared to ACURATE neo group, 45.5% (430 of 945); (RR 1.60, 95% CI, (1.40, 1.84) P < 0.00001; I^2 = 14%) (Figure 4a). Moderate-to-severe PVL was uncommon in the entire series (6.5%); however, there was a significant 3.7-fold increase in moderate-to-severe PVL risk with ACURATE neo implantation: (RR 3.70, 95% CI, (2.04, 6.70) P < 0.0001; I^2 = 53%) (Figure 4b) and corresponding incidence of 11.7% (147/1,256) and 2.3% (36/1,562) in ACURATE neo and SAPIEN 3 valves.

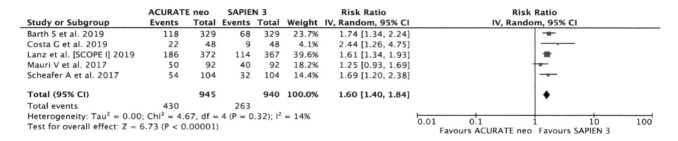

(a)

(b)

Figure 4. Individual and summary risk ratios with corresponding 95% confidence intervals for the comparison of ACURATE neo vs. SAPIEN 3 in the analysis of functional outcomes: (**a**) mild and (**b**) moderate-to-severe paravalvular leak.

Data regarding postprocedural transaortic gradient came from all six studies with 2818 patients. Mauri et al. [18] reported on 1-year transaortic gradients as well. (Figure 2). Mean postprocedural transaortic gradients were higher in SAPIEN 3 patients both at discharge and at 30 days post-op: 12.4 ± 4.7 vs. 8.7 ± 4.5 mmHg (P < 0.00001) and 11.5 ± 4.9 vs. 7.5 ± 3.4 mmHg (P < 0.00001) respectively.

3.6. All-Cause Mortality

Six studies reported on 30-day all-cause mortality. Overall, 61 (2.2%) patients died within the first 30 days, with respective rates of 2.9% and 1.6% in ACURATE neo and SAPIEN 3 groups; ACURATE neo was associated with 77% higher 30-day mortality risk (RR 1.77, 95% CI, (1.03, 3.04); $P = 0.04$; $I^2 = 0$% (Figure 5a and Appendix Figure 12). A random-effects meta-regression was fitted, counter-opposing all-cause mortality risk ratio against the risk difference of moderate-to-severe PVL; there was a trend for higher 30-day mortality rates with higher incidence of moderate-to-severe PVL (beta = 0.023; $P = 0.093$) (Figure 5b); similarly, a meta-regression was fitted with all-cause mortality risk ratio against the mean annulus area in the ACURATE neo arm showing a trend for lower between devices mortality ratio in smaller annuli (beta = 22.078; $P = 0.098$) (Figure 5c).

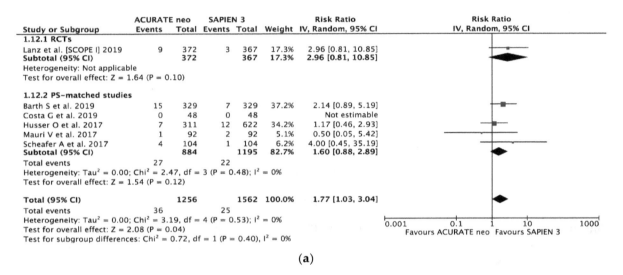

(a)

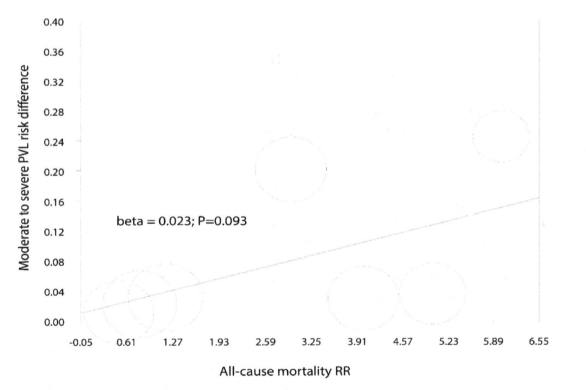

(b)

Figure 5. *Cont.*

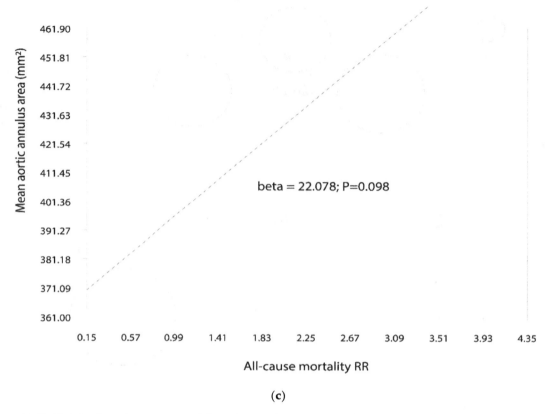

(c)

Figure 5. Individual and summary risk ratios with corresponding 95% confidence intervals for the comparison of ACURATE neo vs. SAPIEN 3 in the analysis of (**a**) 30-day all-cause mortality; (**b,c**) meta regression analyses.

4. Discussion

To the best of our knowledge, this is the first systematic review and meta-analysis of observational trials comparing major procedural, short-term clinical and functional outcomes between the ACURATE neo and SEPIEN 3, the next-generation transcatheter valves designed to minimize shortcomings of the earlier-generation devices. Our analysis, by pooling data from one RCT and five PS-matched studies, demonstrated excellent data regarding short-term performance of both devices. Compared populations of patients were well balanced with respect to baseline characteristics and severity of underlying valvular disease. Main findings of the current study are that the ACURATE neo implantation as compared to SAPIEN 3 was associated with lower transvalvular gradients and lower risk of permanent pacemaker implantation. Other clinical endpoints which included vascular complications, AKI, as well as life threatening and major bleeding; stroke and MIs did not differ between the two groups. The use of ACURATE neo procedures were significantly longer and required a greater amount of contrast volume. Device success and early safety combined endpoints, as defined by VARC-2 criteria, were, however, similar regardless the type of valve implanted. Importantly, the current study revealed significantly higher rates of both mild and moderate-to-severe PVL with ACURATE neo as compared to SAPIEN 3 and the latter were indirectly associated with worse survival observed in ACURATE neo group.

Previous observational studies [15–21] and, among them, the SAVI-TF (Symetis ACURATE neo Valve Implantation Using Transfemoral Access) registry [29,30] reported on excellent short-term outcomes with low complications and, in particular, PPI rates in ACURATE neo valve attributable to the design of the prosthesis. The particularly low gradients also contributed to the similar or better rates of device success for ACURATE neo and SAPIEN 3 in propensity matched comparisons. Whether the abovementioned benefits would hold true in randomized populations and further translate into improved clinical outcomes was investigated in the Safety and Efficacy of the Symetis ACURATE

Neo/TF Compared to the Edwards SAPIEN 3 Bioprosthesis trial (SCOPE I) [14]. Interestingly, the ACURATE neo valve failed to meet noninferiority for its primary endpoint of combined at 30 days against the balloon-expandable SAPIEN 3 (Edwards Lifesciences) valve. Moreover, secondary analyses demonstrated SAPIEN 3 to be superior for the composite safety and efficacy endpoint, driven by less stage 2 or 3 acute kidney injury and less paravalvular leak. Valve dysfunction requiring repeat interventions was also less common at 30 days. In particular, findings on device success need to be addressed, since the rates varied largely between RCT and the remaining PS-matched studies driven by higher patient prosthesis mismatch in the SAPIEN 3 group ($P < 0.00001$). Indeed, median mean transvalvular gradient was lower, and the median mean aortic valve area was larger, in the ACURATE neo, compared to the SAPIEN 3 group, at follow-up echocardiography in the SCOPE I trial. This may have been partially due to the fact that sizing and thus the choice of the valve process were different in the SCOPE I and the remaining studies. Some residual bias despite propensity score matching also cannot be excluded. In fact, Mauri et al. [18] reports on the sizing category was based on perimeter for ACURATE neo and annular area for SAPIEN 3, then all patients received ACURATE neo size S or SAPIEN 3 23 mm. In the study by Husser et al. [17] after PS-matching, there remained a $P = 0.003$ difference in aortic annular area; Schaefer et al. [19] reports aortic annulus size to have presented significant differences for area derived aortic annulus diameter (23.9 ± 2.8 vs. 24.8 ± 2.6 mm; $P = 0.02$) and perimeter-derived aortic annulus diameter (24.5 ± 2.5 vs. 25.3 ± 2.6 mm; $P = 0.02$), which, in consequence, led to oversizing in the ACURATE neo and undersizing SAPIEN 3 (1.5 ± 6.6 vs. -0.9 ± 6.4; $P = 0.01$ for cover index). Further, only in the SCOPE I trial, both the clinical events and functional assessment details were adjudicated by independent core lab. Independently, there were fewer PPI necessary after ACURATE neo in the PS-matched studies; since not confirmed in the SCOPE I, the supra-annular positioning of the valve must have had played, however, a much less important role than expected, and the lower PPI rates originating from skewed valve-size selection and positioning of the valve in the annulus [29]. More importantly, though, SCOPE I trial, by design, excluded over 300 patients with excessive calcification of aortic valve or left ventricular outflow tract (LVOT), which was not the case in remaining studies included in the current analysis. Presence of calcifications in both aortic annulus and LVOT could have accounted for much higher rates of PPI in the SAPIEN 3 arms across included PS-matched studies (average PPI incidence rate of 15.8%) as compared to SCOPE I trial with 9.3% rate, similarly to what has been already demonstrated for SAPIEN 3 in another meta-analysis by the same group [30].

Conversely to the abovementioned, yet still contributing to device success rates, was the higher incidence of moderate-to-severe PVL in the ACURATE neo valve, which was confirmed also in the current meta-analysis. In the next-generation devices, improved by addition an external sealing cuff or a skirt, the frequencies of mild and moderate-to-severe PVL became significantly lower as compared with the earlier-generation valves. The pooled occurrence of more than mild PVL decreased from 6.9% SAPIEN XT to 1.6% in SAPIEN 3 valve, as in a meta-analysis by Ando et al. with 2498 patients [31]. The PARTNER II SAPIEN-3 trial, which assessed early outcomes after TAVR in inoperable, high-risk and intermediate-risk patients with severe aortic stenosis, showed moderate-to-severe PVL in 3.4% and mild in 40.7% of the cases [32]. The abovementioned improvements seen in next-generation devices seem not to be the case with ACURATE neo; in the meta-analysis, we found 11.7% incidence of moderate-to-severe PVL in the ACURATE neo arm, nearly fourfold higher than in SAPIEN 3 and mild PVL in 45.5% cases, translating into 60% increased risk. Unlike the current findings, SAVI TF registry showed 4.1% of >mild PVL in 1000 patients treated with ACURATE neo which is within ranges observable for other devices [33–38]. Postdilatation was performed in 44.8% of the patients in that series, and this percentage is also comparable to 40.4%–51.9% in the current analysis, and therefore, theoretically, should not influence the outcome; on the other hand, Barth et al. [15] reports lower >mild PVL rates in one of participating centers (C) that used "zero tolerance of more than mild paravalvular leak" policy and postdilated more frequently than other centers (52.7% as compared to 12.3% and 33.3%), which translated to 3.4% rate of >mild PVL (as compared to 6.0% and 34.1% in the remaining centers). Interestingly, this center was the one to demonstrate highest one-year survival (87.4% (95% CI: 79.6–92.3) compared to 75.4% (95% CI: 60.4–85.3) and 81.3% (95% CI: 70.1–88.6)). Corroborating these estimates on larger scale and also in shorter follow-up, the current meta-analysis found an indirect link between increased rates of >mild PVL and higher mortality in the ACURATE neo arm at 30 days. While the presence of residual >mild PVL has been long shown to be associated with increased mortality in the long-term [39,40], the link between >mild PVL and 30-day mortality appears less clear, particularly for next-generation devices [12]. The abovementioned may be of importance given the fact that acute aortic insufficiency of various degree in patients with prior pure aortic stenosis and diminished LV compliance is often a cause of heart-failure exacerbation early in the sequelae [41].

An indirect link to increased mortality with ACURATE neo, as found also in meta-regression of annular area; indeed, lower between-devices mortality risk ratios between ACURATE neo and SAPIEN 3 were shown in patients with smaller annuli. An important hypothesis generated by present meta-analysis is that ACURATE neo performs differently in this setting; since we could not demonstrate excess of annual ruptures, cardiac tamponades, conversions to surgery or other periprocedural complications in either group, the explanation of this phenomenon remains to be elucidated.

Several inherent limitations to the current analysis need to be acknowledged; firstly, the majority of included studies are of an observational nature. Despite accounting for differences in the patients' baseline populations by propensity matching in all of the non-randomized reports, there remain other confounders, like learning curve, operators' experience and decision as of valve size and type that add to the risk of bias. Indeed, it cannot be refused that ACURATE neo was the preferred valve in smaller aortic annuli in PS-matched studies. Secondly, one study [15] reports on outcomes with both transfemoral ACURATE neo and transapical ACURATE TA systems. While similar in stent design and technological features, there are certain, albeit minor, differences in delivery system and biological tissue used in both devices [42]. Thirdly, only half of included studies reported follow-up longer than one month; paucity of data regarding long-term clinical and functional outcomes significantly impedes interpretation of ACURATE neo and SAPIEN 3 clinical suitability. Lastly, all but one study [14] lacked of an external core lab assessment and adjudication of echocardiographic outcomes. Finally, to better visualize the relative advantages of the contemporary-use valve systems, the results of a second similar study, SCOPE II (NCT03192813), will compare the ACURATE neo to the EVOLUT R system with respect to a composite of all-cause death and stroke at one year.

5. Conclusions

Contemporary evidence shows good short-term implantation outcomes of both ACURATE neo and SAPIEN 3 valves, with no differences in combined endpoints of device success and early safety. Implantation of ACURATE neo was associated with lower transvalvular gradients and lower risk of permanent pacemaker implantation. Moderate-to-severe PVL rates were, however, higher in ACURATE neo valve and were indirectly associated with increased 30-day all-cause mortality.

Author Contributions: Conceptualization, M.G., M.M., D.F., F.J., P.M., G.M.R., P.G.M., A.S. and M.K.; methodology, K.Z., M.P., D.P., J.K., R.L., P.S. and M.K.; software, M.K.; validation, all authors; formal analysis, M.G., G.M.R., P.G.M. and M.K.; investigation, M.G., K.Z., M.P., M.M., D.F., F.J., P.M.; resources, not available; data curation, M.G., G.M.R., P.G.M. and M.K.; writing—original draft preparation, all authors; writing—review and editing, R.L., P.S. and M.K.; visualization, M.K.; supervision, R.L., P.S. and M.K.; project administration, M.K.; funding acquisition, not available. All authors have read and agreed to the published version of the manuscript.

Appendix A

Table A1. Checklist for meta-analyses of observational studies.

Item No.	Recommendation	Reported on Page No.
	Reporting of background should include	
1	Problem definition	2
2	Hypothesis statement	NA
3	Description of study outcome(s)	3–11
4	Type of exposure or intervention used	5
5	Type of study designs used	5
6	Study population	5
	Reporting of search strategy should include	
7	Qualifications of searchers (e.g., librarians and investigators)	Title page
8	Search strategy, including time period included in the synthesis and key words	4, Figure 1
9	Effort to include all available studies, including contact with authors	5
10	Databases and registries searched	5
11	Search software used, name and version, including special features used (e.g., explosion)	NA
12	Use of hand searching (e.g., reference lists of obtained articles)	5
13	List of citations located and those excluded, including justification	NA
14	Method of addressing articles published in languages other than English	NA
15	Method of handling abstracts and unpublished studies	NA
16	Description of any contact with authors	NA
	Reporting of methods should include	
17	Description of relevance or appropriateness of studies assembled for assessing the hypothesis to be tested	NA
18	Rationale for the selection and coding of data (e.g., sound clinical principles or convenience)	NA
19	Documentation of how data were classified and coded (e.g., multiple raters, blinding and interrater reliability)	NA
20	Assessment of confounding (e.g., comparability of cases and controls in studies where appropriate)	Table A2
21	Assessment of study quality, including blinding of quality assessors, stratification or regression on possible predictors of study results	Table A2
22	Assessment of heterogeneity	3
23	Description of statistical methods (e.g., complete description of fixed or random effects models, justification of whether the chosen models account for predictors of study results, dose-response models, or cumulative meta-analysis) in sufficient detail to be replicated	3
24	Provision of appropriate tables and graphics	yes

Table A1. *Cont.*

Item No.	Recommendation	Reported on Page No.
	Reporting of results should include	
25	Graphic summarizing individual study estimates and overall estimate	Figures 3–5
26	Table giving descriptive information for each study included	Table 2
27	Results of sensitivity testing (e.g., subgroup analysis)	NA
28	Indication of statistical uncertainty of findings	13–14
	Reporting of discussion should include	
29	Quantitative assessment of bias (e.g., publication bias)	NA
30	Justification for exclusion (e.g., exclusion of non-English language citations)	Figure 1
31	Assessment of quality of included studies	13, Table A2
	Reporting of conclusions should include	
32	Consideration of alternative explanations for observed results	11–13
33	Generalization of the conclusions (i.e., appropriate for the data presented and within the domain of the literature review)	14
34	Guidelines for future research	NA
35	Disclosure of funding source	Title page

From: Stroup DF, Berlin JA, Morton SC, et al. for the Meta-Analysis of Observational Studies in Epidemiology (MOOSE) Group. Meta-Analysis of Observational Studies in Epidemiology. A Proposal for Reporting. JAMA 2000; 283:2008-2012.

Table A2. Publication bias analysis.

Study (RCT)	Random sequence generation (selection bias)	Allocation concealment (selection bias)	Blinding of participants and personnel (performance bias)	Blinding of outcome assessment (detection bias)	Incomplete outcome data (attrition bias)	Selective reporting (reporting bias)	Other bias
Lanz et al. [SCOPE I] 2019 [14]	Low	Unclear	High	Low	Low	Low	Low

Study (PS-matched studies)	Bias due to confounding	Bias in selection of participants into the study	Bias in measurement of interventions	Bias due to departures from intended interventions	Bias due to missing data	Bias in measurement of outcomes[1]	Bias in selection of reported result	Overall bias
Barth S et al. 2019 [15]	Serious	Serious	Low	Low	Low	Serious	Low	Moderate
Costa G et al. 2019 [16]	Serious	Low	Low	Low	Low	Serious	Low	Moderate
Husser O et al. 2017 [17]	Serious	Low	Low	Low	Low	Serious	Low	Moderate
Mauri V et al. 2017 [18]	Serious	Low	Low	Low	Low	Serious	Low	Moderate
Scheafer A et al. 2017 [19]	Serious	Low	Low	Low	Low	Serious	Low	Moderate

1 When multiple outcomes were reported for a study, the highest level of bias at the outcome level is reported in the table.

Table A3. Inclusion and exclusion criteria. Choice of procedure and valve-type.

Study [ref]	Inclusion criteria	Exclusion criteria	Selection criteria for the procedure	Selection criteria for the valve
Barth S et al. 2019 [15]	Patients received either the ACURATE/ACURATE neo prostheses ($n = 591$) or the SAPIEN 3 prosthesis ($n = 715$).	Through nearest neighborhood matching with exact allocation for access route and center, pairs of 329 patients (250 transfemoral, 79 transapical) per group were determined.	Not reported.	Not reported.
Costa et al. 2019 [16]	All the patients treated with SAPIEN 3, Evolut R, or ACURATE neo, which could have indifferently received all the three devices according to manufacturer sizing indications.	Patients who did not performed pre-TAVI multi-detector computed tomography assessment (n = 169), patients who had a valve-in- valve implantation in a failed aortic bioprosthesis (n = 21), patients with bicuspid aortic valve (n = 28), and pure aortic regurgitation (n = 1).	Not reported.	Not reported.
Husser O et al. 2017 [17]	Patients with symptomatic, severe stenosis of the native aortic valve were treated with transfemoral TAVI using ACURATE neo ($n = 311$) or SAPIEN 3 ($n = 810$) at 3 centers in Germany.	Not reported.	The interdisciplinary heart team discussed all cases and consensus was achieved regarding the therapeutic strategy.	The interdisciplinary heart team discussed all cases and consensus was achieved regarding the therapeutic strategy.

Table A3. *Cont.*

Study [ref]	Inclusion criteria	Exclusion criteria	Selection criteria for the procedure	Selection criteria for the valve
Lanz J et al. 2019 [14]	Patients aged 75 years or older. With severe aortic stenosis defined by an aortic valve area (AVA) < 1 cm^2 or AVA indexed to body surface area of < 0·6 cm^2/m^2. Symptomatic (NYHA functional class > I, angina or syncope). At increased risk for mortality if undergoing SAVR as determined by: - the heart team OR - an STS-PROM score > 10% OR - a Logistic EuroSCORE > 20%. Heart team agrees on eligibility for participation. Aortic annulus perimeter 66–85 mm AND area 338–573 mm^2 based on multi-slice computed tomography. Minimum diameter of arterial aorto-iliac-femoral axis on one side: ≥5·5 mm. Patient understand the purpose, potential risks and benefits of the trial, is able to provide written informed content and willing to participate in all parts of the follow-up.	-Non-valvular, congenital or non-calcific acquired aortic stenosis, uni- or bicuspid aortic valve. -Anatomy not appropriate for transfemoral TAVR due to degree or eccentricity of calcification or tortuosity of aorto- and iliac-femoral arteries. -Pre-existing prosthetic heart valve in aortic or mitral position. -Emergency procedures, cardiogenic shock (vasopressor dependence, mechanical hemodynamic support), or severely reduced left ventricular ejection fraction (< 20%). -Concomitant planned procedure except for percutaneous coronary intervention. -Stroke or myocardial infarction (except type 2) in prior 30 days. -Planned non-cardiac surgery within 30 days after TAVR. -Severe coagulation conditions, inability to tolerate anticoagulation/antiplatelet therapy. -Evidence of intra-cardiac mass, thrombus or vegetation. -Active bacterial endocarditis or other active infection. -Hypertrophic cardiomyopathy with or without obstruction. -Contraindication to contrast media or allergy to nitinol. -Participation in another trial leading to deviations in the preparation and conduction of the intervention or the post-implantation management.	The heart team or an STS-PROM score > 10% or a Logistic EuroSCORE > 20%. Heart team agrees on eligibility for participation.	Patients were randomly assigned in a 1:1 ratio to undergo TAVI with either the ACURATE neo or the SAPIEN 3 system.

Table A3. *Cont.*

Study [ref]	Inclusion criteria	Exclusion criteria	Selection criteria for the procedure	Selection criteria for the valve
Mauri V et al. 2017 [18]	Inclusion criteria were small annular dimension defined as an annulus area <400 mm^2 and transfemoral TAVI with either an ACURATE neo size S or an Edwards SAPIEN 3 size 23 mm.	Not reported.	Eligibility of the individual candidate for TAVI had been decided within the local institutional heart team.	Prosthesis selection was at the discretion of the operating physicians at each center.
Schaefer A et al. 2017 [19]	A consecutive series of 104 patients received transfemoral TAVI using the ACURATE neo for treatment of severe symptomatic calcified aortic stenosis (study group) between 2012 and 2016. For comparative assessment, a matched control group of 104 patients treated by transfemoral TAVI using the Edwards SAPIEN 3 during the same time frame (2014 to 2016) was retrieved from dedicated hospital database containing a total of 1326 TAVI patients (210 SAPIEN 3 patients).	Patients unsuitable for a retrograde transfemoral approach and all valve-in-valve procedures were excluded from analysis.	Allocation of patients to TAVI followed current international recommendations after consensus of the local dedicated heart team.	Not reported.

Table A4. Patients' baseline characteristics.

Study [ref]	Intervention	HT (%)	DM (%)	PVD (%)	CKI (%)	COPD (%)	PM/ICD (%)	AF (%)	CAD (%)	MI history (%)	Stroke history (%)	Heart surgery history (%)	NYHA III/IV (%)	LVEF (%)	Mean aortic gradient (mmHg)	Aortic valve area (cm²)	Aortic annulus diameter (mm)
Barth S et al. 2019 [15]	ACURATE neo	93.3	36.8	NR	2.7	15.8	NR	38.0	NR	NR	14.0	14.9	79.0	53.0 ± 13.0	44.0 ± 15.0	0.68 ± 0.18	21.0 ± 2.0
	SAPIEN 3	93.0	35.0	NR	2.7	14.9	NR	38.7	NR	NR	14.6	14.6	78.1	54.0 ± 15.0	45.0 ± 14.0	0.67 ± 0.17	21.0 ± 3.0
Costa et al. 2019 [16]	ACURATE neo	89.6	18.8	6.3	4.2	20.8	NR	12.5	NR	14.6	2.1	6.3	NR	54.5 ± 9.7	51.3 ± 14.5	NR	NR
	SAPIEN 3	89.6	27.1	4.2	2.1	14.6	NR	12.5	NR	14.6	4.2	2.1	NR	56.1 ± 9.7	51.3 ± 17.2	NR	NR
Husser O et al. 2017 [17]	ACURATE neo	NR	33.1	10.6	2.3	13.5	9.0	24.8	61.1	10.0	13.8	10.6	82.3	NR	45.0 ± 15.0	NR	NR
	SAPIEN 3	NR	32.3	11.3	1.9	17.8	10.0	26.2	62.7	10.1	12.5	8.7	78.6	NR	44.0 ± 16.0	NR	NR
Lanz J et al. 2019 [14]	ACURATE neo	92.0	29.0	12.0	4.0	9.0	12.0	36.0	59.0	10.0	13.0	9.0	77.0	56.4 ± 11.1	42.9 ± 17.2	0.7 ± 0.2	23.6 ± 1.6
	ACURATE neo	91.0	32.0	11.0	5.0	12.0	10.0	37.0	60.0	13.0	13.0	9.0	73.0	57.1 ± 10.7	41.5 ± 15.1	0.7 ± 0.2	23.7 ± 1.6
Mauri V et al. 2017 [18]	SAPIEN 3	NR	NR	NR	NR	NR	NR	NR	NR	NR	NR	NR	NR	59.0 ± 8.0	46.0 ± 16.0	NR	NR
	ACURATE neo	NR	NR	NR	NR	NR	NR	NR	NR	NR	NR	NR	NR	59.0 ± 10.0	47.0 ± 16.0	NR	NR
Schaefer A et al. 2017 [19]	SAPIEN 3	85.6	27.9	16.3	NR	17.3	NR	34.6	59.6	NR	14.4	9.6	86.5	NR	35.9 ± 16.6	0.8 ± 0.2	24.5 ± 2.5
	ACURATE neo	93.3	26.0	13.5	NR	20.2	NR	32.7	57.7	NR	11.5	5.8	88.5	NR	37.6 ± 16.7	0.8 ± 0.2	25.3 ± 2.6

HT, hypertension; DM, diabetes mellitus; PVD, peripheral vascular disease; CKI, chronic kidney injury; COPD, chronic obstructive pulmonary disease; PM/ICD, pacemaker/implantable cardioverter-defibrillator; AF, atrial fibrillation; CAD, coronary artery disease; MI, myocardial infarction; LVEF, left ventricle ejection fraction; NR, not reported. In bold are highlighted the variables that differed significantly.

Table A5. Procedural characteristics.

Study [ref]	Intervention	Anesthesia (%)	Access Site (%)	Valve sizes Implanted (%), (Mean ± SD)	Pre-Dilatation (%)	Post-Dilatation (%)	Contrast Volume (mL)	Fluoroscopy Time (min)	Procedure Duration (min)
Barth S et al. 2019 [15]	ACURATE neo	general 96.0, conscious sedation 4.0	femoral 74.5, apical 25.5	S NR, M NR, L NR (25.0 ± 2.0)	97.6	40.4	128 ± 54	9.2 ± 4.4	62.0 ± 24.0
	SAPIEN 3	general 96.4, conscious sedation 3.6	femoral 75.7, apical 24.3	23 mm NR, 26 mm NR, 29 mm NR (25.0 ± 2.0)	52.1	11.6	106 ± 43	8.5 ± 4.9	59.0 ± 26.0
Costa et al. 2019 [16]	ACURATE neo	NR	femoral 100	NR	NR	NR	NR	NR	NR
	SAPIEN 3		femoral 100	NR	NR	NR	NR	NR	NR
Husser O et al. 2017 [17]	ACURATE neo	general 52.7, conscious sedation 47.3	femoral 100	S 30.9, M 40.2, L 28.9	95.8	42.1	115.0 ± 54.0	10.0 ± 6.0	55.0 ± 30.0
	SAPIEN 3	general 54.0, conscious sedation 46.0	femoral 100	23 mm 43.9, 26 mm 41.6, 29 mm 14.5	74.3	23.8	104.0 ± 53.0	11.0 ± 5.9	54.0 ± 24.0
Lanz J et al. 2019 [14]	ACURATE neo	general 25.0, conscious sedation 75.0	femoral 99.0, other 1.0	S 20.0, M 43.0, L 34.0	88.0	52.0	136.0 ± 55.6	NR	53.2 ± 26.5
	SAPIEN 3	general 23.0, conscious sedation 77.0	femoral 99.0, other 1.0	23 mm 39.0, 26 mm 55.0, 29 mm 5.0	23.0	48.0	110 ± 45.9	NR	46.0 ± 25.9
Mauri V et al. 2017 [18]	ACURATE neo	general 100.0	femoral 100	S 100.0	94.6	31.5	NR	NR	NR
	SAPIEN 3		femoral 100	23 mm 100.0	31.5	6.5	NR	NR	NR
Schaefer A et al. 2017 [19]	ACURATE neo	conscious sedation 47.1% general 52.9%	femoral 100	S 35.6, M 38.5, L 25.9	90.3	47.6	162.6 ± 70.3	19.3 ± 9.4	94.0 ± 46.9
	SAPIEN 3	conscious sedation 34.6% general 65.4%	femoral 100	23mm 40.4, 26mm 49.0, 29mm 10.6	53.8	20.2	154.8 ± 73.0	19.4 ± 9.1	94.8 ± 38.0

NR, not reported.

Table 6. VARC-2 derived permanent pacemaker implantation criteria quality appraisal.

Study [ref]	Presence of Pacemaker at Baseline Reported	Precision of the Indication Reported	Days Post TAVR for PPI Reported
Barth S et al. 2019 [15]	No	no	In-hospital
Costa et al. 2019 [16]	Yes	no	NA
Husser O et al. 2017 [17]	Yes	no	In-hospital and 30 days
Lanz J et al. 2019 [14]	Yes	no	30 days
Mauri V et al 2017 [18]	No	no	30 days
Schaefer A et al. 2017 [19]	No	Atrioventricular block Grade 3 or rapid progressive left bundle branch block	In-hospital

TAVR, transcatheter aortic valve replacement; PPI, permanent pacemaker implantation; NA, not available.

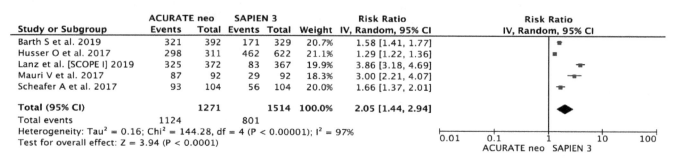

Figure 1. Procedural outcomes. Individual and summary risk ratios with corresponding 95% confidence intervals for the comparison of ACURATE neo vs. SAPIEN 3 in the analysis of predilatation.

Figure 2. Procedural outcomes. Individual and summary risk ratios with corresponding 95% confidence intervals for the comparison of ACURATE neo vs. SAPIEN 3 in the analysis of postdilatation.

Figure 3. Procedural outcomes. Detailed analysis of individual weighted mean differences (MDs) with corresponding 95% CIs on contrast volume used for the comparison of ACURATE neo vs. SAPIEN 3.

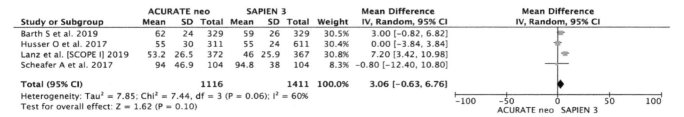

Figure 4. Procedural outcomes. Detailed analysis of individual weighted mean differences (MDs) with corresponding 95% CIs on procedure duration for the comparison of ACURATE neo vs. SAPIEN 3.

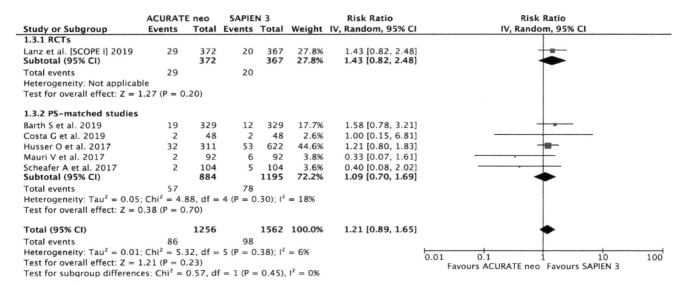

Figure 5. Clinical outcomes. Individual and summary risk ratios with corresponding 95% confidence intervals for the comparison of ACURATE neo and SAPIEN 3 in the analysis of major vascular complications.

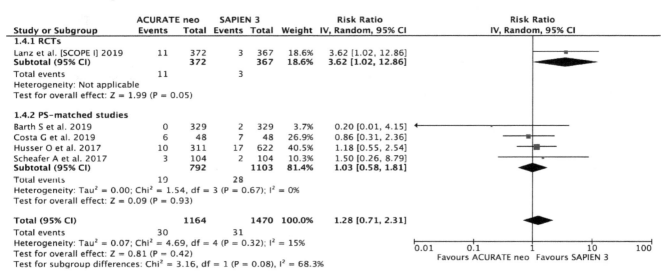

Figure 6. Clinical outcomes. Individual and summary risk ratios with corresponding 95% confidence intervals for the comparison of ACURATE neo and SAPIEN 3 in the analysis of acute kidney injury.

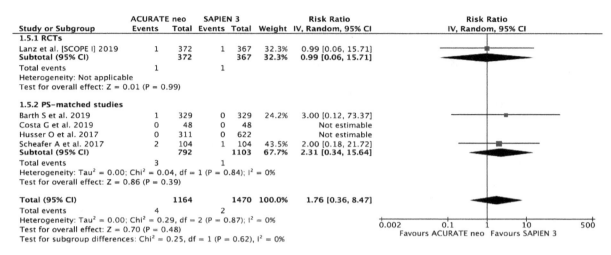

Figure 7. Clinical outcomes. Individual and summary risk ratios with corresponding 95% confidence intervals for the comparison of ACURATE neo and SAPIEN 3 in the analysis of periprocedural myocardial infarction.

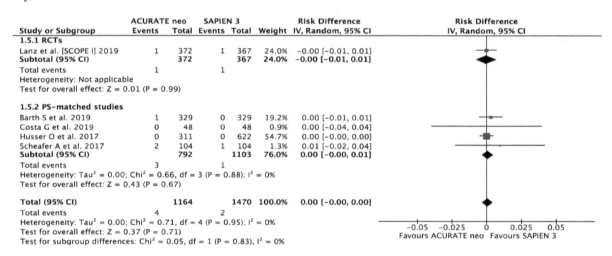

Figure 8. Clinical outcomes. Individual and summary risk ratios with corresponding 95% confidence intervals for the comparison of ACURATE neo and SAPIEN 3 in the analysis of periprocedural myocardial infarction taking into account "0 events".

Study or Subgroup	ACURATE neo Events	Total	SAPIEN 3 Events	Total	Weight	Risk Ratio IV, Random, 95% CI	Risk Ratio IV, Random, 95% CI
1.6.1 RCTs							
Lanz et al. [SCOPE I] 2019	10	372	12	367	37.1%	0.82 [0.36, 1.88]	
Subtotal (95% CI)		372		367	37.1%	0.82 [0.36, 1.88]	
Total events	10		12				
Heterogeneity: Not applicable							
Test for overall effect: Z = 0.46 (P = 0.64)							
1.6.2 PS-matched studies							
Barth S et al. 2019	6	329	3	329	13.4%	2.00 [0.50, 7.93]	
Costa G et al. 2019	0	48	0	48		Not estimable	
Husser O et al. 2017	7	311	19	622	34.6%	0.74 [0.31, 1.73]	
Mauri V et al. 2017	3	92	2	92	8.1%	1.50 [0.26, 8.77]	
Scheafer A et al. 2017	2	104	2	104	6.7%	1.00 [0.14, 6.97]	
Subtotal (95% CI)		884		1195	62.9%	1.03 [0.55, 1.95]	
Total events	18		26				
Heterogeneity: Tau² = 0.00; Chi² = 1.65, df = 3 (P = 0.65); I² = 0%							
Test for overall effect: Z = 0.10 (P = 0.92)							
Total (95% CI)		1256		1562	100.0%	0.95 [0.57, 1.57]	
Total events	28		38				
Heterogeneity: Tau² = 0.00; Chi² = 1.84, df = 4 (P = 0.77); I² = 0%							
Test for overall effect: Z = 0.21 (P = 0.84)							
Test for subgroup differences: Chi² = 0.18, df = 1 (P = 0.67), I² = 0%							

Favours ACURATE neo   Favours SAPIEN 3

Figure 9. Clinical outcomes. Individual and summary risk ratios with corresponding 95% confidence intervals for the comparison of ACURATE neo and SAPIEN 3 in the analysis of stroke.

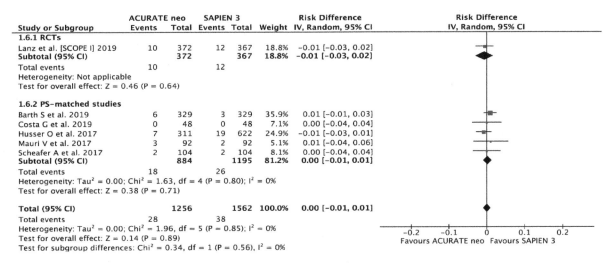

Figure 10. Clinical outcomes. Individual and summary risk ratios with corresponding 95% confidence intervals for the comparison of ACURATE neo and SAPIEN 3 in the analysis of stroke taking into account "0 events".

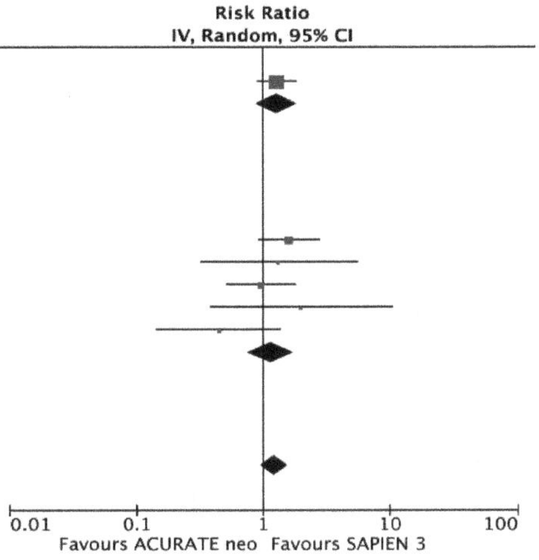

Figure 11. Clinical outcomes. Individual and summary risk ratios with corresponding 95% confidence intervals for the comparison of ACURATE neo and SAPIEN 3 in the analysis serious bleeding events.

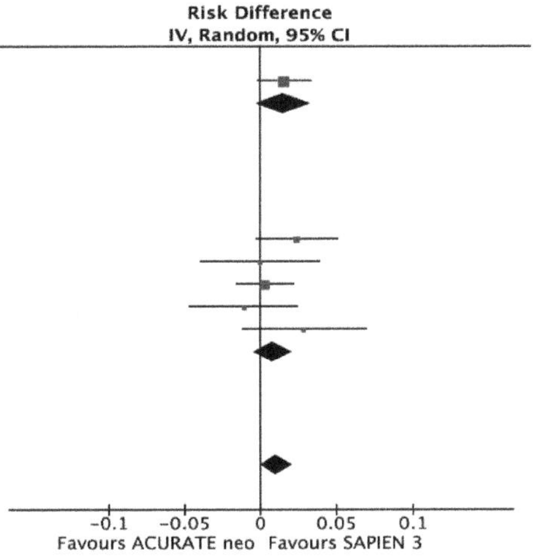

Figure 12. Clinical outcomes. Individual and summary risk ratios with corresponding 95% confidence intervals for the comparison of ACURATE neo and SAPIEN 3 in the analysis of 30-day all-cause mortality taking into account "0 events".

References

1. Cribier, A.; Eltchaninoff, H.; Bash, A.; Borenstein, N.; Tron, C.; Bauer, F.; Derumeaux, G.; Anselme, F.; Laborde, F.; Leon, M.B. Percutaneous transcatheter implantation of an aortic valve prosthesis for calcific aortic stenosis: First human case description. *Circulation* **2002**, *106*, 3006–3008. [CrossRef]

2. Smith, C.R.; Leon, M.B.; Mack, M.J.; Miller, D.C.; Moses, J.W.; Svensson, L.G.; Tuzcu, E.M.; Webb, J.G.; Fontana, G.P.; Makkar, R.R.; et al. Transcatheter versus surgical aortic-valve replacement in high-risk patients. *N. Engl. J. Med.* **2011**, *364*, 2187–2198. [CrossRef] [PubMed]

3. Adams, D.H.; Popma, J.J.; Reardon, M.J.; Yakubov, S.J.; Coselli, J.S.; Deeb, G.M.; Gleason, T.G.; Buchbinder, M.; Hermiller, J., Jr.; Kleiman, N.S.; et al. Transcatheter aortic-valve replacement with a self-expanding prosthesis. *N. Engl. J. Med.* **2014**, *370*, 1790–1798. [CrossRef] [PubMed]

4. Webb, J.G.; Pasupati, S.; Humphries, K.; Thompson, C.; Altwegg, L.; Moss, R.; Sinhal, A.; Carere, R.G.; Munt, B.; Ricci, D.; et al. Percutaneous transarterial aortic valve replacement in selected high-risk patients with aortic stenosis. *Circulation* **2007**, *116*, 755–763. [CrossRef]

5. Leon, M.B.; Smith, C.R.; Mack, M.; Miller, D.C.; Moses, J.W.; Svensson, L.G.; Tuzcu, E.M.; Webb, J.G.; Fontana, G.P.; Makkar, R.R.; et al. Transcatheter aortic-valve implantation for aortic stenosis in patients who cannot undergo surgery. *N. Engl. J. Med.* **2010**, *363*, 1597–1607. [CrossRef]

6. Thourani, V.H.; Kodali, S.; Makkar, R.R.; Herrmann, H.C.; Williams, M.; Babaliaros, V.; Smalling, R.; Lim, S.; Malaisrie, S.C.; Kapadia, S.; et al. Transcatheter aortic valve replacement versus surgical valve replacement in intermediate-risk patients: A propensity score analysis. *Lancet* **2016**, *387*, 2218–2225. [CrossRef]

7. Leon, M.B.; Smith, C.R.; Mack, M.J.; Makkar, R.R.; Svensson, L.G.; Kodali, S.K.; Thourani, V.H.; Tuzcu, E.M.; Miller, D.C.; Herrmann, H.C.; et al. Transcatheter or Surgical Aortic-Valve Replacement in Intermediate-Risk Patients. *N. Engl. J. Med.* **2016**, *374*, 1609–1620. [CrossRef]

8. Reardon, M.J.; Van Mieghem, N.M.; Popma, J.J.; Kleiman, N.S.; Sondergaard, L.; Mumtaz, M.; Adams, D.H.; Deeb, G.M.; Maini, B.; Gada, H.; et al. Surgical or Transcatheter Aortic-Valve Replacement in Intermediate-Risk Patients. *N. Engl. J. Med.* **2017**, *376*, 1321–1331. [CrossRef]

9. Mack, M.J.; Leon, M.B.; Thourani, V.H.; Makkar, R.; Kodali, S.K.; Russo, M.; Kapadia, S.R.; Malaisrie, S.C.; Cohen, D.J.; Pibarot, P.; et al. Transcatheter Aortic-Valve Replacement with a Balloon-Expandable Valve in Low-Risk Patients. *N. Engl. J. Med.* **2019**, *380*, 1695–1705. [CrossRef]

10. Nishimura, R.A.; Otto, C.M.; Bonow, R.O.; Carabello, B.A.; Erwin, J.P., 3rd; Fleisher, L.A.; Jneid, H.; Mack, M.J.; McLeod, C.J.; O'Gara, P.T.; et al. 2017 AHA/ACC Focused Update of the 2014 AHA/ACC Guideline for the Management of Patients With Valvular Heart Disease: A Report of the American College of Cardiology/American Heart Association Task Force on Clinical Practice Guidelines. *Circulation* **2017**, *135*, e1159–e1195. [CrossRef]

11. Van Belle, E.; Juthier, F.; Susen, S.; Vincentelli, A.; Dallongeville, J.; Iung, B.; Eltchaninoff, H.; Laskar, M.; Leprince, P.; Lievre, M.; et al. Response to letter regarding article, "postprocedural aortic regurgitation in balloon-expandable and self-expandable transcatheter aortic valve replacement procedures: Analysis of predictors and impact on long-term mortality: Insights from the FRANCE2 registry". *Circulation* **2015**, *131*, e16–e17. [CrossRef]

12. Kodali, S.K.; Williams, M.R.; Smith, C.R.; Svensson, L.G.; Webb, J.G.; Makkar, R.R.; Fontana, G.P.; Dewey, T.M.; Thourani, V.H.; Pichard, A.D.; et al. Two-year outcomes after transcatheter or surgical aortic-valve replacement. *N. Engl. J. Med.* **2012**, *366*, 1686–1695. [CrossRef]

13. Jones, B.M.; Tuzcu, E.M.; Krishnaswamy, A.; Popovic, Z.; Mick, S.; Roselli, E.E.; Gul, S.; Devgun, J.; Mistry, S.; Jaber, W.A.; et al. Prognostic significance of mild aortic regurgitation in predicting mortality after transcatheter aortic valve replacement. *J. Thorac. Cardiovasc. Surg.* **2016**, *152*, 783–790. [CrossRef]

14. Lanz, J.; Kim, W.K.; Walther, T.; Burgdorf, C.; Mollmann, H.; Linke, A.; Redwood, S.; Thilo, C.; Hilker, M.; Joner, M.; et al. Safety and efficacy of a self-expanding versus a balloon-expandable bioprosthesis for transcatheter aortic valve replacement in patients with symptomatic severe aortic stenosis: A randomised non-inferiority trial. *Lancet* **2019**, *394*, 1619–1628. [CrossRef]

15. Barth, S.; Reents, W.; Zacher, M.; Kerber, S.; Diegeler, A.; Schieffer, B.; Schreiber, M.; Lauer, B.; Kuntze, T.; Dahmer, M.; et al. Multicentre propensity-matched comparison of transcatheter aortic valve implantation using the ACURATE TA/neo self-expanding versus the SAPIEN 3 balloon-expandable prosthesis. *EuroIntervention* **2019**, *15*, 884–891. [CrossRef]

16. Costa, G.; Buccheri, S.; Barbanti, M.; Picci, A.; Todaro, D.; Di Simone, E.; La Spina, K.; D'Arrigo, P.; Criscione, E.; Nastasi, M.; et al. Outcomes of three different new generation transcatheter aortic valve prostheses. *Catheter. Cardiovasc. Interv.* **2019**. [CrossRef]

17. Husser, O.; Kim, W.K.; Pellegrini, C.; Holzamer, A.; Walther, T.; Mayr, P.N.; Joner, M.; Kasel, A.M.; Trenkwalder, T.; Michel, J.; et al. Multicenter Comparison of Novel Self-Expanding Versus Balloon-Expandable Transcatheter Heart Valves. *JACC Cardiovasc. Interv.* **2017**, *10*, 2078–2087. [CrossRef]

18. Mauri, V.; Kim, W.K.; Abumayyaleh, M.; Walther, T.; Moellmann, H.; Schaefer, U.; Conradi, L.; Hengstenberg, C.; Hilker, M.; Wahlers, T.; et al. Short-Term Outcome and Hemodynamic Performance of Next-Generation Self-Expanding Versus Balloon-Expandable Transcatheter Aortic Valves in Patients With Small Aortic Annulus: A Multicenter Propensity-Matched Comparison. *Circ. Cardiovasc. Interv.* **2017**, *10*. [CrossRef]

19. Schaefer, A.; Linder, M.; Seiffert, M.; Schoen, G.; Deuschl, F.; Schofer, N.; Schneeberger, Y.; Blankenberg, S.; Reichenspurner, H.; Schaefer, U.; et al. Comparison of latest generation transfemoral self-expandable and balloon-expandable transcatheter heart valves. *Interact. Cardiovasc. Thorac. Surg.* **2017**, *25*, 905–911. [CrossRef]

20. Moriyama, N.; Vento, A.; Laine, M. Safety of Next-Day Discharge After Transfemoral Transcatheter Aortic Valve Replacement With a Self-Expandable Versus Balloon-Expandable Valve Prosthesis. *Circ. Cardiovasc. Interv.* **2019**, *12*, e007756. [CrossRef]

21. Pagnesi, M.; Kim, W.K.; Conradi, L.; Barbanti, M.; Stefanini, G.G.; Zeus, T.; Pilgrim, T.; Schofer, J.; Zweiker, D.; Testa, L.; et al. Transcatheter Aortic Valve Replacement With Next-Generation Self-Expanding Devices: A Multicenter, Retrospective, Propensity-Matched Comparison of Evolut PRO Versus Acurate neo Transcatheter Heart Valves. *JACC Cardiovasc. Interv.* **2019**, *12*, 433–443. [CrossRef]

22. Stroup, D.F.; Berlin, J.A.; Morton, S.C.; Olkin, I.; Williamson, G.D.; Rennie, D.; Moher, D.; Becker, B.J.; Sipe, T.A.; Thacker, S.B. Meta-analysis of observational studies in epidemiology: A proposal for reporting. Meta-analysis Of Observational Studies in Epidemiology (MOOSE) group. *JAMA* **2000**, *283*, 2008–2012. [CrossRef]

23. Liberati, A.; Altman, D.G.; Tetzlaff, J.; Mulrow, C.; Gotzsche, P.C.; Ioannidis, J.P.; Clarke, M.; Devereaux, P.J.; Kleijnen, J.; Moher, D. The PRISMA statement for reporting systematic reviews and meta-analyses of studies that evaluate health care interventions: Explanation and elaboration. *PLoS Med.* **2009**, *6*, e1000100. [CrossRef]

24. Higgins, J.P.; Altman, D.G.; Gotzsche, P.C.; Juni, P.; Moher, D.; Oxman, A.D.; Savovic, J.; Schulz, K.F.; Weeks, L.; Sterne, J.A.; et al. The Cochrane Collaboration's tool for assessing risk of bias in randomised trials. *BMJ* **2011**, *343*, d5928. [CrossRef]

25. Sterne, J.A.; Hernan, M.A.; Reeves, B.C.; Savovic, J.; Berkman, N.D.; Viswanathan, M.; Henry, D.; Altman, D.G.; Ansari, M.T.; Boutron, I.; et al. ROBINS-I: A tool for assessing risk of bias in non-randomised studies of interventions. *BMJ* **2016**, *355*, i4919. [CrossRef]

26. Kappetein, A.P.; Head, S.J.; Genereux, P.; Piazza, N.; van Mieghem, N.M.; Blackstone, E.H.; Brott, T.G.; Cohen, D.J.; Cutlip, D.E.; van Es, G.A.; et al. Updated standardized endpoint definitions for transcatheter aortic valve implantation: The Valve Academic Research Consortium-2 consensus document. *J. Am. Coll. Cardiol.* **2012**, *60*, 1438–1454. [CrossRef]

27. Higgins, J.P.; Thompson, S.G.; Deeks, J.J.; Altman, D.G. Measuring inconsistency in meta-analyses. *BMJ* **2003**, *327*, 557–560. [CrossRef]

28. Wan, X.; Wang, W.; Liu, J.; Tong, T. Estimating the sample mean and standard deviation from the sample size, median, range and/or interquartile range. *BMC Med. Res. Methodol.* **2014**, *14*, 135. [CrossRef]

29. Sathananthan, J.; Hensey, M.; Fraser, R.; Landes, U.; Blanke, P.; Hatoum, H.; Dasi, L.P.; Sedaghat, A.; Bapat, V.N.; Leipsic, J.; et al. Implications of hydrodynamic testing to guide sizing of self-expanding transcatheter heart valves for valve-in-valve procedures. *Catheter. Cardiovasc. Interv.* **2019**. [CrossRef]

30. Gozdek, M.; Ratajczak, J.; Arndt, A.; Zieliński, K.; Pasierski, M.; Matteucci, M.; Fina, D.; Jiritano, F.; Meani, P.; Raffa, G.M.; et al. Transcatheter aortic valve replacement with Lotus and Sapien 3 prosthetic valves: A systematic review and meta-analysis. *J. Thorac. Dis.* **2020**. (ahead of print).

31. Ando, T.; Briasoulis, A.; Holmes, A.A.; Taub, C.C.; Takagi, H.; Afonso, L. Sapien 3 versus Sapien XT prosthetic valves in transcatheter aortic valve implantation: A meta-analysis. *Int. J. Cardiol.* **2016**, *220*, 472–478. [CrossRef]

32.   Kodali, S.; Thourani, V.H.; White, J.; Malaisrie, S.C.; Lim, S.; Greason, K.L.; Williams, M.; Guerrero, M.; Eisenhauer, A.C.; Kapadia, S.; et al. Early clinical and echocardiographic outcomes after SAPIEN 3 transcatheter aortic valve replacement in inoperable, high-risk and intermediate-risk patients with aortic stenosis. *Eur. Heart J.* **2016**, *37*, 2252–2262. [CrossRef]

33.   Noble, S.; Stortecky, S.; Heg, D.; Tueller, D.; Jeger, R.; Toggweiler, S.; Ferrari, E.; Nietlispach, F.; Taramasso, M.; Maisano, F.; et al. Comparison of procedural and clinical outcomes with Evolut R versus Medtronic CoreValve: A Swiss TAVI registry analysis. *EuroIntervention* **2017**, *12*, e2170–e2176. [CrossRef]

34.   Naber, C.K.; Pyxaras, S.A.; Ince, H.; Frambach, P.; Colombo, A.; Butter, C.; Gatto, F.; Hink, U.; Nickenig, G.; Bruschi, G.; et al. A multicentre European registry to evaluate the Direct Flow Medical transcatheter aortic valve system for the treatment of patients with severe aortic stenosis. *EuroIntervention* **2016**, *12*, e1413–e1419. [CrossRef]

35.   Wendler, O.; Schymik, G.; Treede, H.; Baumgartner, H.; Dumonteil, N.; Ihlberg, L.; Neumann, F.J.; Tarantini, G.; Zamarano, J.L.; Vahanian, A. SOURCE 3 Registry: Design and 30-Day Results of the European Postapproval Registry of the Latest Generation of the SAPIEN 3 Transcatheter Heart Valve. *Circulation* **2017**, *135*, 1123–1132. [CrossRef]

36.   Thomas, M.; Schymik, G.; Walther, T.; Himbert, D.; Lefevre, T.; Treede, H.; Eggebrecht, H.; Rubino, P.; Michev, I.; Lange, R.; et al. Thirty-day results of the SAPIEN aortic Bioprosthesis European Outcome (SOURCE) Registry: A European registry of transcatheter aortic valve implantation using the Edwards SAPIEN valve. *Circulation* **2010**, *122*, 62–69. [CrossRef]

37.   Naber, C.K.; Pyxaras, S.A.; Ince, H.; Latib, A.; Frambach, P.; den Heijer, P.; Wagner, D.; Butter, C.; Colombo, A.; Kische, S. Real-world multicentre experience with the Direct Flow Medical repositionable and retrievable transcatheter aortic valve implantation system for the treatment of high-risk patients with severe aortic stenosis. *EuroIntervention* **2016**, *11*, e1314–e1320. [CrossRef]

38.   Kowalewski, M.; Gozdek, M.; Raffa, G.M.; Slomka, A.; Zielinski, K.; Kubica, J.; Anisimowicz, L.; Kowalewski, J.; Landes, U.; Kornowski, R.; et al. Transcathether aortic valve implantation with the new repositionable self-expandable Medtronic Evolut R vs. CoreValve system: Evidence on the benefit of a meta-analytical approach. *J. Cardiovasc. Med.* **2019**, *20*, 226–236. [CrossRef]

39.   Tamburino, C.; Capodanno, D.; Ramondo, A.; Petronio, A.S.; Ettori, F.; Santoro, G.; Klugmann, S.; Bedogni, F.; Maisano, F.; Marzocchi, A.; et al. Incidence and predictors of early and late mortality after transcatheter aortic valve implantation in 663 patients with severe aortic stenosis. *Circulation* **2011**, *123*, 299–308. [CrossRef]

40.   Kodali, S.; Pibarot, P.; Douglas, P.S.; Williams, M.; Xu, K.; Thourani, V.; Rihal, C.S.; Zajarias, A.; Doshi, D.; Davidson, M.; et al. Paravalvular regurgitation after transcatheter aortic valve replacement with the Edwards sapien valve in the PARTNER trial: Characterizing patients and impact on outcomes. *Eur. Heart J.* **2015**, *36*, 449–456. [CrossRef]

41.   Gilard, M.; Eltchaninoff, H.; Iung, B.; Donzeau-Gouge, P.; Chevreul, K.; Fajadet, J.; Leprince, P.; Leguerrier, A.; Lievre, M.; Prat, A.; et al. Registry of transcatheter aortic-valve implantation in high-risk patients. *N. Engl. J. Med.* **2012**, *366*, 1705–1715. [CrossRef]

42.   Choudhury, T.; Solomonica, A.; Bagur, R. The ACURATE neo transcatheter aortic valve system. *Exp. Rev. Med. Device.* **2018**, *15*, 693–699. [CrossRef]

6

Subclinical Atherosclerosis Imaging in People Living with HIV

Isabella C. Schoepf [1], **Ronny R. Buechel** [2], **Helen Kovari** [3], **Dima A. Hammoud** [4] and **Philip E. Tarr** [1,*]

[1] University Department of Medicine and Infectious Diseases Service, Kantonsspital Baselland, University of Basel, 4101 Bruderholz, Switzerland
[2] Department of Nuclear Medicine, Cardiac Imaging, University Hospital Zurich, University of Zurich, 8091 Zurich, Switzerland
[3] Division of Infectious Diseases and Hospital Epidemiology, University of Zurich, 8091 Zurich, Switzerland
[4] Center for Infectious Disease Imaging, Radiology and Imaging Sciences, National Institutes of Health, Bethesda, MD 20892, USA
* Correspondence: philip.tarr@unibas.ch;

Abstract: In many, but not all studies, people living with HIV (PLWH) have an increased risk of coronary artery disease (CAD) events compared to the general population. This has generated considerable interest in the early, non-invasive detection of asymptomatic (subclinical) atherosclerosis in PLWH. Ultrasound studies assessing carotid artery intima-media thickness (CIMT) have tended to show a somewhat greater thickness in HIV+ compared to HIV−, likely due to an increased prevalence of cardiovascular (CV) risk factors in PLWH. Coronary artery calcification (CAC) determination by non-contrast computed tomography (CT) seems promising to predict CV events but is limited to the detection of calcified plaque. Coronary CT angiography (CCTA) detects calcified and non-calcified plaque and predicts CAD better than either CAC or CIMT. A normal CCTA predicts survival free of CV events over a very long time-span. Research imaging techniques, including black-blood magnetic resonance imaging of the vessel wall and 18F-fluorodeoxyglucose positron emission tomography for the assessment of arterial inflammation have provided insights into the prevalence of HIV-vasculopathy and associated risk factors, but their clinical applicability remains limited. Therefore, CCTA currently appears as the most promising cardiac imaging modality in PLWH for the evaluation of suspected CAD, particularly in patients <50 years, in whom most atherosclerotic coronary lesions are non-calcified.

Keywords: subclinical coronary artery disease; accelerated atherosclerosis; HIV infection; carotid intima-media thickness; coronary calcium scoring; coronary CT angiography; magnetic resonance angiography; fluorodeoxyglucose positron emission tomography

1. Introduction

Cardiovascular disease (CVD) has become one of the leading causes of death in people living with HIV (PLWH) worldwide [1–4]. Reducing the burden of CVD, particularly coronary artery disease (CAD), is therefore emerging as a major public health goal in medical care for PLWH [5,6].

Data is inconsistent with respect to whether PLWH have an increased incidence of CAD events compared to the general population [2,7] or not [8–10]. Early reports have observed a 2- to almost 4-fold increased rate in CAD events as compared to HIV-negative patients [11,12], but traditional risk factors, particularly smoking, and socioeconomic factors were not always adjusted for in those studies [13]. Danish data suggest a 1.5- to 2-fold increase in CAD events in PLWH vs. controls [14]; a 2-fold CAD event increase in PLWH was also the conclusion of a recent systematic review and meta-analysis [2].

Other studies have reported smaller increases [15–17] in cardiovascular (CV) events in PLWH. In a large cohort study from California that evaluated the myocardial infarction (MI) risk from 1996 to 2011, a declining relative risk for MI was observed in PLWH vs. HIV-negative persons over time. Between 2010 and 2011, no increased risk of MI was seen in PLWH [17]. In a cohort of US veterans, a 50% increased risk in acute MI was recorded, after adjusting for Framingham risk score, comorbidities and substance use [16]. In another large North American analysis, HIV infection was associated with only a 21% increased incidence of CV events in comparison with a well-matched HIV-negative control group, and the risk increase was not statistically significant in the age group ≥60 years of age [15]. Moreover, in recent studies from Switzerland and Denmark, no increased risk of CAD events and, in Switzerland, no increased subclinical atherosclerosis prevalence was described, perhaps due to the prevalence of modern antiretroviral therapy (ART) regimens, reliably suppressive ART, decreased smoking prevalence, and access to regular medical follow-up [8,9,18]. Also, the data do not generally suggest that CV events occur earlier in PLWH, contradicting the widely held notion of "accelerated atherosclerosis" or even "accelerated aging". Some reports that CV events occur at a younger age seem to be related to the younger median age of many HIV+ populations compared to the general population [19].

The pathogenesis of CV events in HIV-positive individuals likely represents a complex interaction of different factors that contribute to the development of atherosclerosis [18,20–23]. Studies in multiple countries have consistently recorded an increased prevalence of smoking and drug use in PLWH [11,13]. A link between inflammation related to HIV infection and CAD in PLWH is well documented. Several serum biomarkers that are associated with CV risk or overall mortality may be elevated in PLWH compared to HIV-negative persons, including biomarkers of systemic inflammation (high sensitivity C-reactive protein, interleukin-6, soluble tumor necrosis factor-α receptor 1) [24–27], coagulation (D-dimer, fibrinogen) [24–27], monocyte activation (lipopolysaccharide, soluble CD14, CD163, CC-chemokine ligand 2) [24,28–31], and endothelial dysfunction (intercellular adhesion molecule 1) [24]. Although the exact mechanisms underlying the development of atherosclerosis in PLWH have not been conclusively determined, smooth muscle cell proliferation may play an important role [32]. Moreover, endothelial dysfunction due to adhesion molecules may lead to adhesion of circulating leukocytes, transmigration of monocytes/macrophages to the intima and subsequently to vascular inflammation [20,32,33]. In combination with procoagulatory mechanisms in the setting of increased concentrations of D-dimer and coagulation factors, and in the presence of other metabolic disorders (e.g., dyslipidemia), the progression of atherosclerosis might be enhanced in PLWH [20,32].

It is well accepted that viral suppression, in the setting of adequate ART, is associated with lower levels of inflammatory biomarkers and decreased CV risk [34,35]. Advanced immunosuppression has contributed to CV risk in PLWH in some [15,36,37] but not in other studies [38,39].

Also, certain ART agents have been associated with increased CV risk. This notion is most reliably based on findings from the large, multinational, observational D:A:D study [20,23,39]. Dyslipidemia was among the first described deleterious metabolic effects of ART, most notably in the setting of certain protease inhibitors, i.e., lopinavir, indinavir and darunavir [23,40,41]. Within the drug class of nucleoside reverse transcriptase inhibitors, abacavir and didanosine were found to increase CV risk [42].

The potentially increased CV event rate in PLWH has generated considerable interest in early detection of asymptomatic (subclinical) atherosclerosis, in order to improve CAD event prediction and to allow appropriate CVD prevention by early intervention [21]. Most published literature on noninvasive cardiac imaging for the detection of subclinical atherosclerosis in PLWH has focused on carotid artery intima-media thickness (CIMT), coronary artery calcification (CAC), coronary CT angiography (CCTA) [18,43,44] and, more recently, magnetic resonance imaging of the vessel wall (MRI) and 18F- fluorodeoxyglucose positron emission tomography (FDG-PET).

2. Carotid Artery Intima-Media Thickness (CIMT)

CIMT is an ultrasound technique to measure the thickness of the two layers of the carotid artery wall, the intima and the media [45]. CIMT is well recorded to predict future CV events in the general population [46–49]. According to the results of a 2009 meta-analysis that analyzed six cross-sectional, seven case-control and 13 cohort studies (5456 HIV positive and 3600 HIV negative patients) PLWH tend to show a greater thickness in CIMT (0.04 mm thicker; 95% confidence interval: 0.02–0.06 mm, $p < 0.001$) when compared to HIV-negative controls [50]. However, the findings are not concordant with some studies showing increased CIMT was increased in PLWH compared to HIV-negative controls [12,51–71] while other studies did not show a difference or showed only weakly increased CIMT in PLWH [12,45,50–59,61–68]. Those discordant findings may be attributable to differences in study design, participant characteristics, duration of follow-up, and different approaches of ultrasound measurement [45,50].

The largest differences in CIMT between HIV-positive and HIV-negative participants were noted in studies with the greatest demographic differences between the analyzed groups [45,50]. Moreover, small studies were more likely than larger studies to identify an increase in CIMT in PLWH vs. controls [45,50]. In addition, a large report of repeated CIMT measurements over a median of 7 years did not find accelerated CIMT progression in PLWH (747 women, 530 men) compared to HIV-negative controls (264 women, 284 men), but focal plaque prevalence was increased, after adjusting for traditional CV risk factors [70]. These findings are in accordance with another report that observed no different progression in CIMT over 144 weeks in 133 extensively matched HIV+ and HIV− participants [59].

CIMT has a number of limitations for the prediction of CV events, including a limited correlation with angiographically defined atherosclerosis [72,73], limited improvement in CV event prediction by the addition of CIMT to the Framingham risk score [46], and different results when CIMT findings at the common carotid artery level are compared with results obtained at the carotid bifurcation and/or the internal carotid artery level [45,61,65]. Finally, CIMT measurement is dependent on investigator experience, with the reproducibility of results generally being higher in research settings than in practitioner-based settings [74].

3. Coronary Artery Calcium (CAC) Scoring

CAC scoring using non-contrast enhanced CT is a well-established and easily applicable tool for detection and quantification of coronary calcifications [75–80] (Figure 1). Applying different scoring systems, most frequently the Agatston score, based on the landmark work of Arthur Agatston in the late 1980s [81], CAC scoring has emerged as a robust non-invasive atherosclerosis imaging modality characterized by high inter- and intra-observer reliability [74,80,82].

In the general population, there is a strong correlation between CAC score and future CV endpoints [74,80,83–86]. Persons with no detectable coronary calcium have a very low risk for CV events over the following years [87,88] and a ten-year survival of 99.4% [89]. Longitudinal CAC studies have suggested that annual CAC score change of ≥15% may constitute CVD progression [90]. CV event prediction by CAC and CIMT were similar in one report [91], but CAC was a more reliable CV event predictor than CIMT in several other reports [86,92–94]. CV event prediction may be improved when CAC is added to Framingham risk score [88,89].

Current evidence remains equivocal as to whether the presence of HIV is associated with an increased prevalence of coronary calcifications [18,71,95,96]. An increased vascular age was identified in Italian PLWH compared with age-specific CAC percentiles based on the MESA study done in a general US population [95]. However, these findings were not confirmed in a recent study assessing a large Swiss cohort [18]; other studies have also found similar CAC scores in HIV-positive and HIV-negative persons [18,50,96]. High pre-treatment HIV viremia levels were associated with a CAC score >0 [18]. In the US MACS study, CAC scores were elevated in those with metabolic syndrome but were not altered by HIV serostatus [57,96].

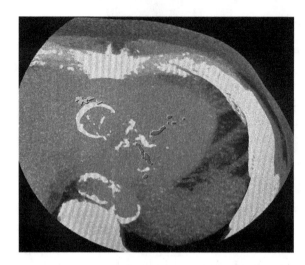

Figure 1. Coronary artery calcium scoring in an asymptomatic 43-year old HIV-positive male patient. Maximum intensity projection depicts extensive calcifications in the left anterior descending artery (purple), in the left circumflex artery (blue), and in the right coronary artery (yellow). The total Agatston score was 1031, classifying this patient as at high risk for future CV events and prompting lifestyle interventions and the initiation of a statin.

A major limitation of CAC is the inability to detect non-calcified plaque. This is of importance because a non-calcified or only partially calcified plaque is more likely to take on morphological features typical of high-risk plaque which is prone to adverse future CV events (e.g., plaque rupture or erosion potentially leading to MI) [97,98]. In addition, coronary artery plaque is predominantly non-calcified in patients <50 years of age [80,99,100]. This point may be particularly relevant to PLWH: as, in Western countries, even though HIV-positive populations are aging, their median age is still relatively low, e.g., 48 years in the Swiss HIV cohort study (www.shcs.ch and [101]). Their Framingham risk scores and CAD event rates have also been relatively low, and the median age at the time of the first CAD event in SHCS participants was 50 years [38].

4. Coronary CT Angiography (CCTA)

CCTA is a non-invasive imaging technique involving contrast-enhanced multi-slice CT for the accurate morphological assessment of the coronary arteries [102] (Figure 2).

Importantly, and in contrast to CIMT and CAC, CCTA can be used to detect calcified and non-calcified plaques, and due to its high spatial resolution also allows for the accurate assessment of plaque composition [74,103] (Figure 3).

CCTA has seen a tremendous development over the last two decades, both in terms of hardware advancements and improvements in image acquisition protocols. Among the latter, the introduction of prospectively electrocardiogram-triggered acquisition has contributed most substantially to lowering radiation dose exposure from 15–20 millisieverts (mSv) [104–106] down to 2–3 mSv [104,107–110]. The addition of sophisticated reconstruction algorithms and widespread use of latest-generation wide-coverage CT devices may now enable routine scanning in the sub-millisievert range [111]. Sensitivity of CCTA in the detection of relevant coronary stenosis is similar to standard invasive coronary angiography [112–114]. However, both modalities inherently lack the ability to predict hemodynamic relevance if a stenosis is found. This is of the utmost importance because the optimal treatment, i.e., the benefit of optimal medical therapy versus revascularization, depends heavily on the presence and extent of myocardial ischemia [115]. While, theoretically, measurement of pressure drops along a vessel and the derivation of the so-called fractional flow reserve constitutes an invasive technique to overcome this limitation, the application of hybrid imaging, that is, the combination and fusion of two non-invasive imaging modalities, has evolved into a robust and elegant technique for the assessment of both coronary anatomy and potential hemodynamical effects of any given lesion, hence providing the non-invasive grounds for optimized patient management decisions (Figure 4).

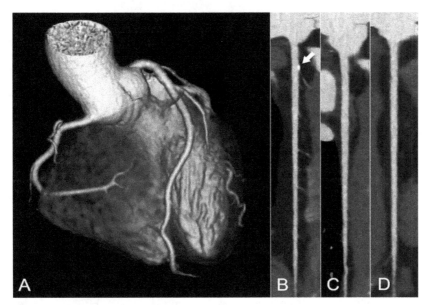

Figure 2. Coronary computed tomography angiography of a 48-year old HIV+ female patient with typical angina. The patient had a positive family history for cardiovascular events and was an active smoker, putting her at intermediate risk for having coronary artery disease. Volume rendering (**A**) of the image datasets depicts normal coronary anatomy, while the curved multiplanar reformats of the left anterior descending (**B**), the left circumflex (**C**), and the right coronary (**D**) arteries reveal only minimal and non-obstructive coronary atherosclerosis in the proximal left anterior descending (white arrow). Coronary artery disease was, therefore, excluded as a cause for her symptoms. BMI 24.2 kg/m^2. Radiation dose exposure 0.57 mSv. Contrast volume 40 mL.

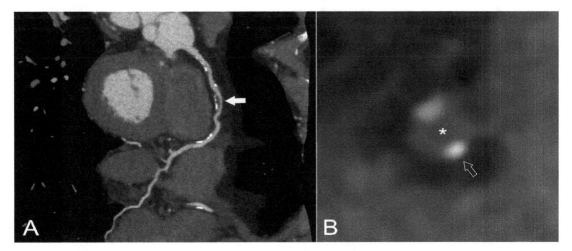

Figure 3. Non-invasive evaluation of an asymptomatic 65-year old HIV+ male patient. The patient had a history of treated arterial hypertension, was an active smoker and suffered from peripheral artery disease with the latter prompting further cardiovascular work-up despite a normal stress-electrocardiogram. Multiplanar curved reconstruction of the coronary computed tomography angiography dataset (**A**) reveals multiple calcified but non-obstructive lesions and 70–90% stenosis (white filled arrow) in the mid-right coronary artery. This obstructive lesion (**B**, cross sectional view) exhibits several morphological high-risk features typical for an event-prone lesion, such as positive remodeling and a low-attenuation core (*) with calcifications only at the edge of the lesion (white empty arrow), constituting the so-called napkin-ring sign.

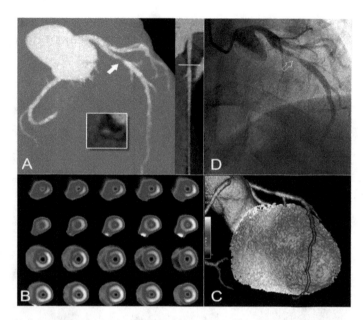

Figure 4. Evaluation of a 49-year old HIV+ male patient with typical angina. The patient had no cardiovascular risk factors and he was referred for exclusion of coronary artery disease with a calculated pre-test probability of 69%. Total cholesterol was 3.6 mmol/L (<5.0), HDL-cholesterol 1.45 mmol/L (>1.0), and LDL-cholesterol 1.8 mmol/L (<3.0). Maximum intensity projection and multiplanar curved reconstruction of the coronary computed tomography angiography (CCTA) datasets (**A**) depict a 70–90% stenosis (white filled arrow) in the proximal left anterior descending artery as shown in the cross-section (inlet). As per clinical routine and in accordance with current guidelines, lesions are primarily graded visually with regard to maximal percent diameter stenosis in our institution. In this particular patient, the qualitative evaluation was complemented by quantitative measurements (using version 2 of CardIQ Xpress/GE Healthcare), because the lesion in the LAD was non-calcified, allowing for more accurate lumen delineation due to the lack of blooming artifacts. The quantitative analysis resulted in a diameter stenosis of 75%. Myocardial perfusion single-photon-computed-emission-tomography (SPECT, (**B**)) confirmed hemodynamical relevance of the lesion, revealing a large perfusion defect during stress (top rows) with reversibility during rest (bottom rows), constituting ischemia in the anteroseptal wall of the left ventricular myocardium. Hybrid CCTA/SPECT imaging (**C**) clearly demonstrates a large area of ischemia in the myocardium subtended by the left anterior descending artery. Finally, obstructive coronary artery disease (white empty arrow) was confirmed during invasive coronary angiography (**D**), and the lesion was treated with a drug-eluting stent.

Compared to intravascular ultrasound, CCTA can precisely detect coronary plaque with a positive and negative predictive value >98% [18,107,116,117]. It is well recorded, however, that CCTA tends to overestimate the degree of coronary stenosis [118,119]. In the general population, among individuals without known CVD, the large scale CONFIRM study documented that the degree of non-obstructive and obstructive coronary artery stenosis and the number of vessels affected in CCTA are closely correlated with CV events and mortality rates over 3 years of follow-up [107]. CCTA improves prediction of future CV events compared to Framingham risk score [120], CAC [107,108,121] or CIMT [108,118].

In early studies, results regarding the presence of subclinical atherosclerosis in CCTA in HIV-positive relative to HIV-negative persons were not uniform. Some investigators recorded an increased [44,100,122–124] prevalence, while others noted a similar [18,43,125] or even lower prevalence in PLWH, compared to HIV-negative controls [18,103]. In a 2015 meta-analysis summarizing initial CCTA studies (1229 HIV-positive and 1029 HIV negative participants), a 3-fold higher prevalence of non-calcified coronary artery plaque on CCTA was recorded in asymptomatic HIV+ compared to HIV-negative subjects [100]. The analyzed studies typically included a small number of participants, that, in addition, were not always matched on CV risk factors [124].

Today, there are three published CCTA studies that enrolled large numbers of HIV+ and HIV-negative participants, with the following key findings: In men who had sex with men that were enrolled in the US-American multicenter AIDS cohort study (MACS), Post et al. [44] recorded a higher prevalence of any coronary plaque and non-calcified plaque in 618 HIV+ compared to 383 HIV-negative men in the baseline CCTA. In a follow-up report, with a median interval of 4.5 years between CCTAs, increased progression of coronary plaques was observed in HIV-positive compared to the HIV-negative MACS participants, but only in men with detectable HIV viremia and, thus, presumably, higher degrees of ongoing systemic inflammation, compared to persons with optimal virological control [44,126].

Lai et al. described the presence of subclinical atherosclerosis in CCTA of 953 HIV+ and 476 HIV-negative African American study participants from Baltimore/USA of whom more than 50% were frequent cocaine users [43]. In this study, there was a trend towards HIV infection being independently associated with non-calcified plaque, however, this association was largely explained by chronic cocaine use.

In addition to these two studies from the US [43,44,126], we recently assessed subclinical atherosclerosis in a cross-sectional study of 428 HIV-positive participants of the Swiss HIV Cohort Study (SHCS) and 276 HIV-negative control individuals with similar Framingham risk scores. HIV-positive participants had similar degrees of non-calcified/mixed plaque and high risk [97] plaque, and, indeed, had less calcified coronary plaque, and lower coronary atherosclerosis involvement and severity scores compared to their negative controls with similar Framingham risk score [18]. These Swiss CCTA results, together with Swiss data showing similar CV incidence rates in HIV+ and HIV-persons [8], attenuate concerns about accelerated atherosclerosis in HIV, and have prompted experts to ask the question whether the prevalent notion of increased CV risk in PLWH amounts to "much ado about nothing" [127].

The different CCTA results in these three large studies [18,43,44] might be related to a number of features. First, CAD rates are lower in southern/central Europe compared to the US [128,129]. Second, we speculate that the low subclinical atherosclerosis prevalence in Swiss PLWH might further be attributable to high rates of successful treatment in the setting of modern ART regimens, regular follow-up, and declining smoking rates in recent years [9,130].

As regards the duration of ART, the Swiss study did not find any association with any type of plaque. This was in line with findings from Lai et al. in the group of non-cocaine users and contrary to MACS [18,43,44]. Concerning the use of antiretroviral agents and subclinical atherosclerosis, the MACS investigators observed no clear association between different ART drugs and any form of coronary artery plaque on CCTA [131]. In contrast, the Swiss study identified an association with exposure to abacavir and an increased prevalence of non-calcified/mixed plaque [132]. This observation seems important, as it may afford a mechanism by which abacavir increases CV risk, i.e., the promotion of atherosclerosis, in addition to putative deleterious effects of abacavir on platelet reactivity [133,134].

Consistent with the MACS findings, the Swiss patients with a low nadir CD4+ cell count had more non-calcified plaque [18,44] and more coronary stenosis greater than 50% [44]. These findings suggest that advanced immunosuppression may contribute to subclinical atherosclerosis in PLWH [100].

In summary, coronary plaque in young persons typically is non-calcified [80,99,100]. CCTA (but not CAC) can detect non-calcified plaque [74] and predicts CVD better than CAC [107] or CIMT [118]. Therefore, and because the median age of most populations of PLWH remains below 50 years today, CCTA is emerging as the preferred research-setting imaging tool to detect subclinical atherosclerosis. There remains a need for additional studies to examine the exact role that CCTA may play in clinical HIV practice.

5. Magnetic Resonance Rmaging (MRI)

Based on CIMT being strongly predictive of CV events [135], multiple studies have reported the use of MRI rather than ultrasound in assessing CVD in PLWH [103,136–139]. Such studies mainly used black-blood MRI (BBMRI), an advanced imaging technique relying on nulling of the MR signal from the vascular lumen while retaining signal from the vascular wall, allowing better visualization of the wall thickness [140,141]. Multiple variations of the BBMRI technique have already been used in extracranial (e.g., aorta, carotid and coronary arteries) as well as intracranial vessel wall imaging [140–146].

In age-related atherosclerosis, BBMRI is generally used to assess the vulnerability characteristics of eccentric, lipid-rich plaques (e.g., lipid core, fibrous cap, hemorrhage). In HIV vasculopathy on the other hand, where intimal smooth muscle hypertrophy occurs in a symmetrical circumferential manner [32,33], BBMRI is more commonly used to assess diffuse wall thickening. This is why the majority of vessel wall imaging studies in HIV have concentrated on measuring the vessel wall thickness (VWT) akin to the measurement of CIMT using ultrasound [103,138,147,148]. In a group of treated HIV+ subjects with low measurable CVD risk, HIV-status was significantly associated with increased wall/outer-wall ratio (W/OW), an index of vascular thickening, after adjusting for age [139]. In another study, increased carotid artery wall thickness was noted in HIV+ subjects on chronic ART compared to controls with similar CVD risk, [137]. Interestingly, while in one study [139], no correlation of CVD with the type of ART was identified, another study [137] found that a longer duration of protease inhibitor therapy was associated with greater wall thickness. Using MRI to assess coronary rather than carotid arteries, subclinical CAD has been documented in ART-treated subjects, with HIV infection being independently associated with increased proximal right coronary artery wall thickness [103].

The connection between HIV-associated inflammation and atherosclerosis burden in HIV infection was also evaluated in a group of HIV+ subjects (treated and untreated) in comparison to a group of demographically similar controls. As expected, HIV-1 viral burden was found to be associated with higher serum levels of the chemokines monocyte chemoattractant protein-1/CC-chemokinligand 2 (MCP-1/CCL2). At the same time, HIV infection correlated with atherosclerosis burden, mainly detectable as increased vessel wall area and thickness in the thoracic aorta [148].

BBMRI has also been important in delineating that traditional CVD risk factors, which seem to disproportionately burden PLWH, need to be controlled. In one study evaluating asymptomatic, young-to-middle-aged African-Americans with and without HIV infection and cocaine use, only total cholesterol (and not HIV status) was significantly associated with the presence of a lipid core in carotid plaques [136]. In another more recent study, carotid VWT was increased in treated PLWH relative to controls with the 10-year ASCVD (atherosclerotic cardiovascular disease) risk score being the only variable significantly associated with VWT whereas HIV status was not. The authors concluded that traditional CVD risk factors in PLWH are adequately captured in the ASCVD risk score which was closely associated with subclinical carotid disease [138].

Over the last few years, there have been significant advances made in MR imaging of the vessel wall, with the ability nowadays of assessing atherosclerotic involvement of the intracranial arteries. To our knowledge, such high-resolution techniques have not yet been applied in the evaluation of PLWH [146,149–153]. At this point, BBMRI of the vessel wall remains a research application rather than a clinically used technique in assessing CVD in PLWH (Figure 5). Whether this would eventually change in the future, as PLWH get older, remains unclear.

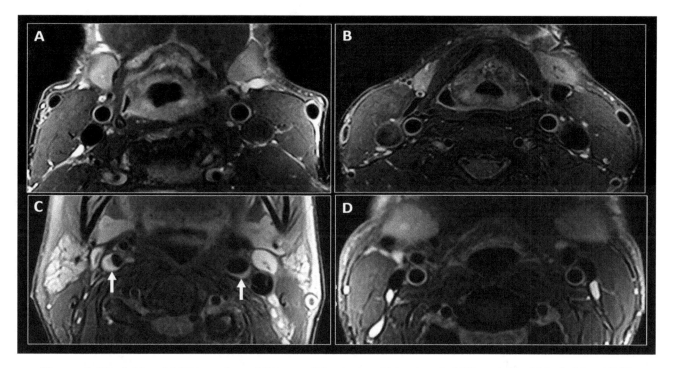

Figure 5. Black-blood MR imaging of the carotid arteries. Fat saturated T2-weighted black-blood MR images at the level of the common carotid arteries in a 56-year-old HIV+ man (**A**) and a 47-year-old HIV− man (**B**). Similar imaging technique at the level of the internal carotid arteries (ICAs) in a 56-year-old HIV+ woman (**C**) shows narrowing of the vascular lumen bilaterally by a plaque (small arrows), more significant on the right side. (**D**) shows similar imaging at the level of ICAs in a 47-year-old HIV negative man with no evidence of atherosclerosis.

6. 18F-Fluorodeoxyglucose Positron Emission Tomography (FDG PET)

The most common application of FDG PET imaging in the clinic is the baseline assessment and follow-up of neoplastic diseases. Applications in imaging infectious and inflammatory diseases using FDG PET, however, have been increasing in the last decade.

One such use is the assessment of vasculitis seen as increased glucose metabolism of the vessel wall, reflecting inflammatory changes [154] (Figure 6).

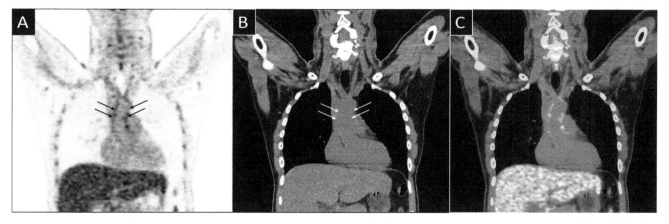

Figure 6. FDG-PET imaging of the major vessels. (**A**) Coronal FDG PET images, (**B**) coronal CT scan images and (**C**) fused PET CT scans show subtle FDG uptake in the vascular wall of the ascending aorta (arrows).

A similar approach has been used by multiple groups to assess HIV-vasculopathy using FDG PET [155–162]. A common presumption is that PLWH will demonstrate increased vessel wall FDG uptake reflecting premature aging and atherosclerotic changes. In fact, in one paper assessing only HIV+ patients, a relationship was found between arterial inflammation on FDG PET and features of high-risk coronary atherosclerotic disease including number of low attenuation plaques and plaque vulnerability characteristics [160].

The results from studies utilizing FDG PET to assess HIV-vasculopathy, however, have been rather inconsistent. In one paper [162], arterial inflammation in the aorta (measured as aortic target to background ratio (TBR)) was higher in the HIV+ group compared to the non-HIV control group matched for CVD, even after adjusting for traditional CV risk factors [162]. More recently, HIV was found to be associated with 0.16 higher aortic TBR compared to controls, independent of traditional risk factors [155]. On the other hand, in one paper assessing virologically controlled HIV+ persons with no known CVD, there was no evidence of increased arterial inflammation on FDG PET compared to healthy volunteers [159]. In a more recent paper looking at a larger group of patients, there was only a marginally higher TBR in PLWH, with significant overlap of TBR values with HIV-negative controls [156]. The discrepancy in the results of those studies could be related to variations in study populations, treatment status of patients and the presence or absence of co-morbid CVD. Another element of variability could also be related to the imaging technique and analysis methods.

Another use for FDG PET is in longitudinally assessing PLWH for changes in arterial inflammation over time. To our knowledge, only one such longitudinal study has been reported, with twelve ART naïve subjects imaged at baseline and again six months after ART initiation. Interestingly, there were no significant changes in TBR between baseline and follow-up scans [157]. This could be due to short interval imaging after ART initiation. Another paper assessing PLWH treated with statins versus placebo found no significant change in arterial inflammation as measured by FDG PET despite the fact that statin therapy reduced non-calcified plaque volume and high-risk coronary plaque features on CCTA [158].

At this point, using FDG PET in PLWH is more likely to be useful in evaluating co-morbidities, specific organ involvement or assessment of central nervous system involvement [163–167]. The role of FDG PET in assessing CVD in individual subjects on the other hand remains uncertain.

7. Outlook

Consistent with Swiss data [8], a nationwide cohort study in Denmark found that after the exclusion of participants with risk factors including illicit drug use or hepatitis B or C co-infections, the mortality rate was similar in HIV-positive and HIV-negative persons [168]. In general, persons with well-controlled HIV infection and a healthy lifestyle appear to have similar survival rates today as do HIV-negative persons, with potentially increased death rates mainly ascribed to traditional risk factors [168,169]. Thus, for efficient primary CAD prevention in PLWH, our aim should be the optimization of traditional risk factor management, early initiation of ART therapy, and regular patient follow-up.

Few studies have simultaneously applied more than one cardiac imaging modality (CIMT and CAC [170], CCTA and MRI [103]) in the same patients, but did not correlate CIMT results with CAC or MRI with CCTA results. Hsue and colleagues found that with or without detectable CAC, PLWH had higher CIMT than HIV-negative controls [171]. Interestingly, among those without detectable CAC, a third of PLWH but no controls had increased CIMT.

CCTA is emerging as an accurate and reliable non-invasive imaging modality for detection of subclinical atherosclerosis in PLWH, especially in persons <50 years who typically have non-calcified or partially calcified plaque. However, in asymptomatic PLWH today, cardiac imaging is not yet indicated to assess coronary atherosclerosis. The exception might be asymptomatic persons with diabetes [172]. Studies that compared coronary imaging to optimization of medical treatment in asymptomatic patients have not yet shown any clinical benefit, but a number of relevant studies are ongoing. Particularly in patients with atypical symptoms suggestive of myocardial ischemia, or in patients with suspected acute coronary syndrome but without ST-segment elevations on EKG, CCTA is now increasingly well established as a valuable diagnostic tool to rule out CAD in the emergency room [173–175], because of its non-invasiveness compared to coronary angiography and its extremely high negative predictive value [176].

Author Contributions: Literature review: I.C.S., D.A.H., P.E.T.; writing—original draft preparation, writing—critical insights during review and editing I.C.S., R.R.B., H.K., D.A.H., P.E.T. Preparation of cardiac imaging figures: R.R.B., D.A.H.

References

1. Mozaffarian, D.; Benjamin, E.J.; Go, A.S.; Arnett, D.K.; Blaha, M.J.; Cushman, M.; Das, S.R.; de Ferranti, S.; Després, J.; Fullerton, H.J.; et al. Heart Disease and Stroke Statistics-2016 Update: A Report From the American Heart Association. *Circulation* **2015**, *133*, 38–360. [CrossRef] [PubMed]

2. Shah, A.S.V.; Stelzle, D.; Lee, K.K.; Beck, E.J.; Alam, S.; Clifford, S.; Longenecker, C.T.; Strachan, F.; Bagchi, S.; Whiteley, W.; et al. Global Burden of Atherosclerotic Cardiovascular Disease in People Living With HIV. *Circulation* **2018**, *138*, 1100–1112. [CrossRef] [PubMed]

3. Weber, R.; Ruppik, M.; Rickenbach, M.; Spoerri, A.; Furrer, H.; Battegay, M.; Cavassini, M.; Calmy, A.; Bernasconi, E.; Schmid, P.; et al. Decreasing mortality and changing patterns of causes of death in the Swiss HIV Cohort Study. *HIV Med.* **2013**, *14*, 195–207. [CrossRef] [PubMed]

4. Smith, C.J.; Ryom, L.; Weber, R.; Morlat, P.; Pradier, C.; Reiss, P.; Kowalska, J.D.; de Wit, S.; Law, M.; el Sadr, W.; et al. Trends over time in underlying causes of death amongst HIV-positive individuals from 1999 to 2011. *Lancet* **2014**, *384*, 241–248. [CrossRef]

5. Frieden, T.R.; Jaffe, M.G. Saving 100 million lives by improving global treatment of hypertension and reducing cardiovascular disease risk factors. *J. Clin. Hypertens.* **2018**, *20*, 208–211. [CrossRef] [PubMed]

6. Patel, P.; Sabin, K.; Godfrey-Faussett, P. Approaches to Improve the Surveillance, Monitoring, and Management of Noncommunicable Diseases in HIV-Infected Persons: Viewpoint. *JMIR Public Heal. Surveill.* **2018**, *4*, e10989. [CrossRef] [PubMed]

7. Hsue, P.Y.; Waters, D.D. Time to Recognize HIV Infection as a Major Cardiovascular Risk Factor. *Circulation* **2018**, *138*, 1113–1115. [CrossRef]

8. Hasse, B.; Tarr, P.E.; Marques-Vidal, P.; Waeber, G.; Preisig, M.; Mooser, V.; Valeri, F.; Djalali, S.; Andri, R.; Bernasconie, E.; et al. Strong Impact of Smoking on Multimorbidity Immunodeficiency Virus-Infected Individuals in and Cardiovascular Risk Among Human Comparison With the General Population. *Open Forum Infect. Dis.* **2015**. [CrossRef]

9. Rasmussen, L.D.; Helleberg, M.; May, M.T.; Afzal, S.; Kronborg, G.; Larsen, C.S.; Pedersen, C.; Gerstoft, J.; Nordestgaard, B.G.; Obel, N. Myocardial infarction among danish HIV-infected individuals: Population-attributable fractions associated with smoking. *Clin. Infect. Dis.* **2015**, *60*, 1415–1423. [CrossRef]

10. Engel, T.; Raffenberg, M.; Marzolini, C.; Cavassini, M.; Kovari, H.; Hasse, B.; Tarr, P.E. HIV and Aging-Perhaps Not as Dramatic as We Feared? *Gerontology* **2018**, *64*, 446–456. [CrossRef]

11. Triant, V.A.; Lee, H.; Hadigan, C.; Grinspoon, S.K. Increased acute myocardial infarction rates and cardiovascular risk factors among patients with human immunodeficiency virus disease. *J. Clin. Endocrinol. Metab.* **2007**, *92*, 2506–2512. [CrossRef] [PubMed]

12. De Lima, L.R.; Petroski, E.L.; Moreno, Y.M.; Silva, D.A.; Trindade, E.B.; de Carvalho, A.P.; de Carlos Back, I. Dyslipidemia, chronic inflammation, and subclinical atherosclerosis in children and adolescents infected with HIV: The PositHIVe Health Study. *PLoS ONE* **2018**' *13*, 1–17.

13. Mallon, P.W.G. Getting to the Heart of HIV and Myocardial Infarction. *JAMA Intern. Med.* **2013**, *173*, 622. [CrossRef] [PubMed]

14. Rasmussen, L.D.; May, M.T.; Kronborg, G.; Larsen, C.S.; Pedersen, C.; Gerstoft, J.; Obel, N. Time trends for risk of severe age-related diseases in individuals with and without HIV infection in Denmark: A nationwide population-based cohort study. *Lancet HIV* **2015**, *2*, e288–e298. [CrossRef]

15. Drozd, D.R.; Kitahata, M.M.; Althoff, K.N.; Zhang, J.; Gange, S.J.; Napravnik, S.; Burkholder, G.A.; Mathews, W.C.; Silverberg, M.J.; Sterling, T.R.; et al. Increased Risk of Myocardial Infarction in HIV-Infected Individuals in North America Compared with the General Population. *J. Acquir. Immune Defic. Syndr.* **2017**, *75*, 568–576. [CrossRef] [PubMed]

16. Freiberg, M.S.; Chang, C.C.H.; Kuller, L.H.; Skanderson, M.; Lowy, E.; Kraemer, K.L.; Butt, A.A.; Goetz, M.B.; Leaf, D.; Oursler, K.A.; et al. HIV infection and the risk of acute myocardial infarction. *JAMA Intern. Med.* **2013**, *173*, 614–622. [CrossRef] [PubMed]

17. Klein, D.B.; Leyden, W.A.; Xu, L.; Chao, C.R.; Horberg, M.A.; Towner, W.J.; Hurley, L.B.; Marcus, J.L.; Quesenberry, C.P.; Silverberg, M.J. Declining relative risk for myocardial infarction among HIV-positive compared with HIV-negative individuals with access to care. *Clin. Infect. Dis.* **2015**, *60*, 1278–1280. [CrossRef] [PubMed]

18. Tarr, P.E.; Ledergerber, B.; Calmy, A.; Doco-Lecompte, T.; Marzel, A.; Weber, R.; Kaufmann, P.A.; Nkoulou, R.; Buechel, R.R.; Kovari, H. Subclinical coronary artery disease in Swiss HIV-positive and HIV-negative persons. *Eur. Heart J.* **2018**, *39*, 2147–2154. [CrossRef] [PubMed]

19. Lang, S.; Mary-Krausea, M.; Cotte, L.; Gilquind, J.; Partisanie, M.; Simonf, A.; Boccarag, F.; Binghamh, A.; Dominique, C.; for the French Hospital Database on HIV-ANRS CO4. Increased risk of myocardial infarction in HIV-infected patients in France, relative to the general population. *Res. Lett.* **2010**, *24*, 1228–1230. [CrossRef]

20. Boccara, F.; Lang, S.; Meuleman, C.; Ederhy, S.; Mary-Krause, M.; Costagliola, D.; Capeau, J.; Cohen, A. HIV and coronary heart disease: Time for a better understanding. *J. Am. Coll. Cardiol.* **2013**, *61*, 511–523. [CrossRef]

21. Vachiat, A.; McCutcheon, K.; Tsabedze, N.; Zachariah, D.; Manga, P. HIV and Ischemic Heart Disease. *J. Am. Coll. Cardiol.* **2017**, *69*, 73–82. [CrossRef]

22. Wang, X.; Chai, H.; Yao, Q.; Chen, C. Molecular Mechanisms of HIV Protease Inhibitor-Induced. *J. Acquir. Immune Defic. Syndr.* **2007**, *44*, 493–499. [CrossRef]

23. Worm, S.W.; Sabin, C.; Weber, R.; Reiss, P.; El-Sadr, W.; Dabis, F.; De Wit, S.; Law, M.; Monforte, A.D.; Friis-Møller, N.; et al. Risk of Myocardial Infarction in Patients with HIV Infection Exposed to Specific Individual Antiretroviral Drugs from the 3 Major Drug Classes: The Data Collection on Adverse Events of Anti-HIV Drugs (D:A:D) Study. *J. Infect. Dis.* **2009**, *201*, 318–330. [CrossRef]

24. Subramanya, V.; McKay, H.S.; Brusca, R.M.; Palella, F.J.; Kingsley, L.A.; Witt, M.D.; Hodis, H.N.; Tracy, R.P.; Post, W.S.; Haberlen, S.A. Inflammatory biomarkers and subclinical carotid atherosclerosis in HIV-infected and HIV-uninfected men in the Multicenter AIDS Cohort Study. *PLoS ONE* **2019**, *14*, e0214735. [CrossRef]

25. Tenorio, A.R.; Zheng, Y.; Bosch, R.J.; Krishnan, S.; Rodriguez, B.; Hunt, P.W.; Plants, J.; Seth, A.; Wilson, C.C.; Deeks, S.G.; et al. Soluble Markers of Inflammation and Coagulation but Not T-Cell Activation Predict Non-AIDS-Defining Morbid Events During Suppressive Antiretroviral Treatment. *J. Infect. Dis.* **2014**, *210*, 1248–1259. [CrossRef]

26. Kuller, L.H.; Tracy, R.; Belloso, W.; De Wit, S.; Drummond, F.; Lane, H.C.; Ledergerber, B.; Lundgren, J.; Neuhaus, J.; Nixon, D.; et al. Inflammatory and Coagulation Biomarkers and Mortality in Patients with HIV Infection. *PLoS Med.* **2008**, *5*, e203. [CrossRef]

27. So-Armah, K.A.; Tate, J.P.; Chang, C.H.; Butt, A.A.; Gerschenson, M.; Gibert, C.L.; Leaf, D.; Rimland, D.; Rodriguez-barradas, M.C.; Budoff, M.J.; et al. Do Biomarkers of Inflammation, Monocyte Activation, and Altered Coagulation Explain Excess Mortality Between HIV Infected and Uninfected People? *J. Acquir. Immune Defic. Syndr.* **2016**, *72*, 206–213. [CrossRef]

28. Sandler, N.G.; Wand, H.; Roque, A.; Law, M.; Nason, M.C.; Nixon, D.E.; Pedersen, C.; Ruxrungtham, K.; Lewin, S.R.; Emery, S.; et al. Plasma Levels of Soluble CD14 Independently Predict Mortality in HIV Infection. 2011, 203, 780–790. *J. Infect. Dis.* **2011**, *203*, 780–790. [CrossRef]

29. Kelesidis, T.; Kendall, M.A.; Yang, O.O.; Hodis, H.N.; Currier, J.S. Biomarkers of Microbial Translocation and Macrophage Activation: Association with Progression of Subclinical Atherosclerosis in HIV-1 Infection. *J. Infect. Dis.* **2012**, *206*, 1558–1567. [CrossRef]

30. Hanna, D.B.; Lin, J.; Post, W.S.; Hodis, H.N.; Xue, X.; Anastos, K.; Cohen, M.H.; Gange, S.J.; Haberlen, S.A.; Heath, S.L.; et al. Association of Macrophage Inflammation Biomarkers With Progression of Subclinical Carotid Artery Atherosclerosis in HIV-Infected Women and Men. *J. Infect. Dis.* **2017**, *10461*, 1352–1361. [CrossRef]

31. Burdo, T.H.; Lo, J.; Abbara, S.; Wei, J.; Delelys, M.E.; Preffer, F.; Rosenberg, E.S.; Williams, K.C.; Grinspoon, S. Soluble CD163, a Novel Marker of Activated Macrophages, Is Elevated and Associated With Noncalcified Coronary Plaque in HIV-Infected Patients. *J. Infect. Dis.* **2011**, *204*, 1227–1236. [CrossRef]

32. Eugenin, E.A.; Morgello, S.; Klotman, M.E.; Mosoian, A.; Lento, P.A.; Berman, J.W.; Schecter, A.D. Human Immunodeficiency Virus (HIV) Infects Human Arterial Smooth Muscle Cells in Vivo and in Vitro Implications for the Pathogenesis of HIV-Mediated Vascular Disease. *Am. J. Pathol.* **2008**, *172*, 1100–1111. [CrossRef]

33. Tabib, A.; Mornex, C.; Leroux, J.-F.; Loire, R. Accelerated coronary atherosclerosis and arteriosclerosis in young human-immunodeficiency-virus-positive patients. *Coron. Artery Dis.* **2000**, *11*, 41–46. [CrossRef]

34. Zanni, M.V.; Schouten, J.; Grinspoon, S.K.; Reiss, P. Risk of coronary heart disease in patients with HIV infection. *Nat. Rev. Cardiol.* **2014**, *11*, 728. [CrossRef]

35. Wolf, K.; Tsakiris, D.A.; Weber, R.; Erb, P.; Battegay, M. Antiretroviral Therapy Reduces Markers of Endothelial and Coagulation Activation in Patients Infected with Human Immunodeficiency Virus Type 1. *J. Infect. Dis.* **2002**, *185*, 456–462. [CrossRef]

36. Lang, S.; Mary-Krause, M.; Simon, A.; Partisani, M.; Gilquin, J.; Cotte, L.; Boccara, F.; Costagliola, D. HIV Replication and Immune Status Are Independent Predictors of the Risk of Myocardial Infarction in HIV-Infected Individuals. *Clin. Infect. Dis.* **2012**, *55*, 600–607. [CrossRef]

37. Michael, S.; Leyden, W.A.; Xu, L.; Horberg, M.A.; Chao, C.R.; Towner, W.J.; Hurley, L.B.; Quesenberry, C.P.; Klein, D.B. Immunodeficiency and risk of myocardial infarction among HIV-positive individuals with access to care. *J. Acquir. Immune Defic. Syndr.* **2014**, *65*, 160–166.

38. Rotger, M.; Glass, T.R.; Junier, T.; Lundgren, J.; Neaton, J.D.; Poloni, E.S.; Van 'T Wout, A.B.; Lubomirov, R.; Colombo, S.; Martinez, R.; et al. Contribution of genetic background, traditional risk factors, and HIV-related factors to coronary artery disease events in HIV-positive persons. *Clin. Infect. Dis.* **2013**, *57*, 112–121. [CrossRef]

39. Sabin, C.A.; Ryom, L.; De Wit, S.; Mocroft, A.; Phillips, A.N.; Worm, S.W.; Weber, R.; Monforte, A.D.; Reiss, P.; Kamara, D.; et al. Associations between immune depression and cardiovascular events in HIV infection. *AIDS* **2013**, *27*, 2735–2748. [CrossRef]

40. Périard, D.; Telenti, A.; Sudre, P.; Cheseaux, J.J.; Halfon, P.; Reymond, M.J.; Marcovina, S.M.; Glauser, M.P.; Nicod, P.; Darioli, R.; et al. Atherogenic dyslipidemia in HIV-infected individuals treated with protease inhibitors. *Circulation* **1999**, *100*, 700–705. [CrossRef]

41. Ryom, L.; Lundgren, J.D.; El-Sadr, W.; Reiss, P.; Kirk, O.; Law, M.; Phillips, A.; Weber, R.; Fontas, E.; d'Arminio Monforte, A.; et al. Cardiovascular disease and use of contemporary protease inhibitors: The D:A:D international prospective multicohort study. *Lancet HIV* **2018**, *5*, e291–e300. [CrossRef]

42. Sabin, C.A.; Worm, S.W.; Weber, R.; Reiss, P.; El-Sadr, W.; Dabis, F.; De Wit, S.; Law, M.; D'Arminio Monforte, A.; Friis-Møller, N.; et al. Use of nucleoside reverse transcriptase inhibitors and risk of myocardial infarction in HIV-infected patients enrolled in the D:A:D study: A multi-cohort collaboration. *Lancet* **2008**, *371*, 1417–1426.

43. Lai, H.; Moore, R.; Celentano, D.D.; Gerstenblith, G.; Treisman, G.; Keruly, J.C.; Kickler, T.; Li, J.; Chen, S.; Lai, S.; et al. HIV infection itself may not be associated with subclinical coronary artery disease among African Americans without cardiovascular symptoms. *J. Am. Heart Assoc.* **2015**, *5*, 1–16. [CrossRef]

44. Post, W.S.; Budoff, M.; Kingsley, L.; Palella, F.J.; Witt, M.D.; Li, X.; George, R.T.; Brown, T.; Jacobson, L.P. Associations between HIV Infection and Subclinical Coronary Atherosclerosis: The Multicenter AIDS Cohort Study (MACS). *Ann. Intern. Med.* **2014**, *160*, 458–467. [CrossRef]

45. Stein, J.H.; Currier, J.S.; Hsue, P.Y. Arterial Disease in Patients With Human Immunodeficiency Virus Infection. *JACC Cardiovasc. Imaging* **2014**, *7*, 515–525. [CrossRef]

46. Inaba, Y.; Chen, J.A.; Bergmann, S.R. Carotid Intima-Media Thickness and Cardiovascular Events. *N. Engl. J. Med.* **2011**, *365*, 1640–1642.

47. Lorenz, M.W.; Polak, J.F.; Kavousi, M.; Mathiesen, E.B.; Völzke, H.; Tuomainen, T.P.; Sander, D.; Plichart, M.; Catapano, A.L.; Robertson, C.M.; et al. Carotid intima-media thickness progression to predict cardiovascular events in the general population (the PROG-IMT collaborative project): A meta-analysis of individual participant data. *Lancet* **2012**, *379*, 2053–2062. [CrossRef]

48. O'Leary, D.H.; Polak, J.F.; Kronmal, R.A.; Manolio, T.A.; Burke, G.L.; Wolfson, S.K. Carotid-Artery Intima and Media Thickness as a Risk Factor for Myocardial Infarction and Stroke in Older Adults. *N. Engl. J. Med.* **2002**, *340*, 14–22. [CrossRef]

49. Den Ruijter, H.M.; Peters, S.A.E.; Anderson, T.J.; Britton, A.R.; Dekker, J.M.; Eijkemans, M.J.; Engström, G.; Evans, G.W.; de Graaf, J.; Grobbee, D.E.; et al. Common carotid intima-media thickness measurements in cardiovascular risk prediction: A meta-analysis. *JAMA* **2012**, *308*, 796–803. [CrossRef]

50. Hulten, E.; Mitchell, J.; Scally, J.; Gibbs, B.; Villines, T.C. HIV positivity, protease inhibitor exposure and subclinical atherosclerosis: A systematic review and meta-analysis of observational studies. *Heart* **2009**, *95*, 1826–1835. [CrossRef]

51. Maggi, P.; Serio, G.; Epifani, G.; Fiorentino, G.; Saracino, A.; Fico, C.; Perilli, F.; Lillo, A.; Ferraro, S.; Gargiulo, M.; et al. Premature lesions of the carotid vessels in HIV-1-infected patients treated with protease inhibitors. *AIDS* **2000**, *14*, F123–F128. [CrossRef]

52. Maggi, P.; Lillo, A.; Perilli, F.; Maserati, R.; Chirianni, A.; Epifani, G.; Fiorentino, G.; Ladisa, N.; Pastore, G.; Angiletta, D.; et al. Colour-Doppler ultrasonography of carotid vessels in patients treated with antiretroviral therapy: A comparative study. *AIDS* **2004**, *18*, 1023–1028. [CrossRef]

53. Hsue, P.Y.; Lo, J.C.; Franklin, A.; Bolger, A.F.; Martin, J.N.; Deeks, S.G.; Waters, D.D. Progression of Atherosclerosis as Assessed by Carotid Intima-Media Thickness in Patients with HIV Infection. *Circulation* **2004**, *109*, 1603–1608. [CrossRef]

54. Mercié, P.; Thiébaut, R.; Aurillac-Lavignolle, V.; Pellegrin, J.L.; Yvorra-Vives, M.C.; Cipriano, C.; Neau, D.; Morlat, P.; Ragnaud, J.M.; Dupon, M.; et al. Carotid intima-media thickness is slightly increased over time in HIV-1-infected patients. *HIV Med.* **2005**, *6*, 380–387. [CrossRef]

55. Hsue, P.Y.; Hunt, P.W.; Sinclair, E.; Bredt, B.; Franklin, A.; Killian, M.; Hoh, R.; Martin, J.N.; McCune, J.M.; Waters, D.D.; et al. Increased carotid intima-media thickness in HIV patients is associated with increased cytomegalovirus-specific T-cell responses. *AIDS* **2006**, *20*, 2275–2283. [CrossRef]

56. Thiebaut, R.; Aurillac-Lavignolleb, V.; Bonnetb, F.; Ibrahimd, N.; Ciprianoc, C.; Neauc, D.; Duponc, M.; Dabisb, F.; Mercie, P.; Groupe d'Epidemiologie Clinique du Sida en Aquitaine (GECSA). Change in atherosclerosis progression in HIV infected patients: ANRS Aquitaine Cohort, 1999–2004. *AIDS* **2005**, *19*, 729–731. [CrossRef]

57. Johnsen, S.; Dolan, S.E.; Fitch, K.V.; Kanter, J.R.; Hemphill, L.C.; Connelly, J.M.; Lees, R.S.; Lee, H.; Grinspoon, S. Carotid intimal medial thickness in human immunodeficiency virus-infected women: Effects of protease inhibitor use, cardiac risk factors, and the metabolic syndrome. *J. Clin. Endocrinol. Metab.* **2006**, *91*, 4916–4924. [CrossRef]

58. Van Wijk, J.P.H.; De Koning, E.J.P.; Cabezas, M.C.; Joven, J.; Op't Roodt, J.; Rabelink, T.J.; Hoepelman, A.M. Functional and structural markers of atherosclerosis in human immunodeficiency virus-infected patients. *J. Am. Coll. Cardiol.* **2006**, *47*, 1117–1123. [CrossRef]

59. Currier, J.S.; Kendall, M.A.; Henry, W.K.; Alston-Smith, B.; Torriani, F.J.; Tebas, P.; Li, Y.; Hodis, H.N. Progression of carotid artery intima-media thickening in HIV-infected and uninfected adults. *AIDS* **2007**, *21*, 1137–1145. [CrossRef]

60. Jericó, C.; Knobel, H.; Calvo, N.; Sorli, M.L.; Guelar, A.; Gimeno-Bayón, J.L.; Saballs, P.; López-Colomés, J.L.; Pedro-Botet, J. Subclinical carotid atherosclerosis in HIV-infected patients: Role of combination antiretroviral therapy. *Stroke* **2006**, *37*, 812–817. [CrossRef]

61. Lorenz, M.W.; Stephan, C.; Harmjanz, A.; Staszewski, S.; Buehler, A.; Bickel, M.; von Kegler, S.; Ruhkamp, D.; Steinmetz, H.; Sitzer, M. Both long-term HIV infection and highly active antiretroviral therapy are independent risk factors for early carotid atherosclerosis. *Atherosclerosis* **2008**, *196*, 720–726. [CrossRef]

62. Coll, B.; Parra, S.; Alonso-Villaverde, C.; Aragonés, G.; Montero, M.; Camps, J.; Joven, J.; Masana, L. The role of immunity and inflammation in the progression of atherosclerosis in patients with HIV infection. *Stroke* **2007**, *38*, 2477–2484. [CrossRef]

63. Depairon, M.; Chessex, S.; Sudre, P.; Rodondi, N.; Doser, N.; Chave, J.P.; Riesen, W.; Nicod, P.; Darioli, R.; Telenti, A.; et al. Premature atherosclerosis in hiv-infected individuals focus on protease inhibitor therapy. *AIDS* **2001**, *15*, 329–334. [CrossRef]

64. Maggi, P.; Perilli, F.; Lillo, A.; Gargiulo, M.; Ferraro, S.; Grisorio, B.; Ferrara, S.; Carito, V.; Bellacosa, C.; Pastore, G.; et al. Rapid progression of carotid lesions in HAART-treated HIV-1 patients. *Atherosclerosis* **2007**, *192*, 407–412. [CrossRef]

65. Grunfeld, C.; Delaney, J.A.; Wanke, C.; Currier, J.S.; Scherzer, R.; Biggs, M.L.; Tien, P.C.; Shlipak, M.G.; Sidney, S.; Polak, J.F.; et al. Preclinical atherosclerosis due to HIV infection: Carotid intima-medial thickness measurements from the FRAM study. *AIDS* **2009**, *23*, 1841–1849. [CrossRef]

66. Hsue, P.Y.; Hunt, P.W.; Schnell, A.; Kalapus, S.C.; Hoh, R.; Ganz, P.; Martin, J.N.; Deeks, S.G. Role of viral replication, antiretroviral therapy, and immunodeficiency in HIV-associated atherosclerosis. *AIDS* **2009**, *23*, 1059–1067. [CrossRef]

67. Cabello, C.M.; Bair, W.B.; Lamore, S.D.; Ley, S.; Alexandra, S.; Azimian, S.; Wondrak, G.T. Silencing of germline-expressed genes by DNA elimination in somatic cells. *Dev. Cell* **2010**, *46*, 220–231.

68. Kaplan, R.C.; Sinclair, E.; Landay, A.L.; Lurain, N.; Sharrett, A.R.; Gange, S.J.; Xue, X.; Hunt, P.; Karim, R.; Kern, D.M.; et al. T Cell Activation and Senescence Predict Subclinical Carotid Artery Disease in HIV-Infected Women. *J. Infect. Dis.* **2011**, *203*, 452–463. [CrossRef]

69. Sainz, T.; Álvarez-Fuente, M.; Navarro, M.L.; Díaz, L.; Rojo, P.; Blázquez, D.; De José, M.I.; Ramos, J.T.; Serrano-Villar, S.; Martínez, J.; et al. Subclinical atherosclerosis and markers of immune activation in hiv-infected children and adolescents: The carovih study. *J. Acquir. Immune Defic. Syndr.* **2014**, *65*, 42–49. [CrossRef]

70. Hanna, D.B.; Post, W.S.; Deal, J.A.; Hodis, H.N.; Jacobson, L.P.; Mack, W.J.; Anastos, K.; Gange, S.J.; Landay, A.L.; Lazar, J.M.; et al. HIV Infection Is Associated with Progression of Subclinical Carotid Atherosclerosis. *Clin. Infect. Dis.* **2015**, *61*, 640–650. [CrossRef]

71. Hsue, P.Y.; Scherzer, R.; Hunt, P.W.; Schnell, A.; Bolger, A.F.; Kalapus, S.C.; Maka, K.; Martin, J.N.; Ganz, P.; Deeks, S.G. Carotid Intima-Media Thickness Progression in HIV-Infected Adults Occurs Preferentially at the Carotid Bifurcation and Is Predicted by Inflammation. *J. Am. Heart Assoc.* **2012**, *1*, 1–12. [CrossRef]

72. Bots, M.L.; Baldassarre, D.; Simon, A.; De Groot, E.; O'Leary, D.H.; Riley, W.; Kastelein, J.J.; Grobbee, D.E. Carotid intima-media thickness and coronary atherosclerosis: Weak or strong relations? *Eur. Heart J.* **2007**, *28*, 398–406. [CrossRef]

73. Hodis, H.N.; Mack, W.J.; Labree, L.; Selzer, R.H. The Role of Carotid Arterial Intima-Media Thickness in Predicting Clinical Coronary Events Methods Study Design. *Annals Intern. Med.* **2006**, *128*, 262–269. [CrossRef]

74. Greenland, P.; Alpert, J.S.; Beller, G.; Benjamin, E.J.; Budoff, M.J.; Fayad, Z.A.; Foster, E.; Hlatky, M.A.; Hodgson, J.M.; Kushner, F.G.; et al. 2010 ACCF/AHA Guideline for Assessment of Cardiovascular Risk in Asymptomatic Adults. *J. Am. Coll. Cardiol.* **2010**, *56*, 50–103. [CrossRef]

75. Callister, T.Q.; Cooil, B.; Raya, S.; Lippolis, N.J.; Russo, D.J.; Raggi, P. Coronary artery disease: improved reproducibility of calcium scoring with an electron-beam CT volumetric method. *Radiology* **2014**, *208*, 807–814. [CrossRef]

76. Callister, T.Q.; Raggi, P.; Cooil, B.; Lippolis, N.J.; Russo, D.J. Effect of HMG-CoA Reductase Inhibitors on Coronary Artery Disease as Assessed by Electron-Beam Computed Tomography. *N. Engl. J. Med.* **2002**, *339*, 1972–1978. [CrossRef]

77. Raggi, P.; Callister, T.Q.; Shaw, L.J. Progression of coronary artery calcium and risk of first myocardial infarction in patients receiving cholesterol-lowering therapy. *Arterioscler. Thromb. Vasc. Biol.* **2004**, *24*, 1272–1277. [CrossRef]

78. Raggi, P.; Davidson, M.; Callister, T.Q.; Welty, F.K.; Bachmann, G.A.; Hecht, H.; Rumberger, J.A. Aggressive Versus Moderate Lipid-Lowering Therapy in Hypercholesterolemic Postmenopausal Women. *Circulation* **2005**, *112*, 563–571. [CrossRef]

79. Achenbach, S.; Ropers, D.; Pohle, K.; Leber, A.; Thilo, C.; Knez, A.; Menendez, T.; Maeffert, R.; Kusus, M.; Regenfus, M.; et al. Influence of lipid-lowering therapy on the progression of coronary artery calcification: A prospective evaluation. *Circulation* **2002**, *106*, 1077–1082. [CrossRef]

80. Bonow, R.O. Should Coronary Calcium Screening Be Used in Cardiovascular Prevention Strategies? *N. Engl. J. Med.* **2009**, *361*, 990–997. [CrossRef]

81.   Hoffmann, U.; Brady, T.J.; Muller, J. Use of New Imaging Techniques to Screen for Coronary Artery Disease. *Circulation* **2003**, *108*, 1–4. [CrossRef]

82.   Polonsky, T.S.; Mcclelland, R.L.; Jorgensen, N.W.; Bild, D.E.; Burke, G.L.; Guerci, A.D.; Greenland, P. Coronary artery calcium score and risk classification for coronary heart disease prediction. *JAMA* **2011**, *303*, 1610–1616. [CrossRef]

83.   Schmermund, A.; Baumgart, D.; Möhlenkamp, S.; Kriener, P.; Pump, H.; Grönemeyer, D.; Seibel, R.; Erbel, R. Natural History and Topographic Pattern of Progression of Coronary Calcification in Symptomatic Patients. *Arterioscler. Thromb. Vasc. Biol.* **2011**, *21*, 421–426. [CrossRef]

84.   Detrano, R.; Guerci, A.D.; Carr, J.J.; Bild, D.E.; Burke, G.; Folsom, A.R.; Liu, K.; Shea, S.; Szklo, M.; Bluemke, D.A.; et al. Coronary Calcium as a Predictor of Coronary Events in Four Racial or Ethnic Groups. *N. Engl. J. Med.* **2008**, *358*, 1336–1345. [CrossRef]

85.   Pletcher, M.; Tice, J.; Pignone, M.; Browner, W. Using the Coronary Artery Calcium Score to Predict Coronary Heart Disease Events. *Arch. Intern. Med.* **2004**, *164*, 1285–1292. [CrossRef]

86.   Folsam, A.; Kronmal, R.A.; Detrano, R.; O'Leary, D.; Bild, D.E.; Bluemke, D.A.; Budoff, M.J.; Liu, K.; Shea, S.; Szklo, M.; et al. Coronary Artery Calcification Compared With Carotid Intima-Media Thickness in the Prediction of Cardiovascular Disease Incidence. *Arch. Intern. Med.* **2008**, *168*, 1333–1339. [CrossRef]

87.   Taylor, A.J.; Bindeman, J.; Feuerstein, I.; Cao, F.; Brazaitis, M.; O'Malley, P.G. Coronary Calcium Independently Predicts Incident Premature Coronary Heart Disease Over Measured Cardiovascular Risk Factors. *J. Am. Coll. Cardiol.* **2005**, *46*, 807–814. [CrossRef]

88.   Arad, Y.; Goodman, K.J.; Roth, M.; Newstein, D.; Guerci, A.D. Coronary calcification, coronary disease risk factors, C-reactive protein, and atherosclerotic cardiovascular disease events: The St. Francis heart study. *J. Am. Coll. Cardiol.* **2005**, *46*, 158–165. [CrossRef]

89.   Budoff, M.J.; Shaw, L.J.; Liu, S.T.; Weinstein, S.R.; Mosler, T.P.; Tseng, P.H.; Flores, F.R.; Callister, T.Q.; Raggi, P.; Berman, D.S. Long-Term Prognosis Associated With Coronary Calcification. Observations From a Registry of 25,253 Patients. *J. Am. Coll. Cardiol.* **2007**, *49*, 1860–1870. [CrossRef]

90.   Raggi, P.; Cooil, B.; Shaw, L.J.; Aboulhson, J.; Takasu, J.; Budoff, M.; Callister, T.Q. Progression of coronary calcium on serial electron beam tomographic scanning is greater in patients with future myocardial infarction. *Am. J. Cardiol.* **2003**, *92*, 827–829. [CrossRef]

91.   Newman, A.B.; Naydeck, B.; Ives, D.; Boudreau, R.; Sutton-Tyrrell, K.; O'Leary, D.H.; Kuller, L.H. Coronary Artery Calcium, Carotid Artery Wall Thickness and Cardiovascular Disease Outcomes in Adults 70 to 99 Years Old. *Am. J. Cardiol.* **2010**, *46*, 220–231. [CrossRef]

92.   Vliegenthart, R.; Oudkerk, M.; Hofman, A.; Oei, H.-H.; van Dijck, W.; Van Rooij, F.J.A.; Witteman, J.C.M. Coronary Calcification Improves Cardiovascular Risk Prediction in the Elderly. *Circulation* **2005**, 572–577. [CrossRef]

93.   Jain, A.; McClelland, R.L.; Polak, J.F.; Shea, S.; Burke, G.L.; Bild, D.E.; Watson, K.E.; Budoff, M.J.; Liu, K.; Post, W.S.; et al. Cardiovascular imaging for assessing cardiovascular risk in asymptomatic men versus women the Multi-Ethnic Study of Atherosclerosis (MESA). *Circ. Cardiovasc. Imaging* **2011**, *4*, 8–15. [CrossRef]

94.   Yeboah, J.; Mcclelland, R.L.; Polonsky, T.S.; Burke, G.L.; Sibley, C.T.; O'Leary, D.H.; Carr, J.J.; Goff, D.C.; Greenland, P.; Herrington, D.M. Comparison of novel risk markers for improvement in cardiovascular risk assessment in intermediate-risk individuals. *JAMA* **2012**, *308*, 788–795. [CrossRef]

95.   Guaraldi, G.; Zona, S.; Alexopoulos, N.; Orlando, G.; Carli, F.; Ligabue, G.; Fiocchi, F.; Lattanzi, A.; Rossi, R.; Modena, M.G.; et al. Coronary Aging in HIV-Infected Patients. *Clin. Infect. Dis.* **2009**, *49*, 1756–1762. [CrossRef]

96.   Kingsley, L.A.; Cuervo-Rojas, J.; Muñoz, A.; Palella, F.J.; Post, W.; Witt, M.D.; Budoff, M.; Kuller, L. Subclinical coronary atherosclerosis, HIV infection and antiretroviral therapy: Multicenter AIDS Cohort Study. *AIDS* **2008**, *22*, 1589–1599. [CrossRef]

97.   Motoyama, S.; Ito, H.; Sarai, M.; Kondo, T.; Kawai, H.; Nagahara, Y.; Harigaya, H.; Kan, S.; Anno, H.; Takahashi, H.; et al. Plaque characterization by coronary computed tomography angiography and the likelihood of acute coronary events in mid-term follow-up. *J. Am. Coll. Cardiol.* **2015**, *66*, 337–346. [CrossRef]

98.   Giannopoulos, A.A.; Benz, D.C.; Gräni, C.; Buechel, R.R. Imaging the event-prone coronary artery plaque. *J. Nucl. Cardiol.* **2019**, *26*, 141–153. [CrossRef]

99. Monroe, A.K.; Haberlen, S.A.; Post, W.S.; Palella, F.; Kingsley, L.A.; Witts, M.D.; Budoff, M.; Jacobson, L.; Brown, T.T. Cardiovascular Disease Risk Scores' Relationship to Subclinical Cardiovascular Disease Among HIV-Infected and HIV-Uninfected Men. *AIDS* **2015**, *155*, 1683–1695. [CrossRef]

100. Ascenzo, F.D.; Cerrato, E.; Calcagno, A.; Grossomarra, W.; Montefusco, A.; Veglia, S.; Barbero, U.; Gili, S.; Cannillo, M.; Pianelli, M.; et al. High prevalence at computed coronary tomography of non-calcified plaques in asymptomatic HIV patients treated with HAART: A meta-analysis. *Atherosclerosis* **2015**, *240*, 197–204. [CrossRef]

101. Schoeni-Affolter, F.; Ledergerber, B.; Rickenbach, M.; Rudin, C.; Günthard, H.F.; Telenti, A.; Furrer, H.; Yerly, S.; Francioli, P. Cohort profile: The Swiss HIV cohort study. *Int. J. Epidemiol.* **2010**, *39*, 1179–1189.

102. Min, J.K.; Shaw, L.J.; Devereux, R.B.; Okin, P.M.; Weinsaft, J.W.; Russo, D.J.; Lippolis, N.J.; Berman, D.S.; Callister, T.Q. Prognostic Value of Multidetector Coronary Computed Tomographic Angiography for Prediction of All-Cause Mortality. *J. Am. Coll. Cardiol.* **2007**, *50*, 1161–1170. [CrossRef]

103. Abd-Elmoniem, K.Z.; Unsal, A.B.; Eshera, S.; Matta, J.R.; Muldoon, N.; McAreavey, D.; Purdy, J.B.; Hazra, R.; Hadigan, C.; Gharib, A.M. Increased coronary vessel wall thickness in HIV-infected young adults. *Clin. Infect. Dis.* **2014**, *59*, 1779–1786. [CrossRef]

104. Husmann, L.; Valenta, I.; Gaemperli, O.; Adda, O.; Treyer, V.; Wyss, C.A.; Veit-haibach, P.; Tatsugami, F.; Von Schulthess, G.K.; Kaufmann, P.A. Feasibility of low-dose coronary CT angiography: First experience with prospective. *Eur. Heart J.* **2008**, *29*, 191–197. [CrossRef]

105. Buechel, R.R.; Husmann, L.; Herzog, B.A.; Pazhenkottil, A.P.; Nkoulou, R.; Ghadri, J.R.; Treyer, V.; Von Schulthess, P.; Kaufmann, P.A. Low-dose computed tomography coronary angiography with prospective electrocardiogram triggering: Feasibility in a large population. *J. Am. Coll. Cardiol.* **2011**, *57*, 332–336. [CrossRef]

106. Kaufmann, P.A. Low-Dose Computed Tomography Coronary Angiography With Prospective Triggering. A Promise for the Future. *J. Am. Coll. Cardiol.* **2008**, *52*, 1456–1457. [CrossRef]

107. Min, J.K.; Dunning, A.; Lin, F.Y.; Achenbach, S.; Al-Mallah, M.; Budoff, M.J.; Cademartiri, F.; Callister, T.Q.; Chang, H.J.; Cheng, V.; et al. Age- and sex-related differences in all-cause mortality risk based on coronary computed tomography angiography findings: Results from the international multicenter CONFIRM (Coronary CT Angiography Evaluation for Clinical Outcomes: An International Multice. *J. Am. Coll. Cardiol.* **2011**, *58*, 849–860. [CrossRef]

108. Hadamitzky, M.; Freißmuth, B.; Meyer, T.; Hein, F.; Kastrati, A.; Martinoff, S.; Schömig, A.; Hausleiter, J. Prognostic Value of Coronary Computed Tomographic Angiography for Prediction of Cardiac Events in Patients With Suspected Coronary Artery Disease. *JACC Cardiovasc. Imaging* **2009**, *2*, 404–411. [CrossRef]

109. McEvoy, J.W.; Blaha, M.J.; Nasir, K.; Yoon, Y.E.; Choi, E.K.; Cho, I.S.; Chun, E.J.; Choi, S.I.; Rivera, J.J.; Blumenthal, R.S.; et al. Impact of coronary computed tomographic angiography results on patient and physician behavior in a low-risk population. *Arch. Intern. Med.* **2011**, *171*, 1260–1268. [CrossRef]

110. Herzog, B.A.; Wyss, C.A.; Husmann, L.; Gaemperli, O.; Valenta, I.; Treyer, V.; Landmesser, U.; Kaufmann, P.A. First head-to-head comparison of effective radiation dose from low-dose 64-slice CT with prospective ECG-triggering versus invasive coronary angiography. *Heart* **2009**, *95*, 1656–1661. [CrossRef]

111. Benz, D.C.; Gräni, C.; Hirt Moch, B.; Mikulicic, F.; Vontobel, J.; Fuchs, T.; Stehli, J.; Clerc, O.; Possner, M.; Pazhenkottil, A.; et al. A low-dose and an ultra-low-dose contrast agent protocol for coronary CT angiography in a clinical setting: Quantitative and qualitative comparison to a standard dose protocol. *Br. J. Radiolody* **2017**, *90*, 1–10. [CrossRef]

112. Litt, H.; Gatsonis, C.; Snyder, B.; Singh, H.; Miller, C.; Entrikin, D.; Leaming, J.; Gavin, L.; Pacella, C.; Hollander, J. CT Angiography for Safe Discharge of Patients with Possible Acute Coronary Syndromes. *N. Engl. J. Med.* **2012**, *366*, 1393–1403. [CrossRef]

113. Wyler von Ballmoos, M.; Haring, B.; Juillerat, P.; Alkadhi, H. Meta-analysis: Diagnostic Performance of Low-Radiation-Dose Coronary Computed Tomography Angiography. *Ann. Intern. Med.* **2011**, *154*, 413–420. [CrossRef]

114. Goldstein, J.A.; Chinnaiyan, K.M.; Abidov, A.; Achenbach, S.; Berman, D.S.; Hayes, S.W.; Hoffmann, U.; Lesser, J.R.; Mikati, I.A.; Neil, B.J.O.; et al. The CT-STAT (Coronary Computed Tomographic Angiography for Systematic Triage of Acute Chest Pain Patients to Treatment) Trial. *J. Am. Coll. Cardiol.* **2011**, *58*, 1414–1422. [CrossRef]

115. Hachamovitch, R.; Hayes, S.W.; Friedman, J.D.; Cohen, I.; Berman, D.S. Comparison of the short-term survival benefit associated with revascularization compared with medical therapy in patients with no prior coronary artery disease undergoing stress myocardial perfusion single photon emission computed tomography. *Circulation* **2003**, *107*, 2900–2906. [CrossRef]

116. Petoumenos, K.; Law, M. Comment HIV-infection and comorbidities: A complex mix. *Lancet HIV* **2015**, *2*, e265–e266. [CrossRef]

117. Gharib, A.M.; Abd-Elmoniem, K.Z.; Pettigrew, R.I.; Hadigan, C. Noninvasive Coronary Imaging for Atherosclerosis in Human Immunodeficiency Virus Infection. *Curr. Probl. Diagn. Radiol.* **2011**, *40*, 262–267. [CrossRef]

118. Van Velzen, J.E.; Schuijf, J.D.; De Graaf, F.R.; Boersma, E.; Pundziute, G.; Spanó, F.; Boogers, M.J.; Schalij, M.J.; Kroft, L.J.; De Roos, A.; et al. Diagnostic performance of non-invasive multidetector computed tomography coronary angiography to detect coronary artery disease using different endpoints: Detection of significant stenosis vs. detection of atherosclerosis. *Eur. Heart J.* **2011**, *32*, 637–645. [CrossRef]

119. Wijns, W.; Kolh, P.; Danchin, N.; Di Mario, C.; Falk, V.; Folliguet, T.; Garg, S.; Huber, K.; James, S.; Knuuti, J.; et al. Guidelines on myocardial revascularization: The Task Force on Myocardial Revascularization of the European Society of Cardiology (ESC) and the European Association for Cardio-Thoracic Surgery (EACTS). *Eur. Heart J.* **2010**, *31*, 2501–2555.

120. Lin, F.Y.; Shaw, L.J.; Dunning, A.M.; Labounty, T.M.; Choi, J.; Weinsaft, J.W.; Koduru, S.; Gomez, M.J.; Delago, A.J.; Callister, T.Q.; et al. Mortality Risk in Symptomatic Patients with Nonobstructive Coronary Artery Disease. *J. Am. Coll. Cardiol.* **2011**, *58*, 510–519. [CrossRef]

121. Kristensen, T.S.; Kofoed, K.F.; Khl, J.T.; Nielsen, W.B.; Nielsen, M.B.; Kelbæk, H. Prognostic implications of nonobstructive coronary plaques in patients with NonST-segment elevation myocardial infarction: A multidetector computed tomography study. *J. Am. Coll. Cardiol.* **2011**, *58*, 502–509. [CrossRef]

122. Fitch, K.V.; Lo, J.; Abbara, S.; Ghoshhajra, B.; Shturman, L.; Soni, A.; Sacks, R.; Wei, J.; Grinspoon, S. Increased coronary artery calcium score and noncalcified plaque among HIV-infected men: Relationship to metabolic syndrome and cardiac risk parameters. *J. Acquir. Immune Defic. Syndr.* **2010**, *55*, 495–499. [CrossRef]

123. Lai, S.; Bartlett, J.; Lai, H.; Moore, R.; Cofrancesco, J.; Pannu, H.; Tong, W.; Meng, W.; Sun, H.; Fishman, E.K. Long-Term Combination Antiretroviral Therapy Is Associated with the Risk of Coronary Plaques in African Americans with HIV Infection. *AIDS Patient Care STDS* **2009**, *23*, 815–824. [CrossRef]

124. Loa, J.; Abbarab, S.; Shturmanc, L.; Sonic, A.; Weia, J.; Rocha-Filhoc, J.; Nasirc, K.; Grinspoona, S.K. Increased prevalence of subclinical coronary atherosclerosis detected by coronary computed tomography angiography in HIV-infected men. *AIDS* **2010**, *24*, 243–253. [CrossRef]

125. Duarte, H.; Matta, J.R.; Muldoon, N.; Masur, H.; Hadigan, C.; Gharib, A.M. Non-calcified coronary plaque volume inversely related to CD4(+)T-cell count in HIV infection. *Antivir. Ther.* **2012**, *17*, 763–767. [CrossRef]

126. Post, W.S.; Haberlen, S.A.; Zhang, L. HIV infection is associated with progression of high risk coronary plaques in the MACS. In Proceedings of the Conference on Retroviruses and Opportunistic Infections, Boston, MA, USA, 4–7 March 2018.

127. Ma, G.S.; Cotter, B.R. HIV and cardiovascular disease: much ado about nothing? *Eur. Heart J.* **2018**, *39*, 2155–2157. [CrossRef]

128. Tunstall-Pedoe, H.; Kuulasmaa, K.; Amouyel, P.; Arveiler, D.; Rajakangas, A.M.; Pajak, A. Myocardial infarction and coronary deaths in the World Health Organization MONICA Project. Registration procedures, event rates, and case-fatality rates in 38 populations from 21 countries in four continents. *Circulation* **1994**, *90*, 583–612. [CrossRef]

129. Piepoli, M.; Hoes, A.; Agewall, S.; Albus, C.; Brotons, C.; Catapano, A.; Cooney, M.-T.; Corra, U.; Verschuren, W.M.M. New European guidelines for cardiovascular disease prevention in clinical practice. *Clin. Chem. Lab. Med.* **2009**, *47*, 2315–2381.

130. Huber, M.; Ledergerber, B.; Sauter, R.; Young, J.; Fehr, J.; Cusini, A.; Battegay, M.; Calmy, A.; Orasch, C.; Nicca, D.; et al. Outcome of smoking cessation counselling of HIV-positive persons by HIV care physicians. *HIV Med.* **2012**, *13*, 387–397. [CrossRef]

131. Guajira, T.P.; Xiuhong, L.; Post, W.S.; Jacobson, L.P.; Witt, M.D.; Brown, T.T.; Kingsley, L.A.; Phair, J.P.; Palella, F.J. Associations between antiretroviral use and subclinical coronary atherosclerosis. *AIDS* **2016**, *30*, 2477–2486.

132. Kovari, H.; Calmy, A.; Doco-Lecompte, T.; Nkoulou, R.; Marzel, A.; Weber, R.; Kaufmann, P.A.; Buechel, R.R.; Ledergerber, B.; Tarr, P.E. Antiretroviral Drugs Associated with Subclinical Coronary Artery Disease in the Swiss HIV Cohort Study. *Clin. Infect. Dis.* **2019**, *30*, 9.

133. Duprez, D.A.; Neuhaus, J.; Kuller, L.H.; Tracy, R.; Belloso, W.; De Wit, S.; Drummond, F.; Lane, H.C.; Ledergerber, B.; Lundgren, J.; et al. Inflammation, coagulation and cardiovascular disease in HIV-infected individuals. *PLoS ONE* **2012**, *7*, e44454. [CrossRef]

134. Calmy, A.; Gayet-Ageron, A.; Montecucco, F.; Nguyen, A.; Mach, F.; Burger, F.; Ubolyam, S.; Carr, A.; Ruxungtham, K.; Hirschel, B.; et al. HIV increases markers of cardiovascular risk: Results from a randomized, treatment interruption trial. *AIDS* **2009**, *23*, 929–939. [CrossRef]

135. Polak, J.F.; Leary, D.H.O. Carotid Intima-Media Thickness as Surrogate for and Predictor of CVD. *Glob. Heart* **2016**, *11*, 295–312. [CrossRef]

136. Du, J.; Wasserman, A.; Tong, W. Cholesterol Is Associated with the Presence of a Lipid Core in Carotid Plaque of Asymptomatic, Young-to-Middle-Aged African Americans with and without HIV Infection and Cocaine Use Residing in Inner-City Baltimore, Md., USA. *Cerebrovasc. Dis.* **2012**, *21287*, 295–301. [CrossRef]

137. Labounty, T.M.; Hardy, W.D.; Fan, Z.; Yumul, R.; Li, D.; Dharmakumar, R.; Conte, A.H. Carotid artery thickness is associated with chronic use of highly active antiretroviral therapy in patients infected with human immunode fi ciency virus: A 3.0 Tesla magnetic resonance imaging study. *Br. HIV Assoc.* **2016**, *17*, 516–523.

138. Mee, T.C.; Aepfelbacher, J.; Krakora, R.; Chairez, C.; Kvaratskhelia, N.; Smith, B.; Sandfort, V.; Hadigan, C.; Morse, C.; Hammoud, D.A. Carotid magnetic resonance imaging in persons living with HIV and 10-year atherosclerotic cardiovascular disease risk score Short communication Carotid magnetic resonance imaging in persons living with HIV and 10-year atherosclerotic cardiovascular diseas. *Antivir. Ther.* **2018**, *23*, 695–698. [CrossRef]

139. Rose, K.A.M.; Vera, J.H.; Drivas, P.; Banya, W.; Pennell, D.J.; Winston, A. Europe PMC Funders Group Atherosclerosis is evident in treated HIV-infected subjects with low cardiovascular risk by carotid cardiovascular magnetic resonance. *J. Acquir. Immune Defic. Syndr.* **2016**, *71*, 514–521. [CrossRef]

140. Wasserman, B.A. Advanced Contrast-Enhanced MRI for Looking Beyond the Lumen to Predict Stroke Building a Risk Profile for Carotid Plaque. *Stroke* **2010**, *41*, 12–16. [CrossRef]

141. Wasserman, B.A.; Wityk, R.J.; Iii, H.H.T.; Virmani, R. Low-Grade Carotid Stenosis Looking Beyond the Lumen With MRI. *Stroke* **2005**, *36*, 2504–2513. [CrossRef]

142. Fayad, Z.A.; Fuster, V.; Fallon, J.T.; Jayasundera, T.; Worthley, S.G.; Helft, G.; Aguinaldo, J.G.; Badimon, J.J.; Sharma, S.K. Noninvasive In Vivo Human Coronary Artery Lumen and Wall Imaging Using Black-Blood Magnetic Resonance Imaging. *Circulation* **2000**, *102*, 506–510. [CrossRef]

143. U-king-im, J.M.; Trivedi, R.A.; Sala, E.; Graves, M.J.; Higgins, N.J.; Cross, J.C.; Hollingworth, W.; Coulden, R.A.; Kirkpatrick, P.J.; Antoun, N.M.; et al. Evaluation of carotid stenosis with axial high-resolution black-blood MR imaging. *Eur. Radiol.* **2004**, *14*, 1154–1161. [CrossRef]

144. Krishnamurthy, R.; Cheong, B.; Muthupillai, R. Tools for cardiovascular magnetic resonance imaging. *Cardiovasc. Dis. Ther.* **2014**, *4*, 104–125.

145. Saam, T.; Habs, M.; Buchholz, M.; Schindler, A.; Bayer-karpinska, A.; Cyran, C.C.; Yuan, C.; Reiser, M.; Helck, A. Expansive arterial remodeling of the carotid arteries and its effect on atherosclerotic plaque composition and vulnerability: An in-vivo black-blood 3T CMR study in symptomatic stroke patients. *J. Cardiovasc. Magn. Reson.* **2016**, *18*, 11. [CrossRef]

146. Al-Smadi, A.S.; Abdalla, R.N.; Elmokadem, A.H.; Shaibani, A.; Hurley, M.C.; Potts, M.B.; Jahromi, B.S.; Carroll, T.J.; Ansari, S.A. Diagnostic Accuracy of High-Resolution Black-Blood MRI in the Evaluation of Intracranial Large-Vessel Arterial Occlusions. *Am. J. Neuroradiol.* **2019**, *40*, 1–6. [CrossRef]

147. Ripa, R.S.; Knudsen, A.; Hag, A.M.F.; Lebech, A.; Loft, A.; Sune, H. Feasibility of simultaneous PET/MR of the carotid artery: first clinical experience and comparison to PET/CT. *Am. J. Nucl. Med. Mol. Imaging* **2013**, *3*, 361–371.

148. Floris-moore, M.A.; Fayad, Z.A.; Berman, J.W.; Schoenbaum, E.E.; Klein, R.S.; Weinshelbaum, K.B.; Fuster, V.; Howard, A.A.; Lo, Y.; Schecter, D. Association of HIV Viral Load with Monocyte Chemoattractant Protein-1 and Atherosclerosis Burden Measured by Magnetic Resonance Imaging. *AIDS* **2010**, *23*, 941–949. [CrossRef]

149. Bai, X.; Lv, P.; Liu, K.; Li, Q.; Ding, J.; Qu, J.; Lin, J. 3D Black-Blood Luminal Angiography Derived from High-Resolution MR Vessel Wall Imaging in Detecting MCA Stenosis: A Preliminary Study. *Am. J. Neuroradiol.* **2018**, *39*, 1827–1832. [CrossRef]

150. Eiden, S.; Beck, C.; Venhoff, N.; Elsheikh, S.; Id, G.I.; Urbach, H.; Id, S.M. High-resolution contrast-enhanced vessel wall imaging in patients with suspected cerebral vasculitis: Prospective comparison of whole-brain 3D T1 SPACE versus 2D T1 black blood MRI at 3 Tesla. *PLoS Med.* **2019**, *14*, 1–14. [CrossRef]

151. Takano, K.; Hida, K.; Iwaasa, M. Three-Dimensional Spin-Echo-Based Black-Blood MRA in the Detection of Vasospasm Following Subarachnoid Hemorrhage. *J. Magn. Reson. Imaging* **2018**, *49*, 800–887. [CrossRef]

152. Suri, M.; Qiao, Y.; Ma, X.; Guallar, E.; Zhou, J.; Zhang, Y.; Liu, L.; Chu, H.; Qureshi, A.I.; Alonso, A.; et al. Prevalence of Intracranial Atherosclerotic Stenosis Using High-Resolution Magnetic Resonance Angiography in the General Population The Atherosclerosis Risk in Communities Study. *Stroke* **2016**, *47*, 1187–1193. [CrossRef]

153. Dearborn, J.L.; Zhang, Y.; Qiao, Y.; Suri, M.F.; Liu, L.; Gottesman, R.F.; Rawlings, A.M.; Mosley, T.H.; Alonso, A.; Knopman, D.S.; et al. Intracranial atherosclerosis and dementia The Atherosclerosis Risk in Communities (ARIC) Study. *Neurology* **2017**, *88*, 1556–1563. [CrossRef]

154. Jiemy, F.W.; Heeringa, P.; Kamps, J.A.A.M.; van der Laken, C.J.; Slart, R.H.J.A.; Brouwer, E. Positron emission tomography (PET) and single photon emission computed tomography (SPECT) imaging of macrophages in large vessel vasculitis: Current status and future prospects. *Autoimmun. Rev.* **2018**, *17*, 715–726. [CrossRef]

155. Longenecker, C.T.; Sullivan, C.E.; Morrison, J.; Hileman, C.O.; Zidar, D.A.; Gilkeson, R.; O'Donnell, J.; Mc Comsey, G.A. The effects of HIV and smoking on aortic and splenic inflammation. *AIDS* **2019**, *32*, 89–94. [CrossRef]

156. Lawal, I.O.; Ankrah, A.O.; Popoola, G.O. Arterial inflammation in young patients with human immunodeficiency virus infection: A cross-sectional study using F-18 FDG PET/CT. *J. Nucl. Cardiol.* **2018**. [CrossRef]

157. Zanni, M.V.; Toribio, M.; Robbins, G.K.; Burdo, T.H.; Lu, M.T.; Ishai, A.E.; Feldpausch, M.N.; Martin, A.; Melbourne, K.; Triant, V.A.; et al. Effects of Antiretroviral Therapy on Immune Function and Arterial Inflammation in Treatment-Naive Patients With Human Immunodeficiency Virus Infection. *JAMA Cardiol.* **2016**, *1*, 474–480. [CrossRef]

158. Lo, J.; Lu, M.T.; Ihenachor, E.J.; Wei, J.; Looby, S.E.; Fitch, K.V.; Oh, J.; Zimmerman, C.O.; Hwang, J.; Abbara, S.; et al. Effects of Statin Therapy on Coronary Artery Plaque Volume and High Risk Plaque Morphology in HIV-Infected Patients with Subclinical Atherosclerosis: a Randomized Double-Blind Placebo-Controlled Trial. *Lancet HIV* **2016**, *2*, e52–e63. [CrossRef]

159. Knudsen, A.; Fisker, M.; Loft, A.; Lebech, A.; Ripa, S. HIV infection and arterial inflammation assessed by 18 F-fluorodeoxyglucose (FDG) positron emission tomography (PET): A prospective cross-sectional study. *J. Nucl. Cardiol.* **2015**, *22*, 372–380. [CrossRef]

160. Tawakol, A.; Lo, J.; Zanni, M.; Marmarelis, E.; Ihenachor, E.; MacNabb, M.; Wai, B.; Hoffmann, U.; Abbara, S.; Grinspoon, S. Increased Arterial Inflammation Relates to High-risk Coronary Plaque Morphology in HIV-Infected Patients. *J. Acquir. Immune Defic. Syndr.* **2015**, *66*, 164–171. [CrossRef]

161. Yarasheski, K.E.; Laciny, E.; Overton, E.T.; Reeds, D.N.; Harrod, M.; Baldwin, S.; Dávila-román, V.G. 18FDG PET-CT PET-CT imaging detects arterial inflammation and early atherosclerosis in HIV-infected adults with cardiovascular disease risk factors. *J. Inflamm.* **2012**, *9*, 1–9. [CrossRef]

162. Subramanian, S.; Tawakol, A.; Burdo, T.H.; Wei, J.; Corsini, E.; Hoffmann, U.; Williams, K.C.; Lo, J.; Grinspoon, S.K. Arterial Inflammation in Patients With HIV. *JAMA* **2012**, *308*, 379–386. [CrossRef]

163. Mhlanga, J.C.; Durand, D.; Tsai, H.-L.; Durand, C.M.; Leal, J.P.; Wang, H.; Moore, R.; Wahl, R.L. Differentiation of HIV-associated lymphoma from HIV-associated reactive adenopathy using quantitative FDG PET and symmetry. *Eur. J. Nucl. Med. Mol. Imaging* **2014**, *41*, 596–604. [CrossRef]

164. Esmail, H.; Lai, R.P.; Lesosky, M.; Wilkinson, K.A.; Graham, C.M.; Coussens, A.K.; Oni, T. Europe PMC Funders Group Characterization of progressive HIV-associated tuberculosis using 2-deoxy-2-[^{18}F] fluoro-D-glucose positron emission and computed tomography. *Nat. Med.* **2017**, *22*, 1090–1093. [CrossRef]

165. Hammoud, D.A.; Boulougoura, A.; Papadakis, G.Z.; Wang, J.; Dodd, L.E.; Rupert, A.; Higgins, J.; Roby, G.; Metzger, D.; Laidlaw, E.; et al. Increased Metabolic Activity on 18 F-Fluorodeoxyglucose Positron Emission Tomography-Computed Tomography in Human Immunodeficiency Virus-Associated Immune Reconstitution Inflammatory Syndrome. *Clin. Infect. Dis.* **2019**, *68*, 229–238. [CrossRef]

166. Hammoud, D.A.; Sinharay, S.; Steinbach, S.; Wakim, P.G. Global and regional brain hypometabolism on FDG-PET in treated HIV-infected individuals. *Neurology* **2018**, *91*, 1–12. [CrossRef]

167. Schreiber-stainthorp, W.; Sinharay, S.; Srinivasula, S.; Shah, S.; Wang, J.; Dodd, L.; Lane, H.C.; Di Mascio, M.; Hammoud, D.A. Brain ^{18}F-FDG PET of SIV-infected macaques after treatment interruption or initiation. *J. Neuroinflammation* **2018**, *15*, 1–9. [CrossRef]

168. Obel, N.; Omland, L.H.; Kronborg, G.; Larsen, C.S.; Pedersen, C.; Pedersen, G.; Sørensen, H.T.; Gerstoft, J. Impact of Non-HIV and HIV risk factors on survival in HIV-Infected patients on HAART: A Population-Based nationwide cohort study. *PLoS ONE* **2011**, *6*, 5–10. [CrossRef]

169. Gueler, A.; Moser, A.; Calmy, A.; Günthard, H.F.; Bernasconi, E.; Furrer, H.; Fux, C.A.; Battegay, M.; Cavassini, M.; Vernazza, P.; et al. Life expectancy in HIV-positive persons in Switzerland: Matched comparison with general population. *AIDS* **2017**, *31*, 427–436. [CrossRef]

170. Mangili, A.; Gerrior, J.; Tang, A.M.; Leary, D.H.O.; Polak, J.K.; Schaefer, E.J.; Gorbach, S.L.; Wanke, C.A. Risk of Cardiovascular Disease in a Cohort of HIV-Infected Adults: A Study Using Carotid Intima-Media Thickness and Coronary Artery Calcium Score. *Clin. Infect. Dis.* **2006**, *43*, 1482–1489. [CrossRef]

171. Hsue, P.Y.; Ordovas, K.; Lee, T.; Reddy, G.; Gotway, M.; Schnell, A.; Ho, J.E.; Selby, V.; Madden, E.; Martin, J.N.; et al. Carotid Intima-Media Thickness Among Human Immunodeficiency Virus-Infected Patients Without Coronary Calcium. *Am. J. Cardiol.* **2012**, *109*, 742–747. [CrossRef]

172. Andreini, D. Screening CT Angiography in Asymptomatic Diabetes Mellitus? *JACC Cardiovasc. Imaging* **2016**, *9*, 1301–1303. [CrossRef]

173. Roffi, M.; Patrono, C.; Collet, J.P.; Mueller, C.; Valgimigli, M.; Andreotti, F.; Bax, J.J.; Borger, M.A.; Brotons, C.; Chew, D.P.; et al. [2015 ESC Guidelines for the management of acute coronary syndromes in patients presenting without persistent ST-segment elevation. Task Force for the Management of Acute Coronary Syndromes in Patients Presenting without Persistent ST-Segment Elevation of the European Society of Cardiology (ESC)]. *Eur. Heart J.* **2016**, *37*, 267–315.

174. The SCOT Heart Investigators Coronary CT Angiography and 5-Year Risk of Myocardial Infarction. *N. Engl. J. Med.* **2018**, *379*, 924–933. [CrossRef]

175. Hoffmann, U.; Udelson, J.E. Imaging Coronary Anatomy and Reducing Myocardial Infarction. *N. Engl. J. Med.* **2018**, *379*, 977–978. [CrossRef]

176. Ryan, T.; Affandi, J.S.; Gahungu, N.; Dwivedi, G. Noninvasive Cardiovascular Imaging: Emergence of a Powerful Tool for Early Identification of Cardiovascular Risk in People Living With HIV. *Can. J. Cardiol.* **2019**, *35*, 260–269. [CrossRef]

7

Ganglionated Plexi Ablation for the Treatment of Atrial Fibrillation

Sahar Avazzadeh [1,†]⬤, **Shauna McBride** [1,†], **Barry O'Brien** [2], **Ken Coffey** [2], **Adnan Elahi** [3,4]⬤,
Martin O'Halloran [3], **Alan Soo** [5] **and Leo. R Quinlan** [1,*]⬤

[1] Physiology and Human Movement Laboratory, CÚRAM SFI Centre for Research in Medical Devices,
     School of Medicine, Human biology building, National University of Ireland (NUI) Galway,
     H91 TK33 Galway, Ireland; sahar.avazzadeh@nuigalway.ie (S.A.); shauna.mcbride@nuigalway.ie (S.M.)
[2] AtriAN Medical Limited, Unit 204, NUIG Business Innovation Centre, Upper Newcastle, H91 TK33 Galway,
     Ireland; barry.obrien@atrianmedical.com (B.O.); ken.coffey@atrianmedical.com (K.C.)
[3] Translational Medical Devise Lab (TMD Lab), Lambe Institute of Translational Research, University College
     Hospital Galway, H91 ERW1 Galway, Ireland; adnan.elahi@nuigalway.ie (A.E.);
     martin.ohalloran@nuigalway.ie (M.O.)
[4] Electrical & Electronic Engineering, School of Engineering, National University of Ireland Galway,
     H91 TK33 Galway, Ireland
[5] Department of Cardiothoracic Surgery, University Hospital Galway, Saolta Hospital HealthCare Group,
     H91 YR71 Galway, Ireland; Alan.Soo@hse.ie
*   Correspondence: leo.quinlan@nuigalway.ie;
†   Joint first author.

Abstract: Atrial fibrillation (AF) is the most common type of cardiac arrhythmia and is associated with significant morbidity and mortality. The autonomic nervous system (ANS) plays an important role in the initiation and development of AF, causing alterations in atrial structure and electrophysiological defects. The intrinsic ANS of the heart consists of multiple ganglionated plexi (GP), commonly nestled in epicardial fat pads. These GPs contain both parasympathetic and sympathetic afferent and efferent neuronal circuits that control the electrophysiological properties of the myocardium. Pulmonary vein isolation and other cardiac catheter ablation targets including GP ablation can disrupt the fibers connecting GPs or directly damage the GPs, mediating the benefits of the ablation procedure. Ablation of GPs has been evaluated over the past decade as an adjunctive procedure for the treatment of patients suffering from AF. The success rate of GP ablation is strongly associated with specific ablation sites, surgical techniques, localization techniques, method of access and the incorporation of additional interventions. In this review, we present the current data on the clinical utility of GP ablation and its significance in AF elimination and the restoration of normal sinus rhythm in humans.

Keywords: atrial fibrillation; ganglionated plexi; autonomic nervous system; ablation

1. Introduction

Atrial Fibrillation presents clinically as chaotic electrical excitation that is detrimental to normal atrial contractility [1]. AF is the most common form of cardiac dysrhythmia and is categorized as a supraventricular tachyarrhythmia, which will affect 18 million people in Europe and 6–12 million in the United States by 2060 and 2050, respectively [2–5]. AF is generally classified as either paroxysmal, persistent, or long-standing persistent, and its presentation can in fact evolve and change over time [6]. The effects of AF can be life-threatening, as insufficient contraction of the atria results in blood stasis which promotes the formation of thromb-oemboli which effect the heart but can also propagate to other vital organs [7,8]. Despite many advances in recent years, no specific etiological factor has been pinpointed as the main cause of AF. Some epidemiological and clinical factors such as abnormalities associated with metabolism, endocrine function and genetics, are known to predispose patients to AF [6,9]. Furthermore, pathophysiological factors such as electrical and structural remodelling, inflammation, and local autonomic system regulation are also seen with AF [10]. Evidence from the literature highlights the role of the intrinsic and extrinsic autonomic nervous system (ANS) in cardiac function, the underlying mechanism of altered electrical activity in AF is not fully understood [11]. Altered autonomic activity is recognised as a significant component in both the initiation and maintenance of AF [12,13]. The incidence of atrial arrhythmias is reported to reduce when ANS innervation is significantly decreased [14,15]. The activity of the intrinsic cardiac ANS is found to be disrupted in cases of AF, with studies associating vagal interference with networks of GPs [16,17]. GPs are normally found in close proximity with epicardial fat pads and reside in discrete locations on the atria and ventricles, particularly surrounding the pulmonary veins (PV) and great vessels [18]. Numerous trials employing a variety of therapeutic interventions for cardiac disease have been completed to date, with some targeting GPs for AF treatment. The complex anatomical layout and physiological interconnectivity of these GP sites is important in understanding the pathophysiology of AF [19]. Our aim is to address the association of GPs with AF and document the extant literature reporting the impact of GP ablation procedures recorded in human clinical studies.

2. Cardiac Autonomic Nervous System

Components of the peripheral, central and intrinsic cardiac innervation systems form a complex interconnected network that manages cardiovascular function [19,20]. The cardiac ANS is organised into extrinsic and intrinsic components that are supplied by the autonomic nerves. The intrinsic ANS is comprised of clusters of neurons known as GPs that interconnect not only to the atria and ventricles, but also to the extrinsic cardiac ANS. The extrinsic sympathetic innervation arises in the grey matter of the thoracic spinal cord segments T1–T6 and are generally myelinated fibres, that increase heart rate and myocardial contractility by releasing noradrenaline, stimulating inotropy in the heart [18,20] (Figure 1). Noradrenaline (NE) binds to β1-adrenoceptors increasing sodium permeability, thereby increasing heart rate [20]. Parasympathetic fibres arise in the medulla oblongata, pons and midbrain of the brainstem, with some fibres arising from the sacral portion of the spinal cord (S2–S4). The resting heart is dominated by parasympathetic tone, which acts to reduce heart rate and slow cardiac impulses from the atria to the ventricles (Figure 1) through the release of acetylcholine (ACh).The binding of ACh to G-protein coupled muscarinic receptors (M2) activates inhibitory G proteins, reducing both the rate of depolarization and force of contraction of the atria [20]. This is achieved by reducing intracellular cyclic-AMP (cAMP) formation, reversing sympathetic effects on ion channels and Ca^{2+} handling.

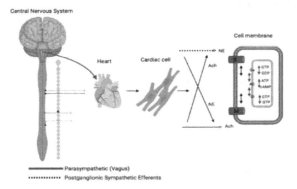

Figure 1. Sympathetic and parasympathetic mechanism in the autonomic nervous system (ANS). Parasympathetic vagal activity (in red) inhibits noradrenaline (NE) which in turn inhibit acetylcholine release (ACh). Released ACh binds to M muscarinic receptors (M) and, through the inhibition of Protein G1, coupled to adenylate cyclase (AC). Released NE from postganglionic sympathetic nerve endings (dotted line) binds to β-adrenergic receptors (β) which activate AC increasing intracellular cyclic-AMP (cAMP).

Role of the ANS in the Pathogenesis of AF

Experimental and clinical studies have reinforced the important role of the ANS in AF pathogenesis, initiation and maintenance [12]. Factors including alteration of ion currents, atrial myocardial metabolism and local autonomic regulation are responsible for the multifactorial induction of AF [21]. Reports show that pulmonary vein (PV) focal firing and AF can arise by GP stimulation at the PV-atrial junctions [22,23]. Less commonly, focal initiation of AF can be seen related to ectopic activity from the muscular sleeves of the Superior vena cava (SVC), ligament of Marshall, or regions elsewhere on the left and right atria which possibly coincide with GPs in those regions [24].

Changes in autonomic tone prior to AF onset have commonly been noted [25]. The underlying mechanism behind this is the effect of inward Ca^{2+} and/or outward K^+ current and the shortening of action potential duration observed in patients with paroxysmal AF [26]. Cervical vagal stimulation causes the release of ACh which activates outward K^+ currents in atrial myocytes, substantially shortening the action potential duration [27,28]. This has been proven to facilitate the onset and maintenance of AF in patients [29–31]. In addition, direct stimulation of GPs is commonly followed by hyperactivity and excess secretion of neurotransmitters, creating ideal conditions for AF initiation and continuation [32]. Excess release of ACh and catecholamines has been shown to result in rapid electrical firing of GPs from both PV and non-PV sites [32,33]. Studies by Po et al. investigated the effects of ACh directly injected into GPs in a canine model of AF and showed it to induce focal firing of PVs and sustained AF [23]. Thus it appears that GP stimulation not only triggers AF in patients, but also directly impacts atrial conduction properties [34]. This influence stems from both sympathetic and parasympathetic branches of the ANS, with the parasympathetic appearing as the predominant branch [34]. GPs provide a site for AF maintenance as autonomic activity was found to increase firing in six-hour rapid atrial pacing recorded from the right anterior GP, showing a decrease in the effective refractory period [35]. A shortening of atrial refractory period (AERP) is commonly seen in AF or rapid atrial pacing [36]. In a canine models of AF, GP ablation reversed electrical remodelling, implying that GP ablation may prove to be a promising strategy for the management of AF in patients [37].

3. Ganglionated Plexi

GPs are localised neural clusters of intrinsic cardiac ganglia, containing local circuits, parasympathetic neurons, and sympathetic afferent and efferent [38]. The variety of neuronal contributions associated with each ganglion reflects their complex synaptology [39]. GPs typically contain 200–1000 neurons and are variable in size, with predominantly oval-shaped soma [17,40]. Histological studies show the mean area of a human ganglia to be 0.07 ± 0.02 mm^2, with few exceeding 0.2 mm^2 [41]. Neurons within GPs vary in their projection orientation (unipolar, multipolar) (Figure 2), neurochemical profiles, and abundance on the atria (approx. 400 per GP) and ventricles (approx. 5–40) [40,42,43].

| Smooth unipolar | Unsmooth unipolar | Multipolar with single long processes | Multipolar with numerous long processes |

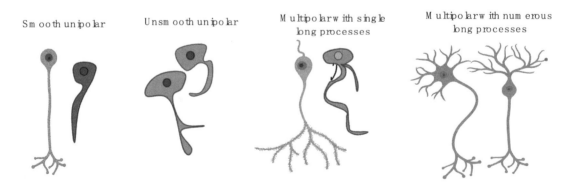

Figure 2. Different morphology of neurons found in ganglionated plexi (GP) sites in humans. There are three types of neurons that are populated in GP sites. These are either unipolar (brown, blue) or multipolar (green, red) having either single (brown, blue, green) or multiple (red) processes.

GPs are typically found embedded in epicardial adipose tissue (EAT) and have been described as having a 'raisin in bread' pattern, forming chain-like extensions onto the atria and ventricles [44]. The degree of EAT coverage varies in quantity and depth, and is generally concentrated along the coronary sulcus and interventricular and atrioventricular grooves [45,46]. The electrophysiological characteristics of three distinct epicardial fat pads have been investigated previously. These are located at the intersection of the right atrium and right superior PV (Right Pulmonary Vein-RPV fat pad), the junction of the left atrium and IVC (IVC-LA fat pad), and between the root of the aorta and SVC (SVC-Ao fat pad) superior to the right pulmonary artery [47–49] (Figure 3).

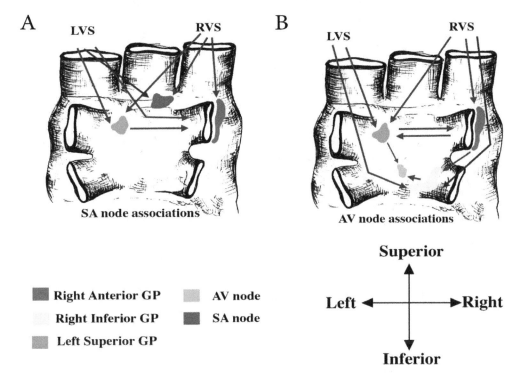

Figure 3. Posterior view of the atria showing the interactions between neural pathways. (**A**): Arrows indicate the direction of impulse and the connections of the left vagosympathetic trunk (LVS) and right vagosympathetic trunk (RVS) with the anterior right (AR) and superior left (SL) GPs. These pathways have been shown to modulate the effects of the sinoatrial node (SA) node and attenuate sinus rate slowing. (**B**): Arrows indicate the direction of impulse and connections involving the LVS and RVS trunks, with the SL, AR and inferior right (IR) GP's. These pathways have been shown to influence atrioventricular node (AV) node function and ventricular rate response. The inferior left GP (ILGP) acts as a pivotal element in the connection pathway to the AV node.

Anatomical Location of GPs

In general, GP locations are concentrated on the posterior regions of the atria and the posterior-superior aspect of the ventricles [39] (Figure 3). Knowledge of GP location and their axonal projection pathways are important when considering targeted therapeutic interventions. GPs are found in the posterior portion of the left and right atria (Figure 4), termed the dorso-atrial region, and at the transition from atria to ventricle at the level of the tricuspid and bicuspid valves, in the annular-ventricular region. They are also found around the aorta and pulmonary trunk in the peri-great vessel region, and between the aorta and superior vena cava in the aorto-caval region [50,51]. It is estimated that 75% of epicardial ganglia reside on the dorsal aspect of the heart [41].

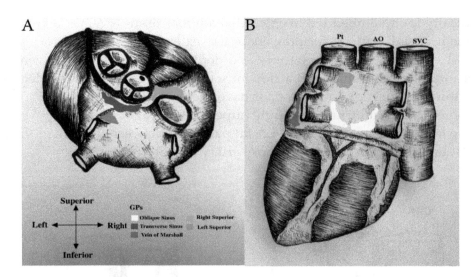

Figure 4. GP's targeted for ablation. A posterior view of the heart showing all the main ganglionated plexi sites essential for ablation. (**A**) These include the transverse sinus (in purple) and superior right (in green) located between aorta (AO) and superior vena cava (SVC). (**B**) The oblique sinus GPs (in yellow) are situated supero-anterior to the right superior pulmonary vein (PV) (ARPV) and infero-posterior region of the right inferior PV (IRPV). The left superior (in orange) can be found medial to the left superior PV (SLPV). Vein of Marshall (in red) is another target ablation region within the ligament of Marshall. Pt, pulmonary trunk.

There are four GP's found in the vicinity of the PVs that are regularly targeted in ablation procedures [52]. Each of these GPs innervate the PVs and the surrounding left atrial myocardium [52]. The superior left GP (SLGP) is located superolateral and medial to the left superior PV and extends around its root [16,44,53] (Figure 3). The SLGP is associated with both the sino-atrial (SA) and atrio-ventricular (AV) nodes, influencing sinus and ventricular rate [54,55]. The anterior right (AR) GP is situated supero-anterior to the right superior PV [52]. This GP has been found to have the most prominent interconnections converging with the SA node, where it acts as an integration center connecting the extrinsic ANS to the SA node [52]. The inferior left GP (ILGP) is located infero-posterior to the left inferior PV and has electrophysiological associations with the AV node, and can induce ventricular slowing caused by left vago-sympathetic stimulation [55]. Finally, the inferior right (IR) ganglion can be found in the infero-posterior region of the right inferior PV. The right inferior ganglion has associations with the AV node [52–54,56]. Together, the ILGPs and IRGPs are retro-atrial and termed the Oblique Sinus GPs [50].

The circuitry connecting the PV ganglia can be categorized according to the region first in contact with the vago-sympathetic trunk [54]. They can be separated into three individual pathways, with the SLGP linked to one circuit and the ARGP linked to two. The neural route, the right vago-sympathetic trunk-ARGP-SA node, is the predominant pathway and is linked to the left and right vago-sympathetic trunks where it modulates sinus rhythm and shortens the atrial refractory period, without disrupting the AV node [54,57] (Figure 3). The IRGP acts primarily on the AV node, and influences ventricular rate slowing responses induced by vago-sympathetic stimulation [54,56]. Ablation studies have shown that the SLGP does not augment sinus rhythm, but stimulation by the AR, IL and IR GPs cause an increase in rate [57].

The morphology of PVs has also been an area of interest to electrophysiologists. As the vein approaches the ostium, atrial tissue doubles over its circumference forming a fragmented myocardial sheath of pacemaker cardiomyocytes and multilayer muscles [58,59]. These myocyte layers are arranged in bundles that are predominantly spiral and circularly orientated [60]. They often associate with other bundles forming a 'mesh-like' assortment of longitudinal and oblique fibers. Ectopic foci have been found to emanate from PVs that can fire at random and induce atrial depolarization [60,61]. A number of groups have shown that the PV sites and the junction between the PVs and left atrium are abundantly enriched with innervation from both sympathetic and parasympathetic nerves, which may contribute to the frequent disruption of signals by GPs in the vicinity [59,62,63]. Experimental and clinical evaluations from some studies have suggested that the formation of spontaneous electrical discharges from PV sites is the result of abnormal automaticity, triggered activity or micro re-entry of electrical signals [60]. Other reports suggest the triggering to be due to PV-associated ganglia rather than the PV itself [64]. An influx of ACh has been touted as central to the stimulation of PV ganglia, inducing PV firing by re-entry pathways in other works [65]. The effect of Ach is to reduce action potential duration in the PV sleeves, causing them to fire until suppressed. Therefore, elimination of PV trigger sites by ablation of the associated ganglia removes the influential vagal drivers which contribute to maintaining AF [65].

The Vein of Marshall (VOM) within the Ligament of Marshall (LOM) contains another common target region for ablation procedures [50,53,66]. The VOM extends from the coronary sinus, between the left PVs and left atrial appendage, then traverses between the base of the left superior PV and pulmonary artery before attaching to the pericardium superiorly [67,68]. In this general region the VOM, myocardial sleeve and autonomic ganglia are found, with the ganglia located in a fat pad between the left PVs and left atrial appendage [67–69] Studies have shown that the LOM may act as a conduit of sympathetic innervation between the ventricles and the left superior ganglia [67]. In some patients, the LOM is an electrically active bypass of the left atrium/PV junction, rendering PV isolation ineffective [53].

There is growing interest in some of the more anatomically inaccessible GPs for ablation purposes. The Transverse Sinus GP (TSGP) resides between the pulmonary artery and base of the aorta, within the transverse sinus. It is sometimes referred to as the Great Artery GP in accordance with its associations [39]. The Aorto-caval or Superior Vena Caval-Aortic ganglion (SVC-Ao) is found along the posteromedial wall of the superior vena cava, the anterolateral wall of the ascending aorta and superior to the right pulmonary artery [70]. It is also referred to as the Superior Right (SR) GP. The SVC-Ao GP was believed to be a large, sprawling GP expanding from the anterolateral aspect of the aorta to the posterior portion of the aorta [71]. However, more recently it is suggested that two separate GPs reside in this area, the TS GP and the SVC-Ao GP. The TS GP and SVC-Ao GP are not as commonly targeted for ablation compared to other GPs and have mainly been targeted in canine studies [72,73] (Table 1).

This is owing primarily to the difficulty in accessing them, with an epicardial approach preferred over an endocardial approach to avoid ablation within the great vessels [66]. The aorto-caval ganglion receives preganglionic parasympathetic innervation from the vagus nerve, while its postganglionic neurons send impulses to the atrium and superior vena cava. The SVC-Ao GP is believed to be the 'head station' for extrinsic cardiac ANS innervation to the heart [73]. Previous studies have shown this GP to shorten the effective refractory period and increase the window of vulnerability to arrhythmias at all atrial and PV sites influenced by stimulation of the vagal trunk [73]. It is also known to act as a trigger of SVC [73] (Figure 4). Hyperactivity of the SVC-Ao GP is also known induce ACh injection which acts as a trigger for SVC firing, but the exact mechanism is not entirely understood and requires further study [72,73] (Figure 4).

Table 1. Ganglionated plexi as main target for AF.

Author, Year	GP Sites Ablated	Localization of GPs	Additional Intervention	Number of Patients	Control Group	Method of Access	Follow Up Period (Max)	Outcome
Iso K et al., 2019	Ligament of Marshall (LOM,) SL, AR, IL, IR	High frequency stimulation (HFS)	Pulmonary vein isolation (PVI)	42	-	Endocardial	N/A	(1) R-R interval was longer in patients with AF. (2) More active GPs were found in patients with AF.
Garabelli P et al., 2018	SL, LL, RL, AR	HFS	PVI	18	-	Endocardial	1.8 ± 0.8 years	(1) 48% freedom from AF in GP ablation alone. (2) 74% freedom of AF in in GP ablation + PVI.
Budera P et al., 2018	LOM, SL, AR, IL, IR	HFS	PVI (Box lesion)	38	-	Epicardial	12 months	(1) 82% AF free using two-staged hybrid ablation of non-paroxysmal AF.
Bagge L et al., 2017	LA GP + LOM (if identified (96%))	HFS	PVI	42	-	Epicardial	12 months	(1) 76% AF free after 12 months.
Budera P et al., 2017	LA GPs	Anatomical	PVI (Box lesion)/cavotricuspid isthmus ablation	41	-	Epicardial/endocardial	507.2 ± 201.1 days	(1) 80% AF free without ADD/re-ablation in 2 staged hybrid procedure after 1.5 years. (2) 65% AF free with ADD/re-ablation at last follow-ups.
Barta J et al., 2017	SL, AR, IR, IL, LOM	HFS	Box lesion, R + L PV isolation, lesion of LA isthmus, resection of LAA + connecting lesion of appendage base with LSIPV	35	65	Epicardial	12 months	(1) GP ablation alone showed 97.5% in NSR with ADD, 50% in NSR without ADD.
Suwalski G et al., 2017	SL, AR, IL, IR	HFS	PVI, LAA	34	-	Epicardial	3 months	(1) 85% success of GP detection based on preoperative heart rate.
Saini A et al., 2017	SL, AR, IL, IR, LOM	HFS	PVI	109	-	Epicardial	5 years	(1) 79.6% AF free without interventions (ADD, cardioversion, CA).
Baykaner T et al., 2017	SL, AR, IL, IR	HFS	N/A	97	-	Endocardial	N/A	(1) Sources of AF were found in: 47% at the SLGP site, 34% at ILGP; 14% at ARGP and 19% at IRGP sites.
Nagamoto Y et al., 2017	SL, AR, IR, IL	HFS	PVI	1	-	Endocardial	Not specified	(1) Inferior GP ablation itself did not eliminate PV potentials. (2) PVI had possibly helped eliminate PV potentials by cumulative effect.
Xhaet O et al., 2017	AR, IR, SL	HFS	PVI	20	-	Epicardial	N/A	(1) GPs are a mandatory link to the right vagus and AV node.
Romanov A et al., 2017	GPs of left atrium	HFS	N/A	1	-	Epicardial	6 months	(1) Using D-SPECTTM SUMO image acquisition created 3D cardiac electro-anatomical mapping system for GP ablation. (2) Patient was AF free with no ADD.
Takahashi K et al., 2016	LOM, SL, AR, IL, IR	HFS	PVI	40	-	Epicardial	18.6 months	(1) >80% Complex fractioned atrial electrograms (CFAE) overlay GP sites while 100% of epicardial adipose tissue (EAT) overlay GP sites.
Sharma P et al., 2016	10 sites each side	HSF + anatomical	Mini maze	67	-	Epicardial	4.5 ± 2.3 years	(1) Selective ablation of right GPs first is linked to higher rate of AF recurrence. (2) Lower number of GPs on the left side observed.
Antoine H.G. et al., 2016	SL, AR, IL, IR, LOM	HFS	PVI	117	123	Epicardial	12 months	(1) GP ablation alone did not reduce the AF occurrence during thoracoscopic surgery (70% vs. 68%).
Jiang et al., 2016	SL, AR, IL, IR	Anatomical	PVI	12	-	Epicardial	Not specified	(1) Majority of PV firing ceased after targeting GP outside of circumferential line or addition ablation along previous circular lesion.
Gelsomino S et al., 2015	SL, AR, IL, IR, LOM + Waterston groove	HSF	PVI (cox maze IV)	306	213	Epicardial	7 years	(1) GP ablations with or without cox maze IV showed no significant difference on AF recurrence NSR.
Sakamoto S et al., 2014	SL, AR, IL, IR, LOM	HSF + anatomical	Modified cox maze	30	-	Endocardial	3 months	(1) Most active GP sites were located in the Right PV antrum. (2) Anatomic GP ablation showed a greater decrease in sympathetic and parasympathetic tone.
Mamchur S et al., 2014	GPs of left atrium	Anatomical	PVI (Hybrid)	10	-	Epicardial & Endocardial	12 months	(1) 100% restoration of sinus rhythm with all patients free from arrhythmia in 6–9 months.
Zheng S et al., 2014	SL, AR, IL, IR,	HFS	PVI	89	-	Epicardial	60 months	(1) Single-procedure success rate is 56.3% for paroxysmal AF, 27.3% for persistent AF, and 25% for long-term persistent AF.
Katrisis D et al., 2013	SL, AR, IL, IR	Anatomic	PVI	242	-	Endocardial	24 months	(1) PVI group 56%, GP 48%, PVI + GP 74% maintained sinus rhythm/free from AF. (2) PVI + GP ablation is best strategy.
Kondo Y et al., 2013	SL, AR, IL, IR	HFS	PVI (Maze IV)	16	-	Epicardial	3 months	(1) 81% maintained NSR. (2) For those with active GPs, 92% maintained SR. (3) IRGP is an important pathway between other GPs and the AV node.
Malcolme-Lawes L et al., 2013	SL, AR, IL, IR	HFS	PVI (Cryoablation)	30	-	Endocardial	N/A	(1) Presence of a LA neural network with a common entry to the AV node via the IRGP.

Table 1. Cont.

Author, Year	GP Sites Ablated	Localization of GPs	Additional Intervention	Number of Patients	Control Group	Method of Access	Follow Up Period (Max)	Outcome
Pokushalov E et al., 2013	SL, AR, IL, IR, LOM	HFS	PVI	132	132	Endocardial	36 months	(1) 34% of patients without GP ablation were in sinus rhythm. (2) 49% of patients with GP ablation were in sinus rhythm.
Kasirajan V et al., 2012	SL, AR, IL, IR	Not specified	PVI	118	-	Epicardial	12 months	(1) Additional ablation needed in 5% of patients. (2) 80% had freedom from AF after single procedure with no need for antiarrhythmics.
Santini M et al., 2012	Left atrial GPs and LOM		PVI	22	-	Epicardial	22 months	(1) Ablation was successful in 73% of patients. (2) Freedom from AF was 91% without ADD.
Calo L et al., 2011	Left & Right atrial GPs	HFSand Anatomic	N/A	34	-	Endocardial	19.7 ± 5.2 months	(1) AF recurred in 29% of patients with anatomic ablation and in 76% of patients with the selective approach.
Krul S et al., 2011	SL, AR	HFS	PVI (Hybrid)	31	-	Epicardial	12 months	(1) 86% AF free after 1 year follow up without use of ADD.
Lim P et al., 2011	SL, AR, IL, IR	HFS	N/A	12	-	Endocardial	N/A	(1) Direct link between activation of the intrinsic cardiac ANS and PV ectopy.
Katritsis D et al., 2011	SL, AR, IL, IR	HFS	PVI	34	33	Endocardial	5 ± 1.3 months	(1) PVI group had 54.5% recurrence rate and re-ablation rate of 21.2%. (2) PVI + GP group had 26.5% recurrence and 17.6% re-ablation.
Mikhaylov E et al., 2011	SL, AR, IL, IR	HFS and Anatomic	PVI	35	35	Endocardial	36 months	(1) Freedom from arrhythmia without drugs at 12 months was 54.3% for GP group and 74.3% for CPVI group. (2) Re-ablation was done in 17% of GP group.
Ware A.L et al., 2011	GPs of Left and Right atrium, LOM	HFS	PVI (Maze)	20	-	Epicardial	25 months	(1) 89% of patients were free of AF. (2) 79% were in NSR. 3) 11% were in a paced rhythm.
Lim et al., 2011	GPs of Left and Right atrium	HFS	N/A	25	-	Endocardial	N/A	(1) 16% reduction in AF cycle length was found in PV adjacent to HFS site. (2) 9% reduction at PV-atrial junction.
Pokushalov E et al., 2010	SL, AR, IL, IR	No specific mapping	N/A	56	-	Endocardial	12 months	(1) 71% of patients free from AF.
Pokushalov E et al., 2010	SL, AR, IL, IR	Anatomic	N/A	89	-	Endocardial	24 ± 3 months	(1) 38.2% freedom from AF after single ablation.
Pokushlov E et al., 2009	SL, AR, IL, IR and Active GP areas	Anatomic and HFS	N/A	80	-	Endocardial	12 months	(1) Recurrence of AF was 57.5% in selective and 22.5% in anatomic.
Po S et al., 2009	SL, AR, IL, IR	HFS	PVI	83	-	Endocardial	22 months	(1) GP ablation alone decreased incidence of spontaneous PV firing from 65.1% to 14.5%. (2) Freedom from AF after first procedure was 80%.
Ohkubo K et al., 2008	SL, AR, IL, IR	HFS	PVI	21	-	Endocardial	8 months	(1) 69% of patients free from AF.
Danik S et al., 2008	SL, AR, IL, IR	HFS	PVI	18	-	Endocardial	6 weeks	(1) Early AF recurrence in 22% of patients.
Onorati F et al., 2008	Left and Right PVs, LOM	HFS	PVI (Maze)	31	44	Epicardial	12 months	(1) Freedom from AF was higher in group with GP ablation (92.9±6.9%) when compared to group without (62.5 ± 6.9%).
Pokushalov E et al., 2008	SL, AR, IL, IR	Anatomic	N/A	58	-	Endocardial	7.2 ± 0.4 months	(1) Transient vagal bradycardia was seen in 93% of patients. (2) 86.2% of patients free from AF.
Matsutani N et al., 2008	GP around Waterson's + left side + LOM	N/A	PVI	17	-	Epicardial	16.6 ± 5.7 months	(1) 90% of patients in NSR. (2) 85% weaned from AADs after 3 months.
Paskas J et al., 2007	LOM	HFS	PVI	1	-	Epicardial	6 months	(1) No AF revealed at months 1, 3 or 6. (2) Patient reported as no symptomatic AF.
Sherlag B et al., 2005	SL, AR, IL, IR	HFS	PVI	33	27	Endocardial	10 months	(1) 91% of patients were free from AF in PVI + GP ablation group, PVI alone group was 70%.

Normal sinus rhythm (NSR), Anti-arrhythmic drugs (ADD), left atrial (LA), left atrial appendage, (LAA), catheter ablation (CA), heart rate variability (HRV).

4. GP Ablation for AF

Therapeutic interventions for AF have been adapted to target the pathophysiological state involved in structural remodeling or to influence the excitation of ion channels and adrenergic receptors [21,74]. Many therapeutic approaches are employed to serve as a preventative measure, aiming to inhibit the primary occurrence of new-onset AF or secondary recurrence of AF, and are less effective in cases of persistent AF or AF with a prolonged duration [21,75,76]. Many invasive techniques have been adapted to target symptomatic drug refractory AF [77]. Surgical ablation such as the classical 'cut and sew' Cox-Maze procedures, claim a 97–99% success rate and have been deemed by some to be more effective than catheter-based approaches [78–80]. The drive to develop less aggressive techniques has encouraged the development of minimally invasive catheter-based procedures [81]. In the last 20 years, catheter cardiac ablation has become an established, fundamental treatment strategy for AF. Catheter ablation aims to relieve symptoms of AF, by eliminating the trigger of AF or altering the arrhythmogenic tissue underlying AF [80,82].

4.1. GP Localization and Its Importance for Effective Ablation

The active area of all GP sites, i.e., the GP areas where the vagal response is mostly elicited, appears significantly higher in AF compared to non-AF patients [83]. Additionally, the maximum R-R interval is significantly longer in AF patients after high frequency stimulation (HFS), when compared to non-AF groups [83]. Active GP areas are more prevalent on the right side of the PVs, with no considerable difference observed between paroxysmal, persistent and long-standing persistent AF patients [84–87] (Table 1). Ablation of active GPs on the right side of the PVs resulted in 92% sinus rhythm maintenance in patients at three month follow-up [86]. Zheng et al. reported that there are a mean of 2.8 active GP sites on the right side (Waterson's grove and LOM) compared to 1.4 on the left side [84]. A reduced number of active GPs is associated with cardiac and neural remodelling and subsequent development of AF [84]. 95% of GPs are cholinergic and when activated a local release of ACh leads to bradycardia [62]. In chronic AF, there is a down regulation in the number of available ACh receptors, weakening the vagal response from GP areas upon stimulation [62]. This suggests that the strength of the vagal response is associated with a number of active GP areas before ablation, and higher numbers of GP sites ablated are significantly correlated with reduced AF recurrence at 12-month follow-up [84]. Similar findings are reported by others where 5 active GPs were identified on the right and 2.7 on the left side [88,89]. Again, this was directly linked to higher long-term success rates in patients with a mean number of active GPs over five [84].

A recent study by Hu et al. indicates that endocardial ablation of the right anterior GPs produced a significant increase in heart rate in 93% of patients [16]. In addition, there appears to be an essential role for the right anterior GP which inhibits positive vagal responses and increases heart rate during pulmonary vein isolation (PVI) [90]. These findings demonstrate the importance of GP ablation of specific sites between the PVs and interatrial groove when targeting AF. While ablation of right-sided GPs is a significant factor in minimizing and reducing AF recurrences, active GPs on the left have also been targeted for ablation in some studies (Table 1).

The modulation of SA and AV nodal function is governed by the extrinsic cardiac ANS. Animal studies have demonstrated that GPs on the right side act as "integration centers" and are capable of modulating the effect of stimulated left-sided GPs on AV and SA nodal responses [91]. HFS of the right inferior GPs has shown how they selectively innervate the AV node in humans [92]. As previously demonstrated in animal studies, ablation and mapping of right-sided GPs in humans with HFS can lower the number and magnitude of GP activity on the left side [93]. Neural pathways between left atrial GPs and the AV node have been shown to pass through the lower right GPs [94]. In support of this, there was significantly higher AF and atrial tachyarrhythmia (AT) recurrence rates reported in patients who underwent selective GP ablation of the right side first [93]. This study also implied that ablation of one active GP out of sequential pacing is insufficient for vagal denervation [95]. It is worth noting that no significant difference was observed between patients who underwent extensive anatomical mapping instead of HFS [93].

Despite our growing understanding of the anatomical map and location of GPs, the extent to which GPs are hyperactive and are viable targets for ablation is still largely unknown. GPs can be identified and targeted by applying HFS [44,96] or by ablating at presumed anatomic sites [97,98] (Table 1). The vagal response of GPs to HFS is found to be very specific, but the sensitivity of HFS in portraying the full extent of GPs is still lacking [52]. The first comparative study was carried out by Pokushalov et al. in which they demonstrated that the AF freedom rate after 13 month follow-up was 42.5% and 77.5% in HFS-induced and anatomical mapping ablation groups, respectively [97]. An explanation for this may be the greater extent to which ablation (RF ablation in this case) targets anatomical GP regions in comparison to specific HFS mapped areas. Synchronized HFS serves as an alternative method and involves the delivery of current during the atrial refractory period. This helps identify GP ablation sites based on the activation of autonomic neural elements and has been associated with better outcomes [94]. However, this technology is only applicable for patients in sinus rhythm and further research is required for its use for persistent AF. A case report study by Romanov et al. showed that using D-SPECTTM SUMO image acquisition after injection of I-mIBG provides a 3D cardiac electro-anatomical map that can be used to identify target sites [99]. This approach can potentially increase the efficacy of the ablation procedure by accurately identifying GPs that are verified by HFS [100]. Furthermore, GPs can be identified with additional complex fractioned atrial electrograms (CFAE) around the GP area [101,102].

An additional factor is that the efficacy of GP ablation can be diminished by the surroundings, e.g., the epicardial adipose tissue (EAT) and epicardial fat pads. The location and amount (>5 mm) of EAT may act as a protective covering of the coronary vessels to prevent vascular damage, serving as an insulating cushion to targeted epicardial sites, and minimizing the efficiency of thermal-based ablation strategies [103]. 80% and 100% of the major five anatomical GP sites are found and overlaid at CFAE sites and left atrium-EAT respectively [104]. GP ablation through positive vagal response by HFS stimulation on CFAE areas has shown sinus rhythm maintenance in 71% of patients with paroxysmal AF [102]. Extensive ablation of these CFAE areas defines the boundaries for GP ablation [102,104]. Left atrium-EAT and CFAE areas have similar distribution, and are adjacent to vagal response sites [101,104]. Ablation of the anterior fat pads has also been investigated, with many contradictory results recorded [105,106].

4.2. Technical Procedures for GP Ablation

RF ablation is a well-established technique for GP ablation and is employed in many ablation procedures (Table 1) [107]. Cryoablation is not as commonly used, despite being found to significantly reduce the surface area of GPs, with the SL and ARGPs most dramatically reduced overall [108]. However, with increased reports of its efficacy in treating AF, interest is growing in cryoablation as a stand-alone ablation modality and in the development of cryoablation devices [109]. Cryoablation can also be used in conjunction with RF to target GPs and achieve PVI [107,108]. One study presented a comparison between a group (35 patients) with PVI treated with cryoablation and an additional GP ablation and a group (65 patients) with only PVI, which showed comparable results of sinus rhythm maintenance at 94% and 89% at 12 months, respectively [107].

The extent to whether GP ablation alone contributes to successful abolition of AF is not clear and early experiments by Pokushalov et al. conducted using RF show freedom from AF in 77.5% of patients with paroxysmal AF [97]. A similar outcome was recorded in another of their studies that included 56 patients with paroxysmal AF which yielded a 71% success rate upon ablation of GPs [110]. Furthermore, the same group demonstrated that GP ablation alone over the course of 24 months resulted in freedom of AF in 38.2% of patients with persistent AF, in comparison to higher success rate in 12 months follow up studies [111]. This work also revealed that the success rate increased substantially (59.6%) after performing additional ablation procedures, suggesting that GP ablation may be most effective when accompanied by other ablative procedures such as PVI, rather than a single-shot approach. Interestingly, comparison of results from a single ablation procedure at 13 months and 24 months in two studies by the Pokushalov group showed success to be 77.5% and 38.2%, respectively. Patient numbers were similar in these two studies which may stand as a good comparison for incorporating the long-term effects of GP ablation; however, the types of AF did vary [97,111]. It is plausible that the different success rates may be influenced by the type of AF with a typically lower success related to persistent AF and a higher rate associated with paroxysmal AF [97,111].

PVI is associated with denervation of the ANS and a significant reduction in AF recurrence [82]. Most studies have incorporated PVI into their GP ablation procedures. Investigation of comparative studies of PVI and GP ablation alone or as combined procedures present intriguing results. Studies have shown that a stand-alone PVI yields higher success rates than GP ablation procedures alone [112,113]. However, in studies comparing PVI alone with PVI + GP, the success rate increases from anywhere between 20% and 28% in short-term follow-up of less than 12 months [114,115]. Success of PVI + GP ablation procedures can range from anywhere between 50% and 91% in studies involving all types of AF (paroxysmal, persistent and long-standing persistent) [116,117]. Higher success rates have been associated with paroxysmal AF patients in comparison to long-standing persistent patients at 86% and 50%, respectively [116]. However, some studies recorded high success rates in patients with persistent and long-standing AF, showing an incoherence between AF subtypes [118]. Typically, PVI with GP ablation are carried out in one session or in two stages, giving the patient time to recover between procedures. Hybrid procedures involving initial endocardial PVI followed by GP ablation at a later stage have been trialed on patients with persistent or long-standing persistent AF. The outcome of these procedures shows a high success rate of 93% and 82% at 12 month follow-up, respectively [119,120]. It is plausible that hybrid procedures may be more appropriate in treating these types of AF. The addition of PVI to GP ablation procedures increases the success rate regardless of AF type; however, more testing would be required throughout AF groups to delineate the most appropriate and efficient procedure.

The 'mini-Maze' procedure and Dallas lesion set are examples of adaptations that have been made to some procedures where epicardial PVI is incorporated into lesion sets, with promising results. RF energy is used as an adaption from the original Cox Maze 'cut and sew' methods. These methods can either intentionally or unintentionally integrate the ablation or intersection of GPs into their lesion sets [93]. Mini-maze procedures with intentional GP ablation has proved to be successful in treating AF in previous work. Outcomes recorded from two studies over sixteen months conducted by Onorati et al. and Matsutani et al. showed 83 ± 7.9% freedom from AF (75 patients) and 90% of (18) patients in sinus rhythm [118,121]. A Dallas lesion set modified from the Cox Maze III procedure also shows some potential for AF treatment [122]. A long-term two year follow-up has shown the Dallas lesion set to bring freedom from AF in 80.6% of patients with long-standing persistent AF [123,124].

These are similar data to those reported in Cox Maze studies that incorporated both paroxysmal and persistent AF in their study population [123]. It is possible that the extensive lesions formed during these procedures may in fact be important for treating particularly difficult and advanced AF cases and may inadvertently have included GPs in the lesions. Endocardial and epicardial access during PVI procedures have been associated with unintentional damage and incidental ablation at GP sites [125].

PVI via thermal epicardial approaches can result in overlap of ablation lesions with numerous GP sites, while the endocardial thermal approaches may induce collateral damage by conductive heating. For PVI with GP ablation, mapping can be used to locate gaps in ablation lines to test for electrical block in targeted areas [124]. Epicardial access for GP ablation with PVI yielded a rate of freedom from AF ranging from anywhere between 65% and 90% [121,126]. Similarly, the endocardial approach yielded 73.5%–91% freedom from AF [115,117]. Success rates involving GP ablation mainly appear to be similar, whether procedures are done via epicardial or endocardial approach.

4.3. GP Ablation for Non-AF Cardiovascular Conditions

GP ablation may offer an alternative way of treating other conditions that are related to an imbalance of cardiac ANS activity. Post operational AF (POAF) typically appears two–five days after cardiac surgery and can be associated with serious complications including cardiac failure, stroke and death [100]. Ablation of GP sites has been shown to significantly lower the incidence of POAF by 93% in a randomized controlled trial after coronary artery bypass grafting [88]. However, this approach is sometimes not clinically desirable. To avoid ablation with its destruction of anatomical structures and capacity for collateral damage, alternative measures have been examined, for example involving the neurotoxin Botulism produced by the bacterium Clostridium Botulinum [127]. Studies have shown that the intraoperative injection of Botulism toxin into epicardial fat pads can significantly reduce instances of POAF [127]. The neurotoxin temporarily blocks the exocytotic release of ACh and diminishes sympathetic and parasympathetic activity, highlighting the involvement of autonomic imbalance and GP activation in the mechanism of POAF. The effects of the Botulism toxin can last anywhere between one and six months and provide a better, untaxing alternative to the use of β-blocker medication. In studies by Pokushalov et al. and Romanov et al. the number of AF recurrences in patients administered Botulism injections showed a decrease of AF instances (7% Botulism group, 30% Placebo group, and 23.3% Botulism group, 50% Placebo group) at 12 and 36 months, respectively [127,128]. The Botulism toxin was found to induce a pronounced alteration of heart rate variability (HRV) in patients at six months, with heart rate parameters remaining significantly reduced during follow-up [127].

5. Discussion

The ablation of GPs appears to be an efficacious technique for improving outcomes of patients with paroxysmal, persistent and long-standing persistent forms of AF. Nonetheless, some very important questions remain unanswered. The long-term outcomes of GP ablation, the precise location and depth of GPs, and the exact mechanism in which GP ablation results in improved outcomes for AF are still not fully understood. Similarly, the ablation techniques used pose a risk of damaging the myocardium and surrounding structures.

Collateral damage is a significant drawback to current thermal ablation techniques. Cardiac tamponade, PV stenosis, oesophageal fistula and thrombi are among the associated risks with current ablation energies [1]. Another drawback to thermal ablation is the difficulty in delivering precise, appropriate energy to GPs. While GPs in association with PVs are accessed with relative ease, others are found in concealed locations. Overall, there is also significant complexity involved in catheter positioning from both within the pericardial space and the heart itself. Additionally a more efficient and effective visualization of GPs using imaging techniques such as SPECT^{TM} SUMO (Spectrum Dynamics Medical Limited, Caesarea, Israel) and I-mIBG may provide additional information for a much better localization before ablation [99]. These advances have significantly propelled research over the last decade. While the understanding of GP location is sometimes obscure, this may be due to the degree of anatomical variability between individuals [125]. However, the specifics in terms of report accuracy of the GPs that are targeted in some research papers remain ambiguous, with some studies not including nor clearly describing which GPs, or where they ablated [123,124]. This causes difficulty when comparing results from different studies targeting specific GPs associated with the maintenance of neural pathways and their subsequent effects on the SA and AV nodes [86,94]. Similarly, in some procedures with PVI + GP ablation, no clear reference is made to which GPs are ablated or whether there is an overlap of PVI lesions with targeted GP sites, making it challenging to compare success rates linked to GP ablation [120].

Augmented success rates (by 21%, 20% or 28%) with combined procedures is evident thus far only in short term follow-up (12 months or under) and with small patient numbers [61,115,118]. The added success of the PVI + GP ablation procedures in comparison to PVI alone is much lower (8%, 2.5% and 5%) in long-term follow ups (two–five years); however these studies include many more patients [107,114,129]. Due to the different techniques and study designs in clinical studies in the literature, it is difficult to assess and make a true comparison of success. HRV has been found to be a predictor of ablation success and is a useful, non-invasive tool for investigating cardiac autonomic tone [130,131]. HRV measures the fluctuations of time intervals between consecutive heartbeats [132]. An increased heart rate has been found to have positive associations with freedom from AF [130]. A recent study by Goff et al. showed a correlation between HRV in patients with paroxysmal AF who previously underwent PVI and the recurrence of AF [130]. While HRV is not always associated with PVI, an average increase of 60.6 ± 11.3 to 70.7 ± 12.0 beats per minute was recorded in 53% of patients at 12 months follow-up in this study [130]. Overall, it is evident that sufficient disruption of vagal responses results in an increased HR and freedom from AF. Coinciding with an adjusted HR is a shortening of AERP [133]. This has been found to facilitate the genesis and coexistence of numerous signals linked to AF [134]. Studies have shown the relationship between shortening of fibrillation intervals and AERP [36,135]. Additionally, the mean AERP has been reported to be shorter in persistent AF than those with paroxysmal AF due to electrical remodelling [136]. Reports by Lee et al. have also linked prolonged AERP with future development of AF with possible induction of remodelling over a twelve year follow-up [133,137]. Dispute remains over the relationship of action potential and refractory period in AF initiation, despite extensive animal and human studies [133]. Despite its importance, AERP is not a common parameter measured by clinicians. This may be owing to the technicalities associated with the recording of AERP in humans, in particular its inability to be recorded during AF [138].

In addition, it is possible that the positive post-procedural effects of GP ablation may only persist for a short amount of time. It may also be plausible that the GPs are not entirely ablated, enabling regeneration and the formation of new re-entrant pathways around the proximity of the GP, due to thermal myocardial damage caused by RF for example. Another reason for a low, long-term success rate may be the internal or external factors influencing remodeling of the heart over time. Concern exists regarding the proarrhythmic relationship between GP ablation without PVI. This approach carries the risk of inducing increased atrial parasympathetic and sympathetic innervation, coupled with a decreased atrial effective refractory period [139]. Similarly, selective GP ablation has been linked to the formation of macro-re-entrant atrial tachycardias which may be associated with autonomic reinnervation [139]. Animal studies have linked reinnervation at four weeks post-GP ablation with the selectivity of the regions targeted [140,141]. Therefore, further study must be carried out to understand what may or may not cause this relapse to AF and what changes can be made to increase the denervation time induced by GP ablation, and reduce the occurrence of pro-arrhythmia. Currently sample size is a major limitation in many studies with numbers ranging from individual case studies to research including up to 306 patients [142,143]. Evidently, variation in patient population will significantly influence success percentages, making it difficult to draw accurate comparisons.

Despite our evolving understanding of the physiology and success associated with GP ablation in AF treatment, the complications and challenges are not yet fully understood. Most patients involved in GP ablation procedures experience paroxysmal, persistent or long-standing persistent AF with some studies comparing all three [116]. Patients with symptomatic AF or AF associated with valvular disease are also included in research studies [95,144]. Similarly, investigations into specific AF types are not consistent, which leads to difficulty in assessing the extent to which GP ablation is effective. In a large randomized control during thoracoscopic surgery, there were no reported benefits of GP ablation in patients exhibiting advanced AF [114]. This may further suggest that the role of the ANS in the disease progression of AF may diminish over time [64]. Therefore, while varying degrees of AF have been examined, the true success of GP ablation for each type remains ambiguous. Nevertheless, from the expansive research and meta-analysis undergone on GP ablation, results show that it does give relief from AF in most cases, both initially and in the long term [145,146]. While much work is required to provide consistency between experiments, it is evident that the potential exists for significant advances in the treatment of AF through targeted ablation of GP sites.

Author Contributions: S.A. and S.M. for Conceptualization, investigation, resources, writing—original draft preparation, writing—review and editing. B.O. for writing—review and editing, funding acquisition. K.C. for writing—review and editing, funding acquisition. A.E., M.O. and A.S. for writing—review and editing. L.R.Q. for Conceptualization, investigation, resources, writing—review and editing, supervision. All authors have read and agreed to the published version of the manuscript.

References

1.   Safaei, N.; Montazerghaem, H.; Azarfarin, R.; Alizadehasl, A.; Alikhah, H. Radiofrequency ablation for treatment of atrial fibrillation. *BioImpacts* **2011**, *1*, 171–177.

2.   De Bakker, J.M.T.; Ho, S.Y.; Hocini, M. Basic and clinical electrophysiology of pulmonary vein ectopy. *Cardiovasc. Res.* **2002**, *54*, 287–294. [CrossRef]

3.   Wang, T.J.; Parise, H.; Levy, D.; D'Agostino, R.B.; Wolf, P.A.; Vasan, R.S.; Benjamin, E.J. Obesity and the risk of new-onset atrial fibrillation. *J. Am. Med. Assoc.* **2004**, *292*, 2471–2477. [CrossRef] [PubMed]

4.   Kim, M.H. Concepts in Disease Progression of Atrial Fibrillation and Implications for Medical Management. *J. Innov. Card. Rhythm Manag.* **2012**, *3*, 697–712.

5.   Morillo, C.A.; Banerjee, A.; Perel, P.; Wood, D.; Jouven, X. Atrial fibrillation: The current epidemic. *J. Geriatr. Cardiol.* **2017**, *14*, 195–203. [PubMed]

6.   Fuster, V.; Rydén, L.E.; Cannom, D.S.; Crijns, H.J.; Curtis, A.B.; Ellenbogen, K.A.; Halperin, J.L.; Kay, G.N.; Le Huezey, J.Y.; Lowe, J.E.; et al. 2011 ACCF/AHA/HRS focused updates incorporated into the ACC/AHA/ESC 2006 guidelines for the management of patients with atrial fibrillation: A report of the American College of Cardiology Foundation/American Heart Association Task Force on Practice Guidel. *Circulation* **2011**, *123*, e269–e367. [CrossRef]

7.   Nattel, S. New ideas about atrial fibrillation 50 years on. *Nature* **2002**, *415*, 219–226. [CrossRef]

8.   Patten, M.; Pecha, S.; Aydin, A. Atrial fibrillation in hypertrophic cardiomyopathy: Diagnosis and considerations for management. *J. Atr. Fibrillation* **2018**, *10*, 1556. [CrossRef]

9.   Allessie, M.A.; Boyden, P.A.; Camm, A.J.; Kléber, A.G.; Lab, M.J.; Legato, M.J.; Rosen, M.R.; Schwartz, P.J.; Spooner, P.M.; Van Wagoner, D.R.; et al. Pathophysiology and prevention of atrial fibrillation. *Circulation* **2001**, *103*, 769–777. [CrossRef]

10.   Kourliouros, A.; Savelieva, I.; Kiotsekoglou, A.; Jahangiri, M.; Camm, J. Current concepts in the pathogenesis of atrial fibrillation. *Am. Heart J.* **2009**, *157*, 243–252. [CrossRef]

11.   Calkins, H.; Hindricks, G.; Cappato, R.; Kim, Y.H.; Saad, E.B.; Aguinaga, L.; Akar, J.G.; Badhwar, V.; Brugada, J.; Camm, J.; et al. 2017 HRS/EHRA/ECAS/APHRS/SOLAECE expert consensus statement on catheter and surgical ablation of atrial fibrillation. *Heart Rhythm* **2017**, *14*, e275–e444. [CrossRef] [PubMed]

12.   Schauerte, P.; Scherlag, B.J.; Patterson, E.; Scherlag, M.A.; Matsudaria, K.; Nakagawa, H.; Lazzara, R.; Jackman, W.M. Focal atrial fibrillation: Experimental evidence for a pathophysiologic role of the autonomic nervous system. *J. Cardiovasc. Electrophysiol.* **2001**, *12*, 592–599. [CrossRef] [PubMed]

13.   Shen, M.J.; Choi, E.K.; Tan, A.Y.; Lin, S.F.; Fishbein, M.C.; Chen, L.S.; Chen, P.S. Neural mechanisms of atrial arrhythmias. *Nat. Rev. Cardiol.* **2012**, *9*, 30–39. [CrossRef]

14.   Shen, M.J.; Shinohara, T.; Park, H.-W.; Frick, K.; Ice, D.S.; Choi, E.-K.; Han, S.; Maruyama, M.; Sharma, R.; Shen, C.; et al. Continuous Low-Level Vagus Nerve Stimulation Reduces Stellate Ganglion Nerve Activity and Paroxysmal Atrial Tachyarrhythmias in Ambulatory Canines. *Circulation* **2011**, *123*, 2204–2212. [CrossRef] [PubMed]

15.   Leiria, T.L.L.; Glavinovic, T.; Armour, J.A.; Cardinal, R.; de Lima, G.G.; Kus, T. Longterm effects of cardiac mediastinal nerve cryoablation on neural inducibility of atrial fibrillation in canines. *Auton. Neurosci. Basic Clin.* **2011**, *161*, 68–74. [CrossRef]

16.   Hu, F.; Zheng, L.; Liang, E.; Ding, L.; Wu, L.; Chen, G.; Fan, X.; Yao, Y. Right anterior ganglionated plexus: The primary target of cardioneuroablation? *Heart Rhythm* **2019**, *16*, 1545–1551. [CrossRef]

17.   Choi, E.K.; Zhao, Y.; Everett, T.H.; Chen, P.S. Ganglionated plexi as neuromodulation targets for atrial fibrillation. *J. Cardiovasc. Electrophysiol.* **2017**, *28*, 1485–1491. [CrossRef]

18. Hasan, W. Autonomic cardiac innervation: Development and adult plasticity. *Organogenesis* **2013**, *9*, 176–193. [CrossRef]

19. Kapa, S.; Venkatachalam, K.L.; Asirvatham, S.J. The Autonomic Nervous System in Cardiac Electrophysiology. *Cardiol. Rev.* **2010**, *18*, 275–284. [CrossRef]

20. Gordan, R.; Gwathmey, J.K.; Xie, L.-H. Autonomic and endocrine control of cardiovascular function. *World J. Cardiol.* **2015**, *7*, 204. [CrossRef]

21. Savelieva, I.; Kakouros, N.; Kourliouros, A.; Camm, A.J. Upstream Therapies for Management of Atrial Fibrillation: Review of Clinical Evidence and Implications for European Society of Cardiology Guidelines. Part II: Secondary Prevention. *Eurospace* **2011**, *13*, 610–625. [CrossRef] [PubMed]

22. Zhou, J.; Scherlag, B.J.; Edwards, J.; Jackman, W.M.; Lazzara, R.; Po, S.S. Gradients of Atrial Refractoriness and Inducibility of Atrial Fibrillation due to Stimulation of Ganglionated Plexi. *J. Cardiovasc. Electrophysiol.* **2007**, *18*, 83–90. [CrossRef]

23. Po, S.S.; Scherlag, B.J.; Yamanashi, W.S.; Edwards, J.; Zhou, J.; Wu, R.; Geng, N.; Lazzara, R.; Jackman, W.M. Experimental model for paroxysmal atrial fibrillation arising at the pulmonary vein-atrial junctions. *Heart Rhythm* **2006**, *3*, 201–208. [CrossRef] [PubMed]

24. Markides, V.; Schilling, R.J. Atrial fibrillation: Classification, pathophysiology, mechanism and drug treatment. *Heart* **2003**, *89*, 939–943. [CrossRef] [PubMed]

25. Bettoni, M.; Zimmermann, M. Autonomic tone variations before the onset of paroxysmal atrial fibrillation. *Circulation* **2002**, *105*, 2753–2759. [CrossRef]

26. Patterson, E.; Po, S.S.; Scherlag, B.J.; Lazzara, R. Triggered firing in pulmonary veins initiated by in vitro autonomic nerve stimulation. *Heart Rhythm* **2005**, *2*, 624–631. [CrossRef]

27. Zaza, A.; Malfatto, G.; Schwartz, P.J. Effects on atrial repolarization of the interaction between K^+ channel blockers and muscarinic receptor stimulation. *J. Pharmacol. Exp. Ther.* **1995**, *273*, 1095–1104.

28. Krapivinsky, G.; Gordon, E.A.; Wickman, K.; Velimirović, B.; Krapivinsky, L.; Clapham, D.E. The G-protein-gated atrial K^+ channel IKAch is a heteromultimer of two inwardly rectifying K^+-channel proteins. *Nature* **1995**, *374*, 135–141. [CrossRef]

29. Krummen, D.E.; Bayer, J.D.; Ho, J.; Ho, G.; Smetak, M.R.; Clopton, P.; Trayanova, N.A.; Narayan, S.M. Mechanisms of human atrial fibrillation initiation clinical and computational studies of repolarization restitution and activation latency. *Circ. Arrhythm. Electrophysiol.* **2012**, *5*, 1149–1159. [CrossRef]

30. Roney, C.H.; Siong Ng, F.; Debney, M.T.; Eichhorn, C.; Nachiappan, A.; Chowdhury, R.A.; Qureshi, N.A.; Cantwell, C.D.; Tweedy, J.H.; Niederer, S.A.; et al. Determinants of new wavefront locations in cholinergic atrial fibrillation. *Europace* **2018**, *20*, iii3–iii15. [CrossRef]

31. Quan, K.J.; Lee, J.H.; Geha, A.S.; Biblo, L.A.; Hare, G.F.; Mackall, J.A.; Carlson, M.D. Characterization of Sinoatrial Parasympathetic Innervation in Humans. *J. Cardiovasc. Electrophysiol.* **1999**, *10*, 1060–1065. [CrossRef] [PubMed]

32. Kurotobi, T.; Shimada, Y.; Kino, N.; Ito, K.; Tonomura, D.; Yano, K.; Tanaka, C.; Yoshida, M.; Tsuchida, T.; Fukumoto, H. Features of intrinsic ganglionated plexi in both atria after extensive pulmonary isolation and their clinical significance after catheter ablation in patients with atrial fibrillation. *Heart Rhythm* **2015**, *12*, 470–476. [CrossRef] [PubMed]

33. Ogawa, M.; Zhou, S.; Tan, A.Y.; Song, J.; Gholmieh, G.; Fishbein, M.C.; Luo, H.; Siegel, R.J.; Karagueuzian, H.S.; Chen, L.S.; et al. Left Stellate Ganglion and Vagal Nerve Activity and Cardiac Arrhythmias in Ambulatory Dogs with Pacing-Induced Congestive Heart Failure. *J. Am. Coll. Cardiol.* **2007**, *50*, 335–343. [CrossRef]

34. Krul, S.P.J.; Meijborg, V.M.F.; Berger, W.R.; Linnenbank, A.C.; Driessen, A.H.G.; Van Boven, W.J.; Wilde, A.A.M.; De Bakker, J.M.; Coronel, R.; De Groot, J.R. Disparate response of high-frequency ganglionic plexus stimulation on sinus node function and atrial propagation in patients with atrial fibrillation. *Heart Rhythm* **2014**, *11*, 1743–1751. [CrossRef] [PubMed]

35. Yu, L.; Scherlag, B.J.; Sha, Y.; Li, S.; Sharma, T.; Nakagawa, H.; Jackman, W.M.; Lazzara, R.; Jiang, H.; Po, S.S. Interactions between atrial electrical remodeling and autonomic remodeling: How to break the vicious cycle. *Heart Rhythm* **2012**, *9*, 804–809. [CrossRef]

36. Wijffels, M.C.E.F.; Kirchhof, C.J.H.J.; Dorland, R.; Allessie, M.A. Atrial fibrillation begets atrial fibrillation: A study in awake chronically instrumented goats. *Circulation* **1995**, *92*, 1954–1968. [CrossRef] [PubMed]

37. Lu, Z.; Scherlag, B.J.; Lin, J.; Niu, G.; Fung, K.M.; Zhao, L.; Ghias, M.; Jackman, W.M.; Lazzara, R.; Jiang, H.; et al. Atrial fibrillation begets atrial fibrillation: Autonomic mechanism for atrial electrical remodeling induced by short-term rapid atrial pacing. *Circ. Arrhythm. Electrophysiol.* **2008**, *1*, 184–192. [CrossRef]

38. Hanna, P.; Shivkumar, K. Targeting the Cardiac Ganglionated Plexi for Atrial Fibrillation: Modulate or Destroy? *JACC Clin. Electrophysiol.* **2018**, *4*, 1359–1361. [CrossRef]

39. Armour, J.A.; Murphy, D.A.; Yuan, B.X.; Macdonald, S.; Hopkins, D.A. Gross and microscopic anatomy of the human intrinsic cardiac nervous system. *Anat. Rec.* **1997**, *247*, 289–298. [CrossRef]

40. Pauza, D.H.; Pauziene, N.; Pakeltyte, G.; Stropus, R. Comparative quantitative study of the intrinsic cardiac ganglia and neurons in the rat, guinea pig, dog and human as revealed by histochemical staining for acetylcholinesterase. *Ann. Anat.* **2002**, *184*, 125–136. [CrossRef]

41. Pauza, D.H.; Skripka, V.; Pauziene, N.; Stropus, R. Morphology, distribution, and variability of the epicardiac neural ganglionated subplexuses in the human heart. *Anat. Rec.* **2000**, *259*, 353–382. [CrossRef]

42. Mesiano Maifrino, L.B.; Liberti, E.A.; Castelucci, P.; Rodrigues de Souza, R. NADPH-diaphorase positive cardiac neurons in the atria of mice. A morphoquantitative study. *BMC Neurosci.* **2006**, *7*, 10. [CrossRef]

43. Jurgaitienė, R.; Paužienė, N.; Aželis, V.; Žurauskas, E. Morphometric study of age-related changes in the human intracardiac ganglia. *Medicina* **2004**, *40*, 574–581.

44. Po, S.S.; Nakagawa, H.; Jackman, W.M. Localization of left atrial ganglionated plexi in patients with atrial fibrillation: Techniques and technology. *J. Cardiovasc. Electrophysiol.* **2009**, *20*, 1186–1189. [CrossRef]

45. D'Avila, A.; Scanavacca, M.; Sosa, E.; Ruskin, J.N.; Reddy, V.Y. Pericardial anatomy for the interventional electrophysiologist. *J. Cardiovasc. Electrophysiol.* **2003**, *14*, 422–430. [CrossRef]

46. Abbara, S.; Desai, J.C.; Cury, R.C.; Butler, J.; Nieman, K.; Reddy, V. Mapping epicardial fat with multi-detector computed tomography to facilitate percutaneous transepicardial arrhythmia ablation. *Eur. J. Radiol.* **2006**, *57*, 417–422. [CrossRef]

47. Randall, W.C.; Ardell, J.L. Selective parasympathectomy of automatic and conductile tissues of the canine heart. *Am. J. Physiol.-Heart Circ. Physiol.* **1985**, *248*, H61–H68. [CrossRef]

48. Ardell, J.L.; Randall, W.C. Selective vagal innervation of sinoatrial and atrioventricular nodes in canine heart. *Am. J. Physiol.-Heart Circ. Physiol.* **1986**, *251*, H764–H773. [CrossRef]

49. Chiou, C.W.; Eble, J.N.; Zipes, D.P. Efferent vagal innervation of the canine atria and sinus and atrioventricular nodes: The third fat pad. *Circulation* **1997**, *95*, 2573–2584. [CrossRef]

50. Lachman, N.; Syed, F.F.; Habib, A.; Kapa, S.; Bisco, S.E.; Venkatachalam, K.L.; Asirvatham, S.J. Correlative anatomy for the electrophysiologist, part II: Cardiac ganglia, phrenic nerve, coronary venous system. *J. Cardiovasc. Electrophysiol.* **2011**, *22*, 104–110. [CrossRef]

51. Kapa, S.; DeSimone, C.V.; Asirvatham, S.J. Innervation of the heart: An invisible grid within a black box. *Trends Cardiovasc. Med.* **2016**, *26*, 245–257. [CrossRef] [PubMed]

52. Stavrakis, S.; Po, S. Ganglionated plexi ablation: Physiology and clinical applications. *Arrhythm. Electrophysiol. Rev.* **2017**, *6*, 186–190. [CrossRef] [PubMed]

53. Zipes, D.P.; Knope, R.F. Electrical properties of the thoracic veins. *Am. J. Cardiol.* **1972**, *29*, 372–376. [CrossRef]

54. Hou, Y.; Scherlag, B.J.; Lin, J.; Zhang, Y.; Lu, Z.; Truong, K.; Patterson, E.; Lazzara, R.; Jackman, W.M.; Po, S.S. Ganglionated Plexi Modulate Extrinsic Cardiac Autonomic Nerve Input. Effects on Sinus Rate, Atrioventricular Conduction, Refractoriness, and Inducibility of Atrial Fibrillation. *J. Am. Coll. Cardiol.* **2007**, *50*, 61–68. [CrossRef]

55. Lin, J.; Scherlag, B.J.; Niu, G.; Lu, Z.; Patterson, E.; Liu, S.; Lazzara, R.; Jackman, W.M.; Po, S.S. Autonomic elements within the ligament of marshall and inferior left ganglionated plexus mediate functions of the atrial neural network. *J. Cardiovasc. Electrophysiol.* **2009**, *20*, 318–324. [CrossRef]

56. Chen, P.S.; Chen, L.S.; Fishbein, M.C.; Lin, S.F.; Nattel, S. Role of the autonomic nervous system in atrial fibrillation: Pathophysiology and therapy. *Circ. Res.* **2014**, *114*, 1500–1515. [CrossRef]

57. Qin, M.; Zhang, Y.; Liu, X.; Jiang, W.F.; Wu, S.H.; Po, S. Atrial Ganglionated Plexus Modification: A Novel Approach to Treat Symptomatic Sinus Bradycardia. *JACC Clin. Electrophysiol.* **2017**, *3*, 950–959. [CrossRef]

58. Jiang, R.-H.; Hu, G.-S.; Liu, Q.; Sheng, X.; Sun, Y.-X.; Yu, L.; Zhang, P.; Zhang, Z.-W.; Chen, S.-Q.; Ye, Y.; et al. Impact of Anatomically Guided Ganglionated Plexus Ablation on Electrical Firing from Isolated Pulmonary Veins. *Pacing Clin. Electrophysiol.* **2016**, *39*, 1351–1358. [CrossRef]

59. Chevalier, P.; Tabib, A.; Meyronnet, D.; Chalabreysse, L.; Restier, L.; Ludman, V.; Aliès, A.; Adeleine, P.; Thivolet, F.; Burri, H.; et al. Quantitative study of nerves of the human left atrium. *Heart Rhythm* **2005**, *2*, 518–522. [CrossRef]

60. Kircher, S.; Sommer, P. Electrophysiological Evaluation of Pulmonary Vein Isolation. *J. Atr. Fibrillation* **2013**, *6*, 934. [CrossRef]

61. Scherlag, B.J.; Yamanashi, W.; Patel, U.; Lazzara, R.; Jackman, W.M. Autonomically induced conversion of pulmonary vein focal firing into atrial fibrillation. *J. Am. Coll. Cardiol.* **2005**, *45*, 1878–1886. [CrossRef] [PubMed]

62. Tan, A.Y.; Li, H.; Wachsmann-Hogiu, S.; Chen, L.S.; Chen, P.S.; Fishbein, M.C. Autonomic Innervation and Segmental Muscular Disconnections at the Human Pulmonary Vein-Atrial Junction. Implications for Catheter Ablation of Atrial-Pulmonary Vein Junction. *J. Am. Coll. Cardiol.* **2006**, *48*, 132–143. [CrossRef] [PubMed]

63. Chou, C.C.; Nihei, M.; Zhou, S.; Tan, A.; Kawase, A.; Macias, E.S.; Fishbein, M.C.; Lin, S.F.; Chen, P.S. Intracellular calcium dynamics and anisotropic reentry in isolated canine pulmonary veins and left atrium. *Circulation* **2005**, *111*, 2889–2897. [CrossRef] [PubMed]

64. Stavrakis, S.; Nakagawa, H.; Po, S.S.; Scherlag, B.J.; Lazzara, R.; Jackman, W.M. The role of the autonomic ganglia in atrial fibrillation. *JACC Clin. Electrophysiol.* **2015**, *1*, 1–13. [CrossRef]

65. Lemola, K.; Chartier, D.; Yeh, Y.H.; Dubuc, M.; Cartier, R.; Armour, A.; Ting, M.; Sakabe, M.; Shiroshita-Takeshita, A.; Comtois, P.; et al. Pulmonary vein region ablation in experimental vagal atrial fibrillation: Role of pulmonary veins versus autonomic ganglia. *Circulation* **2008**, *117*, 470–477. [CrossRef]

66. Lachman, N.; Syed, F.F.; Habib, A.; Kapa, S.; Bisco, S.E.; Venkatachalam, K.L.; Asirvatham, S.J. Correlative anatomy for the electrophysiologist, part I: The pericardial space, oblique sinus, transverse sinus. *J. Cardiovasc. Electrophysiol.* **2010**, *21*, 1421–1426. [CrossRef]

67. Rodríguez-Mañero, M.; Schurmann, P.; Valderrábano, M. Ligament and vein of Marshall: A therapeutic opportunity in atrial fibrillation. *Heart Rhythm* **2016**, *13*, 593–601. [CrossRef]

68. Nakagawa, H.; Scherlag, B.J.; Patterson, E.; Ikeda, A.; Lockwood, D.; Jackman, W.M. Pathophysiologic basis of autonomic ganglionated plexus ablation in patients with atrial fibrillation. *Heart Rhythm* **2009**, *6*, S26–S34. [CrossRef]

69. Liu, S.; Yu, X.; Luo, D.; Qin, Z.; Wang, X.; He, W.; Ma, R.; Hu, H.; Xie, J.; He, B.; et al. Ablation of the Ligament of Marshall and Left Stellate Ganglion Similarly Reduces Ventricular Arrhythmias during Acute Myocardial Infarction. *Circ. Arrhythm. Electrophysiol.* **2018**, *11*, e005945. [CrossRef]

70. Hu, T.Y.; Kapa, S.; Cha, Y.M.; Asirvatham, S.J.; Madhavan, M. Swallow-induced syncope: A case report of atrial tachycardia originating from the SVC. *Heart Case Rep.* **2016**, *2*, 83–87. [CrossRef]

71. Padmanabhan, D.; Naksuk, N.; Killu, A.K.; Kapa, S.; Witt, C.; Sugrue, A.; Desimon, C.V.; Madhavan, M.; de Groot, J.R.; O'Brien, B.; et al. Electroporation of epicardial autonomic ganglia: Safety and efficacy in medium-term canine models. *J. Cardiovasc. Electrophysiol.* **2019**, *30*, 607–615. [CrossRef]

72. Lo, L.W.; Scherlag, B.J.; Chang, H.Y.; Lin, Y.J.; Chen, S.A.; Po, S.S. Paradoxical long-term proarrhythmic effects after ablating the head station ganglionated plexi of the vagal innervation to the heart. *Heart Rhythm* **2013**, *10*, 751–757. [CrossRef]

73. Lu, Z.; Scherlag, B.J.; Niu, G.; Lin, J.; Fung, K.M.; Zhao, L.; Yu, L.; Jackman, W.M.; Lazzara, R.; Jiang, H.; et al. Functional properties of the superior Vena Cava (SVC)-aorta ganglionated plexus: Evidence suggesting an autonomic basis for rapid SVC firing. *J. Cardiovasc. Electrophysiol.* **2010**, *21*, 1392–1399. [CrossRef] [PubMed]

74. Pellman, J.; Sheikh, F. Atrial Fibrillation: Mechanisms, Therapeutics, and Future Directions. In *Comprehensive Physiology*; John Wiley & Sons, Inc.: Hoboken, NJ, USA, 2015; Volume 5, pp. 649–665.

75. Hohnloser, S.H.; Kuck, K.H.; Lilienthal, J. Rhythm or rate control in atrial fibrillation—Pharmacological intervention in atrial fibrillation (PIAF): A randomised trial. *Lancet* **2000**, *356*, 1789–1794. [CrossRef]

76. Heist, E.K.; Mansour, M.; Ruskin, J.N. Rate control in atrial fibrillation: Targets, methods, resynchronization considerations. *Circulation* **2011**, *124*, 2746–2755. [CrossRef] [PubMed]

77. Scherr, D.; Khairy, P.; Miyazaki, S.; Aurillac-Lavignolle, V.; Pascale, P.; Wilton, S.B.; Ramoul, K.; Komatsu, Y.; Roten, L.; Jadidi, A.; et al. Five-year outcome of catheter ablation of persistent atrial fibrillation using termination of atrial fibrillation as a procedural endpoint. *Circ. Arrhythm. Electrophysiol.* **2015**, *8*, 18–24. [CrossRef] [PubMed]

78. Khargi, K.; Hutten, B.A.; Lemke, B.; Deneke, T. Surgical treatment of atrial fibrillation; a systematic review. *Eur. J. Cardio-Thorac. Surg.* **2005**, *27*, 258–265. [CrossRef] [PubMed]

79. Cox, J.; Ad, N.; Palazzo, T.; Fitzpatrick, S.; Suyderhoud, J.P.; DeGroot, K.W.; Pirovic, E.A.; Lou, H.G.; Duvall, W.Z.; Kim, Y.D. Current status of the Maze procedure for the treatment of atrial fibrillation. *Elsevier* **2000**, *12*, 15–19. [CrossRef]

80. Kearney, K.; Stephenson, R.; Phan, K.; Chan, W.Y.; Huang, M.Y.; Yan, T.D. A systematic review of surgical ablation versus catheter ablation for atrial fibrillation. *Ann. Cardiothorac. Surg.* **2014**, *3*, 15–29. [CrossRef]

81. Marescaux, J.; Rubino, F. The ZEUS robotic system: Experimental and clinical applications. *Surg. Clin. N. Am.* **2003**, *83*, 1305–1315. [CrossRef]

82. Pappone, C.; Santinelli, V.; Manguso, F.; Vicedomini, G.; Gugliotta, F.; Augello, G.; Mazzone, P.; Tortoriello, V.; Landoni, G.; Zangrillo, A.; et al. Pulmonary Vein Denervation Enhances Long-Term Benefit after Circumferential Ablation for Paroxysmal Atrial Fibrillation. *Circulation* **2004**, *109*, 327–334. [CrossRef] [PubMed]

83. Iso, K.; Okumura, Y.; Watanabe, I.; Nagashima, K.; Takahashi, K.; Arai, M.; Watanabe, R.; Wakamatsu, Y.; Otsuka, N.; Yagyu, S.; et al. Is vagal response during left atrial ganglionated plexi stimulation a normal phenomenon? Comparison between patients with and without atrial fibrillation. *Circ. Arrhythm. Electrophysiol.* **2019**, *12*, 1–9. [CrossRef]

84. Zheng, S.; Zeng, Y.; Li, Y.; Han, J.; Zhang, H.; Meng, X. Active ganglionated plexi is a predictor of atrial fibrillation recurrence after minimally invasive surgical ablation. *J. Card. Surg.* **2014**, *29*, 279–285. [CrossRef] [PubMed]

85. Bagge, L.; Blomström, P.; Jidéus, L.; Lönnerholm, S.; Blomström-Lundqvist, C. Left atrial function after epicardial pulmonary vein isolation in patients with atrial fibrillation. *J. Interv. Card. Electrophysiol.* **2017**, *50*, 195–201. [CrossRef]

86. Kondo, Y.; Ueda, M.; Watanabe, M.; Ishimura, M.; Kajiyama, T.; Hashiguchi, N.; Kanaeda, T.; Nakano, M.; Hiranuma, Y.; Ishizaka, T.; et al. Identification of left atrial ganglionated plexi by dense epicardial mapping as ablation targets for the treatment of concomitant atrial fibrillation. *PACE—Pacing Clin. Electrophysiol.* **2013**, *36*, 1336–1341. [CrossRef]

87. Suwalski, G.; Marczewska, M.M.; Kaczejko, K.; Mróz, J.; Gryszko, L.; Cwetsch, A.; Skrobowski, A. Left atrial ganglionated plexi detection is related to heart rate and early recurrence of atrial fibrillation after surgical ablation. *Braz. J. Cardiovasc. Surg.* **2017**, *32*, 118–124. [CrossRef]

88. Al-Atassi, T.; Toeg, H.; Malas, T.; Lam, B.K. Mapping and ablation of autonomic ganglia in prevention of postoperative atrial fibrillation in coronary surgery: Maappafs atrial fibrillation randomized controlled pilot study. *Can. J. Cardiol.* **2014**, *30*, 1202–1207. [CrossRef]

89. Mehall, J.R.; Kohut, R.M.; Schneeberger, E.W.; Taketani, T.; Merrill, W.H.; Wolf, R.K. Intraoperative Epicardial Electrophysiologic Mapping and Isolation of Autonomic Ganglionic Plexi. *Ann. Thorac. Surg.* **2007**, *83*, 538–541. [CrossRef]

90. Hu, F.; Zheng, L.; Liu, S.; Shen, L.; Liang, E.; Ding, L.; Wu, L.; Chen, G.; Fan, X.; Yao, Y. Avoidance of Vagal Response during Circumferential Pulmonary Vein Isolation: Effect of Initiating Isolation From Right Anterior Ganglionated Plexi. *Circ. Arrhythm. Electrophysiol.* **2019**, *12*, e007811. [CrossRef]

91. Hou, Y.; Scherlag, B.J.; Lin, J.; Zhou, J.; Song, J.; Zhang, Y.; Patterson, E.; Lazzara, R.; Jackman, W.M.; Po, S.S. Interactive atrial neural network: Determining the connections between ganglionated plexi. *Heart Rhythm* **2007**, *4*, 56–63. [CrossRef]

92. Xhaet, O.; De Roy, L.; Floria, M.; Deceuninck, O.; Blommaert, D.; Dormal, F.; Ballant, E.; La Meir, M. Integrity of the Ganglionated Plexi Is Essential to Parasympathetic Innervation of the Atrioventricular Node by the Right Vagus Nerve. *J. Cardiovasc. Electrophysiol.* **2017**, *28*, 432–437. [CrossRef] [PubMed]

93. Sharma, P.S.; Kasirajan, V.; Ellenbogen, K.A.; Koneru, J.N. Interconnections between Left Atrial Ganglionic Plexi: Insights from Minimally Invasive Maze Procedures and Their Outcomes. *PACE—Pacing Clin. Electrophysiol.* **2016**, *39*, 427–433. [CrossRef] [PubMed]

94. Malcolme-Lawes, L.C.; Lim, P.B.; Wright, I.; Kojodjojo, P.; Koa-Wing, M.; Jamil-Copley, S.; Dehbi, H.M.; Francis, D.P.; Davies, D.W.; Peters, N.S.; et al. Characterization of the left atrial neural network and its impact on autonomic modification procedures. *Circ. Arrhythm. Electrophysiol.* **2013**, *6*, 632–640. [CrossRef]

95. Sakamoto, S.I.; Fujii, M.; Watanabe, Y.; Hiromoto, A.; Ishii, Y.; Morota, T.; Nitta, T. Exploration of theoretical ganglionated plexi ablation technique in atrial fibrillation surgery. *Ann. Thorac. Surg.* **2014**, *98*, 1598–1604. [CrossRef]

96. Lim, P.B.; Malcolme-Lawes, L.C.; Stuber, T.; Wright, I.; Francis, D.P.; Davies, D.W.; Peters, N.S.; Kanagaratnam, P. Intrinsic cardiac autonomic stimulation induces pulmonary vein ectopy and triggers atrial fibrillation in humans. *J. Cardiovasc. Electrophysiol.* **2011**, *22*, 638–646. [CrossRef] [PubMed]

97. Pokushalov, E.; Romanov, A.; Shugayev, P.; Artyomenko, S.; Shirokova, N.; Turov, A.; Katritsis, D.G. Selective ganglionated plexi ablation for paroxysmal atrial fibrillation. *Heart Rhythm* **2009**, *6*, 1257–1264. [CrossRef]

98. Katritsis, D.; Giazitzoglou, E.; Sougiannis, D.; Goumas, N.; Paxinos, G.; Camm, A.J. Anatomic Approach for Ganglionic Plexi Ablation in Patients with Paroxysmal Atrial Fibrillation. *Am. J. Cardiol.* **2008**, *102*, 330–334. [CrossRef]

99. Romanov, A.; Minin, S.; Breault, C.; Pokushalov, E. Visualization and ablation of the autonomic nervous system corresponding to ganglionated plexi guided by D-SPECT 123I-mIBG imaging in patient with paroxysmal atrial fibrillation. *Clin. Res. Cardiol.* **2017**, *106*, 76–78. [CrossRef]

100. Stirrup, J.; Gregg, S.; Baavour, R.; Roth, N.; Breault, C.; Agostini, D.; Ernst, S.; Underwood, S.R. Hybrid solid-state SPECT/CT left atrial innervation imaging for identification of left atrial ganglionated plexi: Technique and validation in patients with atrial fibrillation. *J. Nucl. Cardiol.* **2019**. [CrossRef]

101. Katritsis, D.; Giazitzoglou, E.; Sougiannis, D.; Voridis, E.; Po, S.S. Complex fractionated atrial electrograms at anatomic sites of ganglionated plexi in atrial fibrillation. *Europace* **2009**, *11*, 308–315. [CrossRef]

102. Pokushalov, E.; Romanov, A.; Artyomenko, S.; Shirokova, N.; Turov, A.; Karaskov, A.; Katritsis, D.G.; Po, S.S. Ganglionated Plexi Ablation Directed by High-Frequency Stimulation and Complex Fractionated Atrial Electrograms for Paroxysmal Atrial Fibrillation. *Pacing Clin. Electrophysiol.* **2012**, *35*, 776–784. [CrossRef] [PubMed]

103. D'Avila, A.; Gutierrez, P.; Scanavacca, M.; Reddy, V.; Lustgarten, D.L.; Sosa, E.; Ramires, J.A.F. Effects of radiofrequency pulses delivered in the vicinity of the coronary arteries: Implications for nonsurgical transthoracic epicardial catheter ablation to treat ventricular tachycardia. *PACE—Pacing Clin. Electrophysiol.* **2002**, *25*, 1488–1495. [CrossRef] [PubMed]

104. Takahashi, K.; Okumura, Y.; Watanabe, I.; Nagashima, K.; Sonoda, K.; Sasaki, N.; Kogawa, R.; Iso, K.; Kurokawa, S.; Ohkubo, K.; et al. Anatomical proximity between ganglionated plexi and epicardial adipose tissue in the left atrium: Implication for 3D reconstructed epicardial adipose tissue-based ablation. *J. Interv. Card. Electrophysiol.* **2016**, *47*, 203–212. [CrossRef] [PubMed]

105. White, C.M.; Sander, S.; Coleman, C.I.; Gallagher, R.; Takata, H.; Humphrey, C.; Henyan, N.; Gillespie, E.L.; Kluger, J. Impact of Epicardial Anterior Fat Pad Retention on Postcardiothoracic Surgery Atrial Fibrillation Incidence: The AFIST-III Study. *J. Am. Coll. Cardiol.* **2007**, *49*, 298–303. [CrossRef]

106. Cummings, J.E.; Gill, I.; Akhrass, R.; Dery, M.; Biblo, L.A.; Quan, K.J. Preservation of the anterior fat pad paradoxically decreases the incidence of postoperative atrial fibrillation in humans. *J. Am. Coll. Cardiol.* **2004**, *43*, 994–1000. [CrossRef]

107. Bárta, J.; Brát, R. Assessment of the effect of left atrial cryoablation enhanced by ganglionated plexi ablation in the treatment of atrial fibrillation in patients undergoing open heart surgery. *J. Cardiothorac. Surg.* **2017**, *12*, 69. [CrossRef]

108. Garabelli, P.; Stavrakis, S.; Kenney, J.F.A.; Po, S.S. Effect of 28-mm Cryoballoon Ablation on Major Atrial Ganglionated Plexi. *JACC Clin. Electrophysiol.* **2018**, *4*, 831–838. [CrossRef]

109. Baust, J.M.; Robilotto, A.; Snyder, K.; Van Buskirk, R.; Baust, J.G. Evaluation of a new epicardial cryoablation system for the treatment of Cardiac Tachyarrhythmias. *Trends Med.* **2018**, *18*. [CrossRef]

110. Pokushalov, E.; Romanov, A.; Artyomenko, S.; Turov, A.; Shirokova, N.; Katritsis, D.G. Left atrial ablation at the anatomic areas of ganglionated plexi for paroxysmal atrial fibrillation. *PACE—Pacing Clin. Electrophysiol.* **2010**, *33*, 1231–1238. [CrossRef]

111. Pokushalov, E.; Romanov, A.; Artyomenko, S.; Turov, A.; Shugayev, P.; Shirokova, N.; Katritsis, D.G. Ganglionated plexi ablation for longstanding persistent atrial fibrillation. *Europace* **2010**, *12*, 342–346. [CrossRef]

112. Mikhaylov, E.; Kanidieva, A.; Sviridova, N.; Abramov, M.; Gureev, S.; Szili-Torok, T.; Lebedev, D. Outcome of anatomic ganglionated plexi ablation to treat paroxysmal atrial fibrillation: A 3-year follow-up study. *Europace* **2011**, *13*, 362–370. [CrossRef]

113. Pantos, I.; Katritsis, G.; Zografos, T.; Camm, A.J.; Katritsis, D.G. Temporal stability of atrial electrogram fractionation in patients with paroxysmal atrial fibrillation. *Am. J. Cardiol.* **2013**, *111*, 863–868. [CrossRef]

114. Driessen, A.H.G.; Berger, W.R.; Krul, S.P.J.; van den Berg, N.W.E.; Neefs, J.; Piersma, F.R.; Yin, D.R.C.P.; de Jong, J.S.S.G.; van Boven, W.J.P.; de Groot, J.R. Ganglion Plexus Ablation in Advanced Atrial Fibrillation: The AFACT Study. *J. Am. Coll. Cardiol.* **2016**, *68*, 1155–1165. [CrossRef]

115. Katritsis, D.G.; Giazitzoglou, E.; Zografos, T.; Pokushalov, E.; Po, S.S.; Camm, A.J. Rapid pulmonary vein isolation combined with autonomic ganglia modification: A randomized study. *Heart Rhythm* **2011**, *8*, 672–678. [CrossRef]

116. Edgerton, J.R.; McClelland, J.H.; Duke, D.; Gerdisch, M.W.; Steinberg, B.M.; Bronleewe, S.H.; Prince, S.L.; Herbert, M.A.; Hoffman, S.; Mack, M.J. Minimally invasive surgical ablation of atrial fibrillation: Six-month results. *J. Thorac. Cardiovasc. Surg.* **2009**, *138*, 109–114. [CrossRef]

117. Scherlag, B.J.; Nakagawa, H.; Jackman, W.M.; Yamanashi, W.S.; Patterson, E.; Po, S.; Lazzara, R. Electrical stimulation to identify neural elements on the heart: Their role in atrial fibrillation. *J. Interv. Card. Electrophysiol.* **2005**, *13*, 37–42. [CrossRef]

118. Onorati, F.; Curcio, A.; Santarpino, G.; Torella, D.; Mastroroberto, P.; Tucci, L.; Indolfi, C.; Renzulli, A. Routine ganglionic plexi ablation during Maze procedure improves hospital and early follow-up results of mitral surgery. *J. Thorac. Cardiovasc. Surg.* **2008**, *136*, 408–418. [CrossRef]

119. Budera, P.; Osmancik, P.; Talavera, D.; Kraupnerova, A.; Fojt, R.; Zdarska, J.; Vanek, T.; Straka, Z. Two-staged hybrid ablation of non-paroxysmal atrial fibrillation: Clinical outcomes and functional improvements after 1 year. *Interact. Cardiovasc. Thorac. Surg.* **2018**, *26*, 77–83. [CrossRef]

120. Kurfirst, V.; Mokráček, A.; Bulava, A.; Čanádyová, J.; Haniš, J.; Pešl, L. Two-staged hybrid treatment of persistent atrial fibrillation: Short-term single-centre results. *Interact. Cardiovasc. Thorac. Surg.* **2014**, *18*, 451–456. [CrossRef]

121. Matsutani, N.; Takase, B.; Ozeki, Y.; Maehara, T.; Lee, R. Minimally Invasive Cardiothoracic Surgery for Atrial Fibrillation. *Circ. J.* **2008**, *72*, 434–436. [CrossRef]

122. Edgerton, J.R.; Jackman, W.M.; Mack, M.J. A New Epicardial Lesion Set for Minimal Access Left Atrial Maze: The Dallas Lesion Set. *Ann. Thorac. Surg.* **2009**, *88*, 1655–1657. [CrossRef]

123. Wang, J.G.; Xin, M.; Han, J.; Li, Y.; Luo, T.G.; Wang, J.; Meng, F.; Meng, X. Ablation in selective patients with long-standing persistent atrial fibrillation: Medium-term results of the Dallas lesion set. *Eur. J. Cardio-Thorac. Surg.* **2014**, *46*, 213–220. [CrossRef] [PubMed]

124. Lockwood, D.; Nakagawa, H.; Peyton, M.D.; Edgerton, J.R.; Scherlag, B.J.; Sivaram, C.A.; Po, S.S.; Beckman, K.J.; Abedin, M.; Jackman, W.M. Linear left atrial lesions in minimally invasive surgical ablation of persistent atrial fibrillation: Techniques for assessing conduction block across surgical lesions. *Heart Rhythm* **2009**, *6*, S50–S63. [CrossRef] [PubMed]

125. Zdarska, J.; Osmancik, P.; Budera, P.; Herman, D.; Prochazkova, R.; Talavera, D.; Straka, Z. The absence of effect of ganglionated plexi ablation on heart rate variability parameters in patients after thoracoscopic ablation for atrial fibrillation. *J. Thorac. Dis.* **2017**, *9*, 4997–5007. [CrossRef]

126. Han, F.T.; Kasirajan, V.; Kowalski, M.; Kiser, R.; Wolfe, L.; Kalahasty, G.; Shepard, R.K.; Wood, M.A.; Ellenbogen, K.A. Results of a minimally invasive surgical pulmonary vein isolation and ganglionic plexi ablation for atrial fibrillation: Single-center experience with 12-month follow-up. *Circ. Arrhythm. Electrophysiol.* **2009**, *2*, 370–377. [CrossRef]

127. Pokushalov, E.; Kozlov, B.; Romanov, A.; Strelnikov, A.; Bayramova, S.; Sergeevichev, D.; Bogachev-Prokophiev, A.; Zheleznev, S.; Shipulin, V.; Lomivorotov, V.V.; et al. Long-Term Suppression of Atrial Fibrillation by Botulinum Toxin Injection into Epicardial Fat Pads in Patients Undergoing Cardiac Surgery: One-Year Follow-Up of a Randomized Pilot Study. *Circ. Arrhythm. Electrophysiol.* **2015**, *8*, 1334–1341. [CrossRef]

128. Romanov, A.; Pokushalov, E.; Ponomarev, D.; Bayramova, S.; Shabanov, V.; Losik, D.; Stenin, I.; Elesin, D.; Mikheenko, I.; Strelnikov, A.; et al. Long-term suppression of atrial fibrillation by botulinum toxin injection into epicardial fat pads in patients undergoing cardiac surgery: Three-year follow-up of a randomized study. *Heart Rhythm* **2019**, *16*, 172–177. [CrossRef]

129. Katritsis, D.G.; Pokushalov, E.; Romanov, A.; Giazitzoglou, E.; Siontis, G.C.M.; Po, S.S.; Camm, A.J.; Ioannidis, J.P.A. Autonomic denervation added to pulmonary vein isolation for paroxysmal atrial fibrillation: A randomized clinical trial. *J. Am. Coll. Cardiol.* **2013**, *62*, 2318–2325. [CrossRef]

130. Goff, Z.D.; Laczay, B.; Yenokyan, G.; Sivasambu, B.; Sinha, S.K.; Marine, J.E.; Ashikaga, H.; Berger, R.D.; Akhtar, T.; Spragg, D.D.; et al. Heart rate increase after pulmonary vein isolation predicts freedom from atrial fibrillation at 1 year. *J. Cardiovasc. Electrophysiol.* **2019**, *30*, 2818–2822. [CrossRef]

131. Vesela, J.; Osmancik, P.; Herman, D.; Prochazkova, R. Changes in heart rate variability in patients with atrial fibrillation after pulmonary vein isolation and ganglionated plexus ablation. *Physiol. Res.* **2019**, *68*, 49–57. [CrossRef]

132. Shaffer, F.; Ginsberg, J.P. An Overview of Heart Rate Variability Metrics and Norms. *Front. Public Health* **2017**, *5*. [CrossRef]

133. Lee, J.M.; Lee, H.; Janardhan, A.H.; Park, J.; Joung, B.; Pak, H.N.; Lee, M.H.; Kim, S.S.; Hwang, H.J. Prolonged atrial refractoriness predicts the onset of atrial fibrillation: A 12-year follow-up study. *Heart Rhythm* **2016**, *13*, 1575–1580. [CrossRef]

134. Tamargo, J.; Delpón, E. Vagal Stimulation and Atrial Electrical Remodeling. *Rev. Española Cardiol.* **2009**, *62*, 729–732. [CrossRef]

135. Daoud, E.G.; Bogun, F.; Goyal, R.; Harvey, M.; Man, K.C.; Strickberger, S.A.; Morady, F. Effect of Atrial Fibrillation on Atrial Refractoriness in Humans. *Circulation* **1996**, *94*, 1600–1606. [CrossRef]

136. Uhm, J.-S.; Mun, H.-S.; Wi, J.; Shim, J.; Joung, B.; Lee, M.-H.; Pak, H.-N. Prolonged Atrial Effective Refractory Periods in Atrial Fibrillation Patients Associated with Structural Heart Disease or Sinus Node Dysfunction Compared with Lone Atrial Fibrillation. *Pacing Clin. Electrophysiol.* **2013**, *36*, 163–171. [CrossRef]

137. Li, D.; Fareh, S.; Leung, T.K.; Nattel, S. Promotion of Atrial Fibrillation by Heart Failure in Dogs. *Circulation* **1999**, *100*, 87–95. [CrossRef]

138. Sahadevan, J.; Ryu, K.; Matsuo, K.; Khrestian, C.M.; Waldo, A.L. Characterization of Atrial Activation (A-A) Intervals during Atrial Fibrillation Due to a Single Driver: Do They Reflect Atrial Effective Refractory Periods? *J. Cardiovasc. Electrophysiol.* **2011**, *22*, 310–315. [CrossRef]

139. Mao, J.; Yin, X.; Zhang, Y.; Yan, Q.; Dong, J.; Ma, C.; Liu, X. Ablation of epicardial ganglionated plexi increases atrial vulnerability to arrhythmias in dogs. *Circ. Arrhythm. Electrophysiol.* **2014**, *7*, 711–717. [CrossRef]

140. Sakamoto, S.I.; Schuessler, R.B.; Lee, A.M.; Aziz, A.; Lall, S.C.; Damiano, R.J. Vagal denervation and reinnervation after ablation of ganglionated plexi. *J. Thorac. Cardiovasc. Surg.* **2010**, *139*, 444–452. [CrossRef]

141. Oh, S.; Zhang, Y.; Bibevski, S.; Marrouche, N.F.; Natale, A.; Mazgalev, T.N. Vagal denervation and atrial fibrillation inducibility: Epicardial fat pad ablation does not have long-term effects. *Heart Rhythm* **2006**, *3*, 701–708. [CrossRef]

142. Puskas, J.; Lin, E.; Bailey, D.; Guyton, R. Thoracoscopic Radiofrequency Pulmonary Vein Isolation and Atrial Appendage Occlusion. *Ann. Thorac. Surg.* **2007**, *83*, 1870–1872. [CrossRef] [PubMed]

143. Gelsomino, S.; Lozekoot, P.; La Meir, M.; Lorusso, R.; Lucà, F.; Rostagno, C.; Renzulli, A.; Parise, O.; Matteucci, F.; Gensini, G.F.; et al. Is ganglionated plexi ablation during Maze IV procedure beneficial for postoperative long-term stable sinus rhythm? *Int. J. Cardiol.* **2015**, *192*, 40–48. [CrossRef] [PubMed]

144. Mamchur, S.E.; Mamchur, I.N.; Khomenko, E.A.; Gorbunova, E.V.; Sizova, I.N.; Odarenko, Y.N. Catheter ablation for atrial fibrillation after an unsuccessful surgical ablation and biological prosthetic mitral valve replacement: A pilot study. *J. Chin. Med. Assoc.* **2014**, *77*, 409–415. [CrossRef] [PubMed]

145. Kampaktsis, P.N.; Oikonomou, E.K.; Choi, D.Y.; Cheung, J.W. Efficacy of ganglionated plexi ablation in addition to pulmonary vein isolation for paroxysmal versus persistent atrial fibrillation: A meta-analysis of randomized controlled clinical trials. *J. Interv. Card. Electrophysiol.* **2017**, *50*, 253–260. [CrossRef]

146. Zhang, Y.; Wang, Z.; Zhang, Y.; Wang, W.; Wang, J.; Gao, M.; Hou, Y. Efficacy of Cardiac Autonomic Denervation for Atrial Fibrillation: A Meta-Analysis. *J. Cardiovasc. Electrophysiol.* **2012**, *23*, 592–600. [CrossRef] [PubMed]

8

Real-Life Incident Atrial Fibrillation in Outpatients with Coronary Artery Disease

Sandro Ninni [1,2,*], Gilles Lemesle [1,2], Thibaud Meurice [3], Olivier Tricot [4], Nicolas Lamblin [1,5] and Christophe Bauters [1,5]

[1] CHU Lille, Department of Cardiology, University of Lille, F-59000 Lille, France; gilles.lemesle@chru-lille.fr (G.L.); nicolas.lamblin@chru-lille.fr (N.L.); christophe.bauters@chru-lille.fr (C.B.)
[2] Institut Pasteur de Lille, U1011, F-59000 Lille, France
[3] Hôpital Privé Le Bois, 59003 Lille, France; tmeurice@me.com
[4] Centre Hospitalier de Dunkerque, 59240 Dunkerque, France; oliviertricot@gmail.com
[5] Institut Pasteur de Lille, U1167, F-59000 Lille, France
* Correspondence: sandro.ninni@chru-lille.fr;

Abstract: Background: The risk, correlates, and consequences of incident atrial fibrillation (AF) in patients with chronic coronary artery disease (CAD) are largely unknown. **Methods and results:** We analyzed incident AF during a 3-year follow-up in 5031 CAD outpatients included in the prospective multicenter CARDIONOR registry and with no history of AF at baseline. Incident AF occurred in 266 patients (3-year cumulative incidence: 4.7% (95% confidence interval (CI): 4.1 to 5.3)). Incident AF was diagnosed during cardiology outpatient visits in 177 (66.5%) patients, 87 of whom were asymptomatic. Of note, 46 (17.3%) patients were diagnosed at time of hospitalization for heart failure, and a few patients ($n = 5$) at the time of ischemic stroke. Five variables were independently associated with incident AF: older age ($p < 0.0001$), heart failure ($p = 0.003$), lower left ventricle ejection fraction ($p = 0.008$), history of hypertension ($p = 0.010$), and diabetes mellitus ($p = 0.033$). Anticoagulant therapy was used in 245 (92%) patients and was associated with an antiplatelet drug in half ($n = 122$). Incident AF was a powerful predictor of all-cause (adjusted hazard ratio: 2.04; 95% CI: 1.47 to 2.83; $p < 0.0001$) and cardiovascular mortality (adjusted hazard ratio: 2.88; 95% CI: 1.88 to 4.43; $p < 0.0001$). **Conclusions:** In CAD outpatients, real-life incident AF occurs at a stable rate of 1.6% annually and is frequently diagnosed in asymptomatic patients during cardiology outpatient visits. Anticoagulation is used in most cases, often combined with antiplatelet therapy. Incident AF is associated with increased mortality.

Keywords: coronary artery disease; atrial fibrillation; prognosis; anticoagulation; antiplatelet therapy

1. Introduction

Atrial fibrillation (AF) is commonly observed in patients with coronary artery disease (CAD) [1–3]. Thanks to major therapeutic advances in recent decades [4,5], survival of patients with CAD has increased considerably, leaving more opportunity for the development of age-dependent diseases such as AF. The presence of concomitant AF in CAD patients is important in daily practice. Indeed, it may target higher risk patients for both ischemic and bleeding events and critically affect patient management, especially regarding antithrombotic strategies [1,3,6]. Although the risk, correlates, and consequences of incident AF have been extensively studied in the general population [7,8], and to the best of our knowledge, data are lacking in patients with chronic CAD. In addition, how antithrombotic drugs are managed in contemporary practice in such a setting is not known. The level of evidence of guidelines is indeed very low and practices may, therefore, widely differ between physicians. Given the specificities of the CAD population (routine follow-up by cardiologists, background secondary medical prevention therapy including antiplatelet drugs, prognostic implications of concomitant diseases), we sought to investigate these issues.

We analyzed data for 5031 CAD outpatients without prevalent AF included in a prospective registry. Here, we report the incidence, correlates, diagnostic circumstances, management, and prognostic impact of a first episode of AF occurring during the 3-year study follow-up.

2. Methods

2.1. Study Population

The CARDIONOR study is a multicenter registry that enrolled 10,517 consecutive outpatients with a diagnosis of CAD, AF, and/or heart failure (HF) between January 2013 and May 2015 [9]. The patients were included by 81 cardiologists from the French Region of Nord-Pas-de-Calais during outpatient visits. Documented CAD was defined as a history of myocardial infarction (MI), coronary revascularization, and/or the presence of coronary stenosis >50% on a coronary angiogram. Documented AF was defined as a history of AF, even if in sinus rhythm at inclusion. The sole exclusion criterion was age < 18 years. Patients with other cardiovascular or non-cardiovascular illnesses or co-morbidities were not excluded.

A case record form was completed at the initial visit with information regarding demographic and clinical details of the patients, including current medications. The treating cardiologists then followed up with the patients, with the number of outpatient visits at clinician discretion. Protocol-specified follow-up was performed at three years using a standardized case record form to report clinical events. In the case of missing information, a research technician contacted general practitioners and/or patients. The identification of patients with events for adjudication was based on interviews with patients/relatives during outpatient visits, discharge summaries for hospitalization during follow-up that were sent to treating cardiologists, and information obtained by the research technician. The events that patients reported were systematically confirmed from the medical reports.

This study was approved by the French medical data protection committee and authorized by the Commission Nationale de l'Informatique et des Libertés for the treatment of personal health data. All patients consented to the study after being informed in writing of the study's objectives and treatment of the data, as well as about their rights to object and about access and rectification.

2.2. Study Design and Definitions

Figure 1 shows the study flow chart. Among the 10517 outpatients included in the CARDIONOR registry, a total of 6313 had documented CAD. We excluded 1282 patients with prevalent AF, leaving 5031 CAD patients with no history of AF at registry inclusion. For the present analysis, we focused on the 5015 patients (99%) for whom follow-up was available. Two investigators adjudicated incident AF, with a third opinion sought in cases of disagreement.

The diagnostic circumstances of AF, as well as the antithrombotic strategy, were systematically assessed and adjudicated. No specific screening was performed for AF detection; documented AF episodes, therefore, represented daily practice. Data on therapeutic management represent the initial cardiologist recommendation, as described in the medical report associated with the AF diagnosis. Patients with implanted devices who had documented atrial high rate episodes and whose treating cardiologists had diagnosed them as having probable AF (as documented in the medical report) were adjudicated as incident AF. HF was defined as a history of hospitalization for HF and/or a history of symptoms and signs of HF associated with echocardiographic evidence of systolic dysfunction, left ventricular hypertrophy, left atrial enlargement, or diastolic dysfunction. Cause of death was determined after a detailed review of the circumstances of death and classified as cardiovascular or non-cardiovascular, as previously defined [10]. Death by an unknown cause was kept as a separate category.

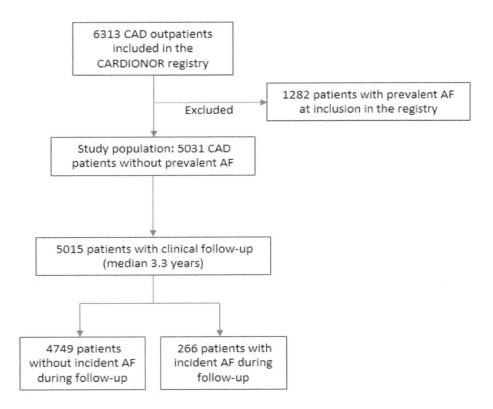

Figure 1. Study flow chart.

2.3. Statistical Analysis

Continuous variables are described as mean ± standard deviation (SD). Categorical variables are presented as absolute numbers and/or percentages. The incidence of AF was estimated with the cumulative incidence function, with death as the competing event. Univariable and multivariable assessments of baseline variables associated with incident AF were performed with the use of a cause-specific hazard model [11,12]. Hazard ratios (HRs) and 95% confidence intervals (CIs) were calculated. The proportional hazards assumption was tested visually using Kaplan–Meier curves and by examining plots of −ln [−ln (survival time)] against the ln (time). For continuous variables, the linearity assumption was assessed by plotting Schoenfeld residuals versus time. Collinearity was excluded by constructing a correlation matrix between candidate predictors. The comparison of baseline variables in patients with incident AF according to antithrombotic treatment was performed using the χ^2 test, the Fisher's exact test for categorical variables, and the Student's unpaired t test for continuous variables. The associations between incident AF and mortality were assessed with Cox analyses, and incident AF was modeled as a time-dependent variable. HRs and 95% CIs were calculated. All statistical analyses were performed using STATA 14.2 software (STATA Corporation, College Station, TX, USA). Significance was assumed at $p < 0.05$.

3. Results

3.1. Study Population

A clinical follow-up was obtained at a median of 3.3 (interquartile range: 3.0 to 3.6) years in 5015 (99%) of the 5031 CAD outpatients without prevalent AF. As shown in Table 1, most patients were male (77.8%), with a mean age of 66.1 ± 11.7 years. A history of MI was documented in 50.7% of the cases, with 72.7% of the patients having had previous percutaneous coronary intervention (PCI) and 19.5% with a previous coronary bypass (CABG). The mean left ventricular ejection fraction (LVEF) was 57 ± 11%, and 18.2% of the patients had LVEF <50%. Secondary prevention medications were widely prescribed (antiplatelet agents 98%, statins 92.5%, angiotensin-converting enzyme inhibitors or angiotensin receptor blockers 83.2%, beta-blockers 82.4%).

Table 1. Baseline characteristics of the study population and correlates of incident atrial fibrillation (AF) according to univariable analysis.

	All Patients with Follow-Up (n = 5015)	No Incident AF (n = 4749)	Incident AF (n = 266)	HR [95% CI]	p
Age, years	66.1 ± 11.7	65.8 ± 11.6	72.6 ± 10.4	1.06 [1.05–1.07]	<0.0001
Women	22.2	21.9	27.8	1.37 [1.05–1.79]	0.021
History of hypertension	59.2	58.4	73.2	1.95 [1.48–2.56]	<0.0001
History of diabetes mellitus	31.7	31.3	39.9	1.46 [1.14–1.86]	0.003
Previous MI	50.7	50.8	49.2	0.96 [0.75–1.22]	0.715
Previous PCI	72.7	73.1	65.8	0.69 [0.53–0.88]	0.004
Previous coronary bypass	19.5	19.3	22.9	1.25 [0.94–1.66]	0.127
Previous stroke	4.7	4.6	6.0	1.39 [0.84–2.30]	0.202
History of peripheral artery disease	23.5	23.3	27.1	1.25 [0.96–1.64]	0.104
Heart failure	14.5	13.8	27.8	2.67 [2.04–3.50]	<0.0001
LVEF, %	57 ± 11	57 ± 10	54 ± 13	0.97 [0.96–0.98]	<0.0001
LVEF < 50%	18.2	17.6	28.2	1.95 [1.49–2.54]	<0.0001
Medications at inclusion:					
Antiplatelet drug	98.0	97.9	98.9	1.80 [0.58–5.62]	0.311
Oral anticoagulant	4.1	4.1	3.4	0.81 [0.42–1.57]	0.533
At least 1 antithrombotic drug	99.3	99.3	99.6	1.82 [0.26–13.0]	0.550
Angiotensin-Converting enzyme inhibitor or angiotensin receptor blocker	83.2	82.9	88.4	1.53 [1.05–2.22]	0.027
Beta-Blocker	82.4	82.2	86.8	1.39 [0.98–1.99]	0.067
Statin	92.5	92.7	90.2	0.72 [0.48–1.07]	0.107

Data are presented as mean ± standard deviation (SD) or %. HR, hazard ratio; CI, confidence interval; MI, myocardial infarction; PCI, percutaneous coronary intervention; LVEF, left ventricular ejection fraction.

3.2. Incident AF

During the follow-up period, there were 495 deaths (cardiovascular deaths: $n = 200$) among the 5015 patients. During the same period, 266 patients experienced real-life incident AF. Risk of AF increased progressively, with cumulative incidences including death as the competing event of 1.6% (95% CI: 1.3 to 1.9), 2.9% (95% CI: 2.4 to 3.3), and 4.7% (95% CI: 4.1 to 5.3) at years 1–3, respectively. Figure 2A shows the cumulative incidence of AF over the time and Figure 2B according to age at inclusion.

We performed univariable and multivariable assessments of baseline variables that might be associated with incident AF (Tables 1 and 2). Five variables determined at registry inclusion were independently associated with incident AF: older age ($p < 0.0001$), heart failure ($p = 0.003$), lower LVEF ($p = 0.008$), history of hypertension ($p = 0.010$), and diabetes mellitus ($p = 0.033$). Of note, a history of MI was not associated with an increased risk for incident AF.

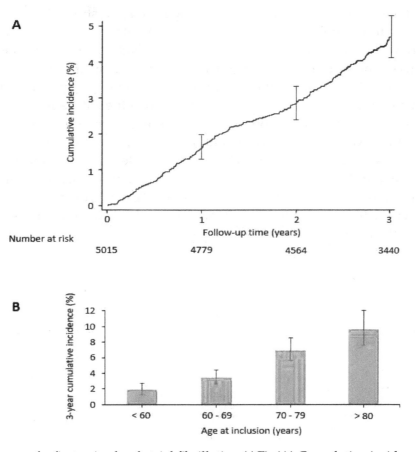

Figure 2. Incidence of a first episode of atrial fibrillation (AF). (**A**) Cumulative incidence of AF during the follow-up period (death as the competing event). (**B**) 3-year cumulative incidence of AF (death as the competing event) according to age at inclusion. Error bars are 95% CI.

Table 2. Independent correlates of incident atrial fibrillation (AF) by multivariable analysis.

	HR [95% CI]	p
Age (per year)	1.05 [1.04–1.07]	<0.0001
Heart failure	1.67 [1.19–2.35]	0.003
LVEF (per %)	0.98 [0.97–0.99]	0.008
History of hypertension	1.45 [1.09–1.93]	0.010
History of diabetes mellitus	1.31 [1.02–1.69]	0.033

HR, hazard ratio; CI, confidence interval; LVEF, left ventricular ejection fraction. The variables included in the model were age, sex, history of hypertension, history of diabetes mellitus, previous myocardial infarction, previous percutaneous coronary intervention, previous coronary bypass, previous stroke, history of peripheral artery disease, heart failure, and LVEF. A stepwise approach was used with forward selection (the p value for entering into the stepwise model was set at 0.05).

3.3. Diagnosis and Management of Incident AF

As shown in Figure 3A, the diagnosis of AF in the 266 patients took place in different settings. In two thirds of cases, incident AF was diagnosed during cardiology outpatient visits. Almost half of the patients in these situations had no evident symptoms of AF. Other relatively frequent diagnostic circumstances included hospitalization for heart failure ($n = 46$) and monitoring of implanted devices ($n = 15$). Of note, the number of patients who had AF diagnosed at the time of hospitalization for ischemic stroke was low ($n = 5$).

We assessed the antithrombotic strategy that was chosen in patients with incident AF. The mean CHA_2DS_2-VASc score in the 266 patients was 4.3 (±1.5). The proportion of women with a CHA_2DS_2-VASc score ≥ 3 was 97%, and the proportion of men with a CHA_2DS_2-VASc score ≥ 2 was 96%. As shown in Figure 3B, most patients were prescribed an anticoagulant (any anticoagulant:

$n = 245$ (92%); direct oral anticoagulant: $n = 127$; vitamin K antagonist: $n = 110$; low-molecular-weight heparin: $n = 8$). When anticoagulation was not used, 12 patients received single-antiplatelet therapy and 8 patients received dual-antiplatelet therapy; one patient had no antithrombotic therapy. When an anticoagulant was used, the antithrombotic regimen also included an antiplatelet drug in half of cases (anticoagulant alone: $n = 123$; anticoagulant + single-antiplatelet therapy: $n = 111$; anticoagulant + dual-antiplatelet therapy: $n = 11$). At time of incident AF, 26 of the 266 patients had a recent (<1 year) history of MI and/or PCI. When focusing on the 240 remaining patients who experienced incident AF in the context of chronic CAD (i.e., previous MI and/or PCI > 12 months) (Figure 3C), an anticoagulant was used in 225 (94%), still often combined with an antiplatelet drug (anticoagulant alone: $n = 121$; anticoagulant + single-antiplatelet therapy: $n = 102$; anticoagulant + dual-antiplatelet therapy: $n = 2$). Apart from higher proportions of previous PCI (75% vs. 54.6%, $p = 0.001$) and previous stroke (8.7% vs. 1.7%, $p = 0.026$), patients who received anticoagulant and antiplatelet therapy had similar characteristics to patients treated with anticoagulant alone (Table 3).

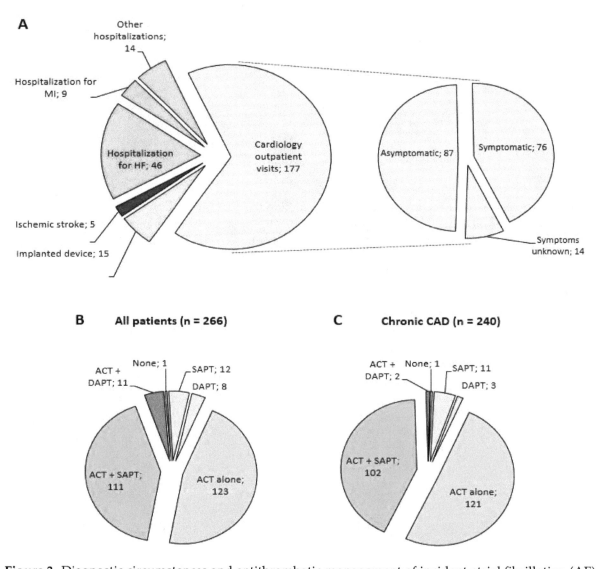

Figure 3. Diagnostic circumstances and antithrombotic management of incident atrial fibrillation (AF) in coronary artery disease (CAD) outpatients. (**A**) Diagnostic circumstances of incident atrial fibrillation (AF) in coronary artery disease (CAD) outpatients. HF, heart failure; MI, myocardial infarction (**B**) Antithrombotic strategy in all coronary artery disease (CAD) outpatients with incident atrial fibrillation (AF); ACT, anticoagulant therapy; DAPT, dual-antiplatelet therapy; SAPT, single-antiplatelet therapy. (**C**) Antithrombotic strategy in patients with incident AF in a context of chronic CAD (i.e., patients without recent (<1 year) history of myocardial infarction and/or percutaneous coronary intervention).

Table 3. Comparison of patients receiving anticoagulant therapy (ACT) alone vs. ACT and antiplatelet therapy (APT) (n = 225 patients with incident atrial fibrillation (AF) and without a recent (<1 year) history of myocardial infarction (MI) or percutaneous coronary intervention (PCI)).

	ACT Alone (n = 121)	ACT + APT (n = 104)	p
Baseline characteristics			
Age, years	73.5 ± 10.0	71.5 ± 10.8	0.137
Women	29.8	25.0	0.426
History of hypertension	69.4	74.8	0.376
History of diabetes mellitus	37.2	44.2	0.283
Previous MI	46.3	52.9	0.323
Previous PCI	54.6	75.0	0.001
Previous coronary bypass	30.6	20.2	0.076
Previous stroke	1.7	8.7	0.026
History of peripheral artery disease	28.9	22.1	0.244
Heart failure	24.8	32.7	0.190
LVEF, %	55 ± 12	53 ± 14	0.149
AF diagnosis			
Cardiology outpatient—asymptomatic	37.2	32.7	0.481
Cardiology outpatient—symptomatic	30.6	28.9	0.777
Hospitalization for heart failure	16.5	19.2	0.597
Implanted device	7.4	3.9	0.391
CHA_2DS_2-VASc score at AF diagnosis	4.3 ± 1.5	4.3 ± 1.3	0.700

Data are presented as mean ± SD or %. LVEF, left ventricular ejection fraction.

3.4. Outcome After Incident AF

For the 266 patients with incident AF, the median clinical follow-up after AF diagnosis was 1.2 (interquartile range: 0.5 to 2.2) years. A total of 42 deaths (cardiovascular deaths: n = 26) occurred during the post-AF period. Table 4 shows the impact of incident AF, analyzed as a time-dependent variable, on all-cause and cardiovascular mortality. In adjusted models, incident AF during follow-up was associated with significant increases in the risk of all-cause mortality (HR: 2.04; 95% CI: 1.47 to 2.83) and cardiovascular mortality (HR: 2.88; 95% CI: 1.88 to 4.43).

Table 4. Association of incident atrial fibrillation (AF) with mortality.

	HR [95% CI]	p
All-Cause Mortality		
unadjusted	3.90 [2.82–5.37]	<0.0001
adjusted	2.04 [1.47–2.83]	<0.0001
Cardiovascular Mortality		
unadjusted	6.49 [4.26–9.89]	<0.0001
adjusted	2.88 [1.88–4.43]	<0.0001

HR, hazard ratio; CI, confidence interval; incident AF was used as a time-dependent variable. Adjusted models included age, sex, history of hypertension, history of diabetes mellitus, heart failure, and LVEF.

4. Discussion

Interest is growing in analyzing outcomes in patients with chronic CAD [13–15]. Incident MI [16] or incident stroke [17] are probably the first events clinicians think of when assessing risk in these patients. However, other cardiovascular events may also affect management and may have significant prognostic implications. Our study documents a relatively high risk of real-life incident AF in chronic CAD patients, with a roughly linear increase of 1.6% per year. This result should be interpreted in the context of an unselected population of consecutive chronic CAD outpatients with a significant proportion of elderly individuals, and frequent history of hypertension, diabetes mellitus, and heart failure, all factors that are associated with incident AF in the present study as well as in the literature [7,18,19]. Incident AF is much less important in general population as reported by Vermond et al. in a large Dutch cohort with a cumulative incidence of 3% after a ten years mean follow-up and 3.3/1000 person-years [7]. In line with this, Wike et al. reported in a larger German cohort an incidence of 4.112/1000 person-years in the general population [20]. Importantly, to the best of our knowledge, no study assessed the incidence of AF in CAD outpatients. Of note, the interpretation of the rate of incident AF implies a need to consider screening strategies in this population. Our study protocol did not require specific screening for AF, so our data document incident AF diagnosed during routine real-life follow-up. Also, from a methodological point of view, we emphasize that our study may differ from earlier literature in that we present cumulative incidences, taking into account death as the competing event. We justify this choice by the high mortality rate of CAD patients at risk for AF. Indeed, inappropriate censoring of competing events may lead the Kaplan–Meier estimator to overestimate the cumulative incidence in the presence of competing risks, especially if the competing risk is frequent [11,12].

As stated above, the real-life design of our study yielded information on the diagnostic circumstances of incident AF. Such data are rarely available in the literature. An integral part of management for patients with chronic CAD is the planning of regular follow-up visits with the cardiologists. Although chronic CAD guidelines recommend an annual resting electrocardiogram (ECG), the level of evidence is acknowledged to be low [4,5]. Our data showed that incident AF was frequently diagnosed by a systematic ECG in the absence of AF-related symptoms. This high proportion of asymptomatic patients could be related to the wide use of betablockers prior to AF occurrence in our population. Moreover, it is plausible (although speculative) that patients with a history of CAD who experienced new symptoms had facilitated access to cardiology advice. This may have had important consequences by minimizing treatment delays. Concordant with these data is the relatively low number of incident AF discovered at time of hospitalization for an ischemic stroke (n = 5 for 5015 CAD patients followed-up during three years; 0.3/1000 patient-years).

International taskforces currently recommend against systematic screening for AF in the general population, citing the cost implications and uncertainty over the benefits of a systematic screening program compared to usual care [21]. However, screening in targeted high-risk groups remains to be questioned. Given the high incidence of AF compared to the general population and the proportion of asymptomatic AF in CAD outpatients reported in our study, extended screening strategies in such patients would be of interest.

One aim of our analysis was to describe the management strategy when incident AF is detected in chronic CAD patients. The present study focused on initial management at the time of AF diagnosis and, as such, clearly differs from previous analyses of registries reporting chronic medications in patients combining CAD and AF [3,22,23]. In addition, the 266 cases of incident AF occurred between 2013 and 2018, so our study describes the modern management of incident AF in patients with a history of CAD. First, we documented a very high use of anticoagulation, which is in accordance with the high thrombotic risk of the study population as documented by the CHA_2DS_2-VASc score. Indeed, according to current guidelines [24], anticoagulation would have to be considered in almost all CAD patients experiencing incident AF in the present study. Second, because almost all patients had a background of antiplatelet therapy before the AF event, the management of combinations of antithrombotic drugs was a matter of interest. When focusing the analysis on chronic patients, we found that cardiologists are still reluctant to stop all antiplatelet therapy in these patients. AF guidelines suggest going with anticoagulation alone if >1 year has passed with no acute events [24]. However, the level of evidence is limited, and expert consensus provides more modulated recommendations [25]. One recent randomized trial and many observational studies have shown that the addition of antiplatelet therapy is associated with a substantially increased risk of bleeding, with no clear benefit on ischemic events [3,22,23,26].

Finally, incident AF has been associated with increased mortality in general populations [7,8]. Our study extends these findings to a large population of outpatients with chronic CAD. In adjusted analyses, CAD patients who developed AF had a two-fold increased risk for all-cause mortality, largely similar to associations previously reported [7,8]. Incident AF should, therefore, be considered as an important warning sign for physicians working with CAD patients, even if anticoagulation is largely used. These data are concordant with previous findings suggesting that next to stroke prevention, further research is needed to improve the prognosis of patients with AF [7,27,28].

Study Limitations

Our study has some limitations. First, our data reflect the practice in a regional area, and we do not know whether these findings are generalizable for practices in other parts of the world. Second, because cardiologists determined inclusion, the data may not be generalizable to the overall population with CAD in the community. Finally, we present here initial management strategies for patients with incident AF and lack details on chronic management and antithrombotic modifications during follow-up. On the other hand, the absence of exclusion criteria, the very high follow-up rate, and the adjudication of clinical events can be considered strengths of the study.

5. Conclusions

Our study shows that real-life incident AF occurs at a stable annual rate of 1.6% in chronic CAD outpatients. Older age, heart failure, low LVEF, hypertension, and diabetes were associated with a higher risk of AF. In patients with chronic CAD, a substantial proportion of incident AF is diagnosed during a systematic cardiology outpatient visit in asymptomatic patients. In patients with chronic CAD and incident AF that were >1 year from their last MI and/or PCI, antiplatelets remain frequently combined with oral anticoagulation. Finally, we found that incident AF in patients with chronic CAD was associated with an increase in all-cause and cardiovascular mortality. Considering the high incidence of AF compared to the general population and the proportion of asymptomatic AF in CAD outpatients, extended screening strategies in such patients would be of interest.

Author Contributions: Conceptualization, S.N., G.L. and C.B.; Data curation, T.M. and O.T.; Formal analysis, S.N.; Funding acquisition, C.B.; Investigation, N.L. and C.B.; Methodology, S.N., G.L., T.M., N.L. and C.B.; Validation, N.L.; Writing—original draft, S.N. and C.B.; Writing—review & editing, G.L. and N.L. All authors have read and agreed to the published version of the manuscript.

Acknowledgments: Michel Deneve for monitoring the CARDIONOR study.

Abbreviations

ACT	anticoagulant therapy
APT	antiplatelet therapy
AF	atrial fibrillation
CAD	coronary artery disease
CI	confidence interval
DAPT	dual antiplatelet therapy
ECG	electrocardiogram
HF	heart failure
HR	hazard ratio
LVEF	left ventricular ejection fraction
MI	myocardial infarction
PCI	percutaneous coronary intervention
SAPT	single antiplatelet therapy

References

1.   Goto, S.; Bhatt, D.L.; Rother, J. Prevalence, clinical profile, and cardiovascular outcomes of atrial fibrillation patients with atherothrombosis. *Am. Heart. J.* **2008**, *156*, 855–863. [CrossRef] [PubMed]
2.   Aguilar, E.; Garcia-Diaz, A.M.; Sanchez Munoz-Torrero, J.F. Clinical outcome of stable outpatients with coronary, cerebrovascular or peripheral artery disease, and atrial fibrillation. *Thromb. Res.* **2012**, *130*, 390–395. [CrossRef] [PubMed]
3.   Hamon, M.; Lemesle, G.; Tricot, O. Incidence, source, determinants, and prognostic impact of major bleeding in outpatients with stable coronary artery disease. *J. Am. Coll. Cardiol.* **2014**, *64*, 1430–1436. [CrossRef] [PubMed]
4.   Fihn, S.D.; Gardin, J.M.; Abrams, J. 2012 ACCF/AHA/ACP/AATS/PCNA/SCAI/STS guideline for the diagnosis and management of patients with stable ischemic heart disease: A report of the American College of Cardiology Foundation/American Heart Association task force on practice guidelines, and the American College of Physicians, American Association for Thoracic Surgery, Preventive Cardiovascular Nurses Association, Society for Cardiovascular Angiography and Interventions, and Society of Thoracic Surgeons. *Circulation* **2012**, *126*, e354–e471. [CrossRef] [PubMed]
5.   Montalescot, G.; Sechtem, U.; Achenbach, S. 2013 ESC guidelines on the management of stable coronary artery disease. *Eur. Heart J.* **2013**, *34*, 2949–3003. [CrossRef] [PubMed]
6.   Schurtz, G.; Bauters, C.; Ducrocq, G. Effect of aspirin in addition to oral anticoagulants in stable coronary artery disease outpatients with an indication for anticoagulation. *Panminerva Med.* **2016**, *58*, 271–285. [PubMed]
7.   Vermond, R.A.; Geelhoed, B.; Verweij, N. Incidence of Atrial Fibrillation and Relationship with Cardiovascular Events, Heart Failure, and Mortality: A Community-Based Study from The Netherlands. *J. Am. Coll. Cardiol.* **2015**, *66*, 1000–1007. [CrossRef]
8.   Andersson, T.; Magnuson, A.; Bryngelsson, I.L. All-cause mortality in 272,186 patients hospitalized with incident atrial fibrillation 1995–2008: A Swedish nationwide long-term case-control study. *Eur. Heart J.* **2013**, *34*, 1061–1067. [CrossRef]
9.   Lamblin, N.; Ninni, S.; Tricot, O. Secondary prevention and outcomes in outpatients with coronary artery disease, atrial fibrillation or heart failure: A focus on disease overlap. *Open Heart* **2020**, *7*, e001165. [CrossRef]
10. Bauters, C.; Tricot, O.; Meurice, T. Long-term risk and predictors of cardiovascular death in stable coronary artery disease: The CORONOR study. *Coron. Artery. Dis.* **2017**, *28*, 636–641. [CrossRef]
11. Wolbers, M.; Koller, M.T.; Stel, V.S. Competing risks analyses: Objectives and approaches. *Eur. Heart J.* **2014**, *35*, 2936–2941. [CrossRef] [PubMed]
12. Austin, P.C.; Lee, D.S.; Fine, J.P. Introduction to the Analysis of Survival Data in the Presence of Competing Risks. *Circulation* **2016**, *133*, 601–609. [CrossRef] [PubMed]
13. Daly, C.; Clemens, F.; Lopez Sendon, J.L. Gender differences in the management and clinical outcome of stable angina. *Circulation* **2006**, *113*, 490–498. [CrossRef] [PubMed]
14. Steg, P.G.; Greenlaw, N.; Tardif, J.C. Women and men with stable coronary artery disease have similar clinical outcomes: Insights from the international prospective CLARIFY registry. *Eur. Heart J.* **2012**, *33*, 2831–2840. [CrossRef]
15. Bauters, C.; Deneve, M.; Tricot, O. Prognosis of patients with stable coronary artery disease (from the CORONOR study). *Am. J. Cardiol.* **2014**, *113*, 1142–1145. [CrossRef]
16. Lemesle, G.; Tricot, O.; Meurice, T. Incident Myocardial Infarction and Very Late Stent Thrombosis in Outpatients with Stable Coronary Artery Disease. *J. Am. Coll. Cardiol.* **2017**, *69*, 2149–2156. [CrossRef]
17. Cordonnier, C.; Lemesle, G.; Casolla, B. Incidence and determinants of cerebrovascular events in outpatients with stable coronary artery disease. *Eur. Stroke J.* **2018**, *3*, 272–280. [CrossRef]
18. Alonso, A.; Krijthe, B.P.; Aspelund, T. Simple risk model predicts incidence of atrial fibrillation in a racially and geographically diverse population: The CHARGE-AF consortium. *J. Am. Heart Assoc.* **2013**, *2*, e000102. [CrossRef]
19. Smith, J.G.; Newton-Cheh, C.; Almgren, P. Assessment of conventional cardiovascular risk factors and multiple biomarkers for the prediction of incident heart failure and atrial fibrillation. *J. Am. Coll. Cardiol.* **2010**, *56*, 1712–1719. [CrossRef]

20. Wilke, T.; Groth, A.; Mueller, S. Incidence and Prevalence of Atrial Fibrillation: An Analysis Based on 8.3 Million Patients. *Europace* **2013**, *4*, 486–493. [CrossRef]

21. Jones, N.R.; Taylor, C.J.; Hobbs, F.D.R. Screening for atrial fibrillation: A call for evidence. *Eur. Heart J.* **2019**, *41*, 1075–1085. [CrossRef] [PubMed]

22. Lamberts, M.; Gislason, G.H.; Lip, G.Y. Antiplatelet therapy for stable coronary artery disease in atrial fibrillation patients taking an oral anticoagulant: A nationwide cohort study. *Circulation* **2014**, *129*, 1577–1585. [CrossRef] [PubMed]

23. Lemesle, G.; Ducrocq, G.; Elbez, Y. Vitamin K antagonists with or without long-term antiplatelet therapy in outpatients with stable coronary artery disease and atrial fibrillation: Association with ischemic and bleeding events. *Clin. Cardiol.* **2017**, *40*, 932–939. [CrossRef] [PubMed]

24. Kirchhof, P.; Benussi, S.; Kotecha, D. 2016 ESC Guidelines for the management of atrial fibrillation developed in collaboration with EACTS. *Eur. Heart J.* **2016**, *37*, 2893–2962. [CrossRef] [PubMed]

25. Angiolillo, D.J.; Goodman, S.G.; Bhatt, D.L. Antithrombotic Therapy in Patients with Atrial Fibrillation Undergoing Percutaneous Coronary Intervention: A North American Perspective-2016 Update. *Circ. Cardiovasc. Interv.* **2016**, *9*, e004395. [CrossRef] [PubMed]

26. Yasuda, S.; Kaikita, K.; Akao, M. Antithrombotic Therapy for Atrial Fibrillation with Stable Coronary Disease. *N. Engl. J. Med.* **2019**, *381*, 1103–1113. [CrossRef] [PubMed]

27. Piccini, J.P.; Hammill, B.G.; Sinner, M.F. Clinical course of atrial fibrillation in older adults: The importance of cardiovascular events beyond stroke. *Eur. Heart J.* **2014**, *35*, 250–256. [CrossRef]

28. Bassand, J.P.; Accetta, G.; Camm, A.J. Two-year outcomes of patients with newly diagnosed atrial fibrillation: Results from GARFIELD-AF. *Eur. Heart J.* **2016**, *37*, 2882–2889. [CrossRef]

9

Assessment of Global Longitudinal and Circumferential Strain Using Computed Tomography Feature Tracking: Intra-Individual Comparison with CMR Feature Tracking and Myocardial Tagging in Patients with Severe Aortic Stenosis

Emilija Miskinyte [1,†], Paulius Bucius [1,2,†], Jennifer Erley [1], Seyedeh Mahsa Zamani [1], Radu Tanacli [1], Christian Stehning [3], Christopher Schneeweis [4], Tomas Lapinskas [2], Burkert Pieske [1,5,6], Volkmar Falk [5,7], Rolf Gebker [1], Gianni Pedrizzetti [8], Natalia Solowjowa [7] and Sebastian Kelle [1,5,6,*]

[1] Department of Internal Medicine/Cardiology, German Heart Center Berlin, 13353 Berlin, Germany
[2] Department of Cardiology, Medical Academy, Lithuanian University of Health Sciences, 50161 Kaunas, Lithuania
[3] Philips Healthcare, 22335 Hamburg, Germany
[4] Klinik für Kardiologie und Internistische Intesivmedizin, Krankenhaus der Augustinerinnen, 50678 Köln, Germany
[5] DZHK (German Centre for Cardiovascular Research), Partner Site Berlin, 10785 Berlin, Germany
[6] Department of Internal Medicine/Cardiology, Charité Campus Virchow Clinic, 13353 Berlin, Germany
[7] Department of Cardiothoracic Surgery, German Heart Center Berlin, 13353 Berlin, Germany
[8] Department of Engineering and Architecture, University of Trieste, 34127 Trieste, Italy
* Correspondence: kelle@dhzb.de;
† Both authors contributted equally.

Abstract: In this study, we used a single commercially available software solution to assess global longitudinal (GLS) and global circumferential strain (GCS) using cardiac computed tomography (CT) and cardiac magnetic resonance (CMR) feature tracking (FT). We compared agreement and reproducibility between these two methods and the reference standard, CMR tagging (TAG). Twenty-seven patients with severe aortic stenosis underwent CMR and cardiac CT examinations. FT analysis was performed using Medis suite version 3.0 (Leiden, The Netherlands) software. Segment (Medviso) software was used for GCS assessment from tagged images. There was a trend towards the underestimation of GLS by CT-FT when compared to CMR-FT (19.4 ± 5.04 vs. 22.40 ± 5.69, respectively; $p = 0.065$). GCS values between TAG, CT-FT, and CMR-FT were similar ($p = 0.233$). CMR-FT and CT-FT correlated closely for GLS ($r = 0.686$, $p < 0.001$) and GCS ($r = 0.707$, $p < 0.001$), while both of these methods correlated moderately with TAG for GCS ($r = 0.479$, $p < 0.001$ for CMR-FT vs. TAG; $r = 0.548$ for CT-FT vs. TAG). Intraobserver and interobserver agreement was excellent in all techniques. Our findings show that, in elderly patients with severe aortic stenosis (AS), the FT algorithm performs equally well in CMR and cardiac CT datasets for the assessment of GLS and GCS, both in terms of reproducibility and agreement with the gold standard, TAG.

Keywords: systemic disease; cardiac computed tomography; cardiac magnetic resonance; feature tracking; tagging; myocardial deformation; strain

1. Introduction

Multiple systemic and neuromuscular diseases can affect the cardiovascular system at some point in their course. A wide variety of pathological processes fall under these definitions, some of which have pathognomonic cardiovascular manifestations [1]. However, non-specific manifestations, such as a subtle decline in regional or global myocardial function, are also common [2]. It can often go unnoticed until the ejection fraction (EF) starts to decline or clinical symptoms of heart failure begin to develop. Recently, myocardial strain has emerged as an imaging technique that adds information about myocardial function beyond the left ventricular ejection fraction (LVEF) [3]. Furthermore, recent studies have shown early reduction in myocardial strain in multiple systemic and neuromuscular disorders, such as amyloidosis [4], systemic sclerosis [5], rheumatoid arthritis [6], and Duchenne muscular dystrophy [7]. These data suggest that deformation imaging could become an important tool for the early identification of cardiac involvement in these patients.

Due to its availability, speckle tracking echocardiography (STE) is the most widely used method for strain assessment. However, the accuracy and feasibility of STE is highly dependent on image quality [8], warranting the need for alternatives in certain patients. Cardiac magnetic resonance (CMR) not only allows for myocardial strain assessment, overcoming the shortcomings of echocardiography, but also offers tissue characterization ability that is second to none. Thus, it is an important tool in the diagnostic work-up of patients with systemic connective tissue disorders [9]. A recently developed cardiac magnetic resonance feature tracking (CMR-FT) technique has been validated against the gold standard myocardial tagging (TAG) and is now considered a preferred CMR tool for strain assessment [10]. The main advantage of CMR-FT is that it can be applied to steady-state free precession (SSFP) cine loops that are used in routine clinical practice, therefore not requiring additional image acquisition. Interestingly, although developed for CMR, the FT algorithm can also be applied to cardiac computed tomography (CT) datasets to assess myocardial strain [11,12]. Naturally, strain assessment from cardiac CT datasets has started to gain popularity.

In this study, we used a single commercially available software solution to acquire global strain parameters via computed tomography feature tracking (CT-FT) and CMR-FT in a cohort of patients with severe aortic stenosis (AS). We compared agreement and reproducibility of global longitudinal (GLS) and global circumferential strain (GCS) between both these methods and the reference standard, TAG.

2. Experimental Section

2.1. Study Population

Twenty-six patients (14 females and 12 males, mean age 80.59 ± 5.87 years) with severe AS referred to our institution for transcathether aortic valve replacement (TAVR) were enrolled in this study. Further demographic and clinical data of the study population are listed in Table 1. AS was diagnosed and graded echocardiographically according to the latest European Society of Cardiology and European Association for Cardiothoracic Surgery guidelines [13]. All subjects underwent clinically indicated CMR and cardiac CT examinations. This study complies with the Declaration of Helsinki. Institutional Review Board approval was not necessary because it was a retrospective analysis of clinical data. According to local law, all individuals signed an informed consent form before entering the clinical CMR and cardiac CT. None of the observers could identify patient information when analyzing the data.

2.2. Cardiac Computed Tomography Acquisition

Contrast-enhanced, retrospectively electrocardiography (ECG)-gated cardiac scans were performed using a 2×128-slice multi-detector computed tomography scanner (Somatom Definition Flash, Siemens AG, Erlangen, Germany). The following study protocol was used: tube voltage 100, 120 kV, tube current 320 ref. mAs/rotation, rotation time 280 ms, slice collimation of 128×0.6 mm, with a temporal resolution of 75 ms, slice width of 0.75 mm, reconstruction increment of 0.4 mm, and reconstruction kernel B30f. Images were acquired in a cranio-caudal direction, from above the aortic sinuses to below the diaphragm.

Table 1. Demographic and clinical data of the study population.

Variables.	$n = 27$ Mean $\pm$ SD or n (%)
Age	22.40 ± 5.69
Male	18.91 ± 5.97
Body mass index (kg/m^2)	26.60 ± 3.60
Heart rate	67.59 ± 10.27
Clinical history	
Hypertension	25 (92.56%)
CAD	16 (59.25%)
Myocardial infarction	6 (22.22%)
History of CABG	5 (18.51%)
Stroke	4 (14.81%)
Diabetes mellitus type 2	6 (22.22%)
COPD	5 (18.51%)

Abbreviations: CAD: coronary artery disease; CABG: coronary artery bypass graft; COPD: chronic obstructive pulmonary disease.

2.3. Cardiac Magnetic Resonance Acquisition

CMR acquisitions were made using a 1.5 Tesla magnetic resonance imaging (MRI) scanner (Achieva, Philips Healthcare, Best, The Netherlands). Signals were received using a five-element phased array cardiac coil. A four-lead vector ECG was used for R-wave triggering. A balanced steady-state free precession (bSSFP) sequence with breath hold was acquired in long-axis (LAX) two-, three-, and four-chamber views, as well as a short-axis (SAX) stack. This was used for volumetric and FT analysis. Acquisition parameters used were a repetition time (TR) of 3.3 ms, echo time (TE) of 1.6 ms, flip angle of 60°, acquisition voxel size of $1.8 \times 1.7 \times 8.0$ mm^3, and 30 phases per cardiac cycle. The complementary spatial modulation of magnetization (CSPAMM) technique was used to acquire tagging images in three short-axis planes (basal, medial, and apical) with a temporal resolution of 35 ms, spatial resolution of 1.4×1.4 mm, and a slice thickness of 8 mm.

2.4. Cardiac CT Data Analysis

Original three-dimensional (3D) datasets were analyzed offline using the commercially available Medis Suite version 3.0 (Leiden, The Netherlands) software package to generate two-dimensional (2D) cine loops of three LAX slices (i.e., two-, three-, and four-chamber), three SAX slices (i.e., basal, mid, and apical), and a SAX stack with a slice thickness of 0.75 mm and a reconstruction increment of 0.4 mm. Images were generated with temporal resolution of 10 phases per cardiac cycle in 10% increments from early systole (0% cardiac cycle) to end-diastole (90% cardiac cycle). Care was taken to make sure that 2D cardiac CT reconstructions closely matched the anatomical locations of the images used for CMR analysis. End-systolic and end-diastolic cardiac phases were chosen visually. Endocardial and epicardial borders in the SAX stack were outlined manually to calculate the volumetric parameters, which were indexed to body surface area (BSA). Left ventricular mass index (LVMi), left ventricular end-diastolic volume index (LVEDVi), left ventricular end-systolic volume index (LVESVi), left ventricular stroke volume index (LVSVi), and left ventricular ejection fraction (LVEF) were calculated. Global longitudinal strain (GLS) was assessed by averaging the peak systolic strain values of 17 segments extracted from three LAX images, while global circumferential strain (GCS) was acquired from three SAX images using a 16-segment model.

2.5. CMR Data Analysis

bSSFP images were analyzed using Medis Suite version 3.0 (Leiden, The Netherlands) software in the same manner as cardiac CT images to determine LVMi, LVEDVi, LVESVi, LVSVi, LVEF, GLS, and GCS. Tagged images were analyzed using commercially available software Segment version 2.2 R6960. Endocardial and epicardial borders were manually outlined at an end-systolic timeframe in three short-axis slices (i.e., basal, mid, and apical). After applying an automatic propagation algorithm, quality of tracking was visually assessed, and changes were made as needed. GCS was derived using a 16-segment model by averaging the peak systolic values. TAG data of one of the subjects could not be analyzed due to breathing artefacts, therefore 26 patients were used for GCS comparisons.

Due to the counter-intuitive increase of strain in more diseased subjects, we chose to report absolute values for easier interpretation.

2.6. Statistics

Data analysis was performed using commercially available software (GraphPad Prism 8, GraphPad Software, San Diego, CA, USA). The Shapiro–Wilk test was used to assess the normality of distribution of continuous variables. Unpaired Student's t-test was used to compare differences between cardiac CT and MRI derived volumetric parameters and GLS. One-way ANOVA was used to compare differences in GCS between the three modalities. Pearson's correlation coefficient and Bland–Altman analysis were used to assess inter-method agreement. Intra- and interobserver variability were assessed using two-way mixed intra-class correlation coefficient (ICC), Bland–Altman analysis, and coefficient of variance (CoV). This was defined as the standard deviation of the differences divided by the mean, in keeping with previous studies [14]. Agreement levels were defined according to previous studies [15] as follows: excellent if ICC > 0.74, good if ICC = 0.6-0.74, fair if ICC = 0.4–0.59, poor if ICC < 0.4. p-values of <0.05 were considered statistically significant.

3. Results

3.1. Volumetric Assessment

Values of volumetric assessment are represented in Table 2. LVEDVi, LVESVi, LVSVi, LVEF, and LVMi values were similar between CMR and cardiac CT. There was excellent correlation between the two techniques in LVEDVi ($r = 0.913$, $p < 0.001$), LVESVi ($r = 0.879$, $p < 0.001$), LVEF ($r = 0.791$, $p < 0.001$), and LVMi ($r = 0.971$, $p < 0.001$), with good correlation for LVSVi ($r = 0.619$, $p < 0.001$). Results of the Bland–Altman analysis of volumetric measurements are shown in the figures (Figures 1a–d and 2).

Table 2. Values of volumetric assessment of the LV by CMR and CCT.

Measurement	CMR	CCT	p-Value
LVEF (%)	64.57 ± 14.55	59.15 ± 14.82	0.181
LVEDVi (mL/m^2)	72.60 ± 27.22	80.35 ± 26.42	0.374
LVESVi (mL/m^2)	28.62 ± 21.21	35.79 ± 23.39	0.293
LVSVi (mL/m^2)	43.98 ± 11.65	44.56 ± 8.13	0.933
LVMi (g/m^2)	62.13 ± 20.51	66.04 ± 19.42	0.471

Values are expressed as mean ± SD. Abbreviations: CCT: cardiac computed tomography; CMR: cardiac magnetic resonance; LVEF: left ventricular ejection fraction; LVEDVi: left ventricular end-diastolic volume index; LVESVi: left ventricular end-systolic volume index; LVMi: left ventricular mass index; LVSVi: left ventricular stroke volume index.

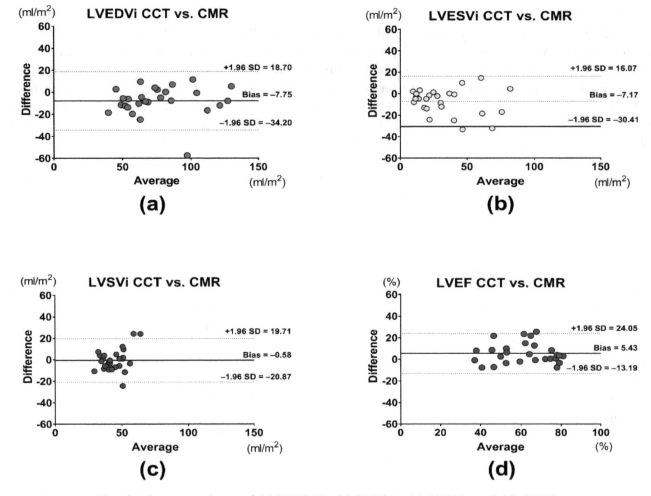

Figure 1. Bland–Altman analyses of (**a**) LVEDVi, (**b**) LVESVi, (**c**) LVSVi, and (**d**) LVEF assessment between CMR and CCT. Abbreviations: CCT: cardiac computed tomography; CMR: cardiac magnetic resonance; LVEF: left ventricular ejection fraction; LVEDVi: left ventricular end-diastolic volume index; LVESVi: left ventricular end-systolic volume index; LVSVi: left ventricular stroke volume index.

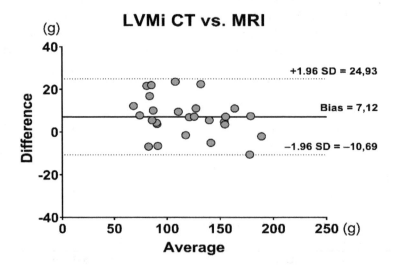

Figure 2. Bland–Altman analysis of LVMi assessment between CMR and CCT. Abbreviations: CCT: cardiac computed tomography; CMR: cardiac magnetic resonance; LVMi: left ventricular mass index.

3.2. Strain Assessment

Figures 3 and 4 show examples of GLS and GCS assessment in the same patient using different strain-assessment techniques. Strain values from each technique are represented in Table 3. GLS showed a trend towards being lower in CT-FT vs. CMR-FT (19.40 ± 5.04 vs. 22.40 ± 5.69, $p = 0.065$). GCS values were similar between all techniques ($p = 0.233$). There was good correlation between CMR-FT and CT-FT derived GLS ($r = 0.686$, $p < 0.001$) and GCS ($r = 0.707$, $p < 0.001$), while both of these methods had moderate correlation with TAG for GCS ($r = 0.479$, $p < 0.001$ for CMR-FT vs. TAG; $r = 0.548$ for CT-FT vs. TAG). Bland–Altman analysis revealed similarly wide limits of agreement (LOA) between all techniques in both GLS and GCS (Figure 5a–d and Table 4).

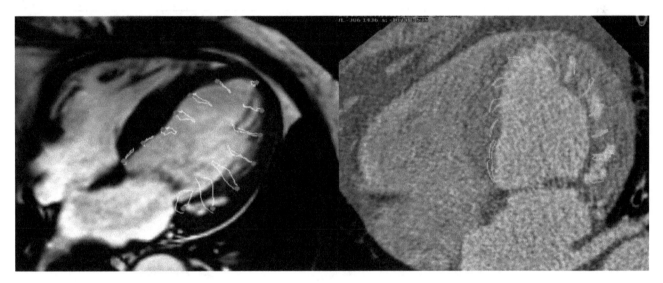

Figure 3. Assessment of GLS from the four-chamber long-axis (LAX) view in the same subject using CMR-FT (**left**) and CT-FT (**right**).

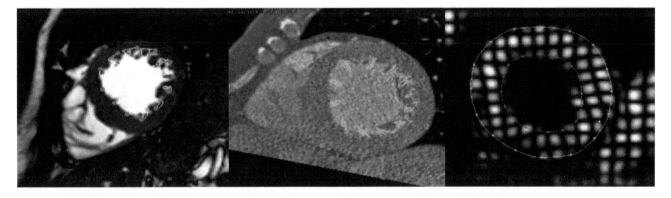

Figure 4. Assessment of GCS in the same subject from the mid-ventricular short-axis (SAX) view using CMR-FT (**left**), CT-FT (**middle**), and TAG (**right**).

Table 3. Values of strain assessment of the LV by CMR and CCT.

Measurement	CMR-FT	CT-FT	TAG
GLS (%)	22.40 ± 5.69	19.4 ± 5.04	N/A
GCS (%)	18.91 ± 5.97	18.13 ± 4.63	16.66 ± 3.38

Values are expressed as mean ± SD. Abbreviations: LV: left ventricular; CCT: cardiac computed tomography; GLS: global longitudinal strain, GCS: global circumferential strain, CMR-FT: cardiac magnetic resonance feature tracking, CT-FT: computed tomography feature tracking; TAG: myocardial tagging.

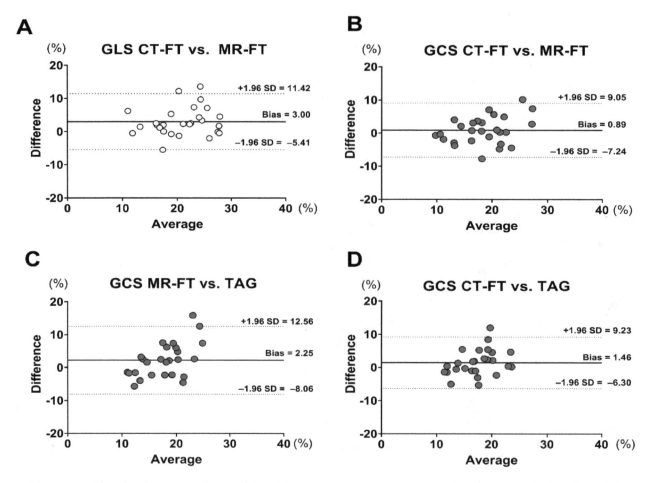

Figure 5. Bland–Altman analysis of the (**a**) GLS assessment between CT-FT and MR-FT; (**b**) GCS assessment between CT-FT and MR-FT; (**c**) GCS assessment between MR-FT and TAG; and (**d**) GCS assessment between CT-FT and TAG. Abbreviations: MR-FT: magnetic resonance feature tracking; CT-FT: computed tomography feature tracking; TAG: myocardial tagging; GLS: global longitudinal strain; GCS: global circumferential strain.

Table 4. Tabular representation of Bland–Altman and Pearson's correlation analyses for strain assessment.

Measurement	Comparison	Bias (%)	LOA (%)	Pearson's R
GLS	CMR-FT vs. CT-FT	3.003	±8.415	0.6860
GCS	CMR-FT vs. CT-FT	0.888	±8.16	0.7067
GCS	CMR-FT vs. TAG	2.250	±10.31	0.4799
GCS	CT-FT vs. TAG	1.468	±7.77	0.5484

Abbreviations: GLS: global longitudinal strain; GCS: global circumferential strain; CMR-FT: cardiac magnetic resonance feature tracking; CT-FT: computed tomography feature tracking; LOA: limits of agreement; TAG: myocardial tagging.

3.3. Intraobserver and Interobserver Reproducibility

The results of the reproducibility analyses are presented in Table 5. Intraobserver and interobserver agreement was excellent for all techniques. CMR-FT had worse intraobserver reproducibility for GLS (LOA ±2.4% vs. ±4.36%; CoV 6.8% vs. 10.1%) but performed better in interobserver comparison (LOA ±3.16% vs. ±5.5%; CoV 7.4% vs. 16.1%). TAG had superior reproducibility compared to the FT-based imaging technique for GCS, while FT-based techniques had similar results in interobserver and intraobserver comparisons.

Table 5. Reproducibility comparison of GLS and GCS between CMR-FT, CT-FT, and TAG.

	Bias (%)	Limits of Agreement (±)	CoV (%)	ICC (95% CI)
		Intraobserver reproducibility		
		CMR-FT		
GLS	0.09	4.36	10.1	0.960 (0.837–0.990)
GCS	−2.44	4.8	13.1	0.931 (0.439–0.985)
		CT-FT		
GLS	−0.08	2.4	6.8	0.983 (0.932–0.996)
GCS	−0.05	5.0	14.4	0.949 (0.801–0.987)
		TAG		
GCS	−0.08	1.26	3.9	0.992 (0.969–0.998)
		Interobserver reproducibility		
		CMR-FT		
GLS	0.03	3.16	7.4	0.982 (0.926–0.995)
GCS	−2.3	6.6	18.1	0.922 (0.629–0.981)
		CT-FT		
GLS	1.25	5.5	16.1	0.866 (0.501–0.966)
GCS	0.39	5.1	14.6	0.940 (0.759–0.985)
		TAG		
GCS	0.48	1.72	5.4	0.981 (0.918–0.995)

Abbreviations: GLS: global longitudinal strain; GCS: global circumferential strain; CMR-FT: cardiac magnetic resonance feature tracking; CT-FT: computed tomography feature tracking; TAG: myocardial tagging; CoV: coefficient of variance; ICC: intra-class correlation coefficient.

4. Discussion

4.1. Main Findings

To our knowledge, this is the first study that compared CT-FT derived strain values to CMR-FT and TAG. The main findings of our study were as follows.

i.   There was good correlation between CMR-FT and CT-FT for GLS and GCS assessment, while GCS derived from both CMR-FT and CT-FT had a moderate correlation with TAG;

ii.   The intra- and interobserver reproducibility of CMR-FT and CT-FT were excellent;

iii.   There were no significant differences between cardiac CT and CMR for the volumetric assessment of the LV.

In the past decade, multiple methods to assess myocardial strain parameters from cardiac CT datasets have emerged. Most use tissue tracking algorithms originally developed for CMR or echocardiography to track either endocardial or epicardial borders of the left ventricular (LV) in 2D cine loops generated from 3D cardiac CT datasets. As with CMR and echocardiography, these methods allow for the quantification of well-studied global strain parameters, GLS, GCS, and global radial strain (GRS). In 2010, Helle-Valle et al. used a multimodality tissue tracking algorithm, originally developed for analysis of echocardiographic images, to assess GRS in a cohort of ischemic heart disease patients ($n = 20$). They demonstrated that the results of this method had good correlation with GRS derived from TAG ($r = 0.68$) and that the method has the ability to discern scarred LV segments [16]. Buss et al. used a similar feature tracking algorithm in a cohort of congestive heart failure patients ($n = 27$) to obtain and compare global strain parameters from cardiac CT and transthoracic echocardiography datasets. They found close correlation for GRS ($r = 0.97$), GCS ($r = 0.94$), and GLS ($r = 0.93$) between these modalities [12]. In the largest study to date ($n = 123$), Fukui et al. compared FT-derived GLS in a cohort of severe AS patients and found moderate correlation between cardiac CT and transthoracic echocardiography (TTE) ($r = 0.62$) [11].

Another method, developed specifically for cardiac CT, allows for the quantification of a cardiac CT-specific 3D principal strain. First, images of neighboring phases are interpolated using a motion coherent algorithm to reduce noise and improve motion coherence. Interpolated images are then analyzed using image and model matching algorithms to create a 3D motion-vector matrix of the LV [17]. Voxels of interest can then be chosen within this matrix to derive either a regional or global principal strain. Unlike 2D strain parameters, 3D principal strain encompasses deformation in all directions. It, thus, incorporates longitudinal, circumferential, and radial components. It is expressed as a positive value [18]. In a recent study, Ammon et al. found a close correlation ($r = -0.8$) between 3D principal strain and STE-derived GLS in a cohort ($n = 35$) of severe AS patients [19].

As previously noted, in the present study, we used a commercially available feature tracking software to measure GLS and GCS from cardiac CT datasets and compared it to CMR-FT and TAG in a cohort of patients with severe AS. We found a strong correlation between CT-FT and CMR-FT, but CT-FT tended to underestimate both GLS (22.40 ± 5.69 vs. 19.4 ± 5.04, $p = 0.065$) and GCS (18.91 ± 5.97 vs. 18.13 ± 4.63, $p = 0.233$). Previous authors have noticed a similar underestimation when comparing cardiac CT-derived strain to STE [12,19]. This underestimation could be driven by low temporal resolution of cardiac CT-derived cine loops. As shown by Rösner et al., accuracy of STE-derived strain measurements is dependent on the temporal resolution of the recordings [20]. They found systematic underestimation of strain parameters at temporal resolutions of less than 30 frames/cardiac cycle. Indeed, our 2D cine cardiac CT reconstructions had a temporal resolution of 10 frames/cardiac cycle, while CMR cine loops were acquired at 30 frames/cardiac cycle. To our knowledge, the performance of feature tracking at lower temporal resolutions has not been investigated yet, thus further studies are needed.

Interestingly, despite having a lower temporal resolution, when compared with TAG (the reference standard strain assessment technique), CT-FT and CMR-FT had similar correlation and LOA for GCS assessment. Additionally, reproducibility analysis revealed similar results for both FT-based techniques. If TAG data are taken as the ground truth, these findings suggest that FT algorithm performs equally well on both CMR and cardiac CT datasets.

Additionally, due to its angle independency and high temporal and spatial resolutions, CMR is the gold standard technique for the functional assessment of the heart [21]. However, despite having the worse temporal resolution, cardiac CT has been shown to have a close correlation and good agreement with CMR for the assessment of LV volumes in multiple studies [22–24], indicating that these methods can be used interchangeably for volumetric assessment. Our results agree with these findings.

4.2. Clinical Implications

There is an increasing number of patients who have implanted cardiac devices, and this decreases the feasibility of CMR due to potential artefacts or the inability to condition these devices. Our results imply that cardiac CT datasets are non-inferior to CMR datasets for the assessment of GLS and GCS using the FT algorithm. Furthermore, ours and multiple previous studies have shown potential interchangeability of volumetric measurements between cardiac CT and CMR. With further advancements in technology and an increase in temporal resolution, a cardiac CT might be used as a convenient follow-up tool to previous CMR assessments for both volumetric and strain measurements in patients with implanted cardiac devices.

4.3. Limitations

Naturally, there are certain limitations in our study. Firstly, this was a small-scale single-center trial. Secondly, we only had TAG acquisitions for short-axis slices, therefore we could not compare FT-derived GLS to a reference standard imaging technique. However, previous studies suggest that

CMR-FT has similar correlation and agreement to TAG for both GCS and GLS [25]. Thirdly, we did not have STE-derived strain parameters for a more comprehensive inter-modality comparison. Finally, given the retrospective nature of this trial and limited availability of high quality CT and CMR acquisitions that were made within a short timeframe in other populations, the trial was performed in a highly selected population of patients with severe AS. Thus, further studies are required to confirm these findings in more diverse cohorts.

5. Conclusions

Our findings show that the FT algorithm performs equally well in both CMR and cardiac CT datasets for the assessment of GLS and GCS, both in terms of reproducibility and agreement with the gold standard, TAG. In the clinical routine, cardiac CT might be used as a convenient follow-up tool to previous CMR assessments for both volumetric and strain measurements in patients with implanted cardiac devices.

Author Contributions: Conceptualization: S.K., B.P., and V.F.; methodology: S.K. and G.P.; validation: E.M., P.B., J.E., S.M.Z., R.T., and C.S. (Christopher Schneeweis); formal analysis: P.B.; investigation: C.S. (Christian Stehning) and N.S.; resources: S.K. and R.G.; data curation: S.M.Z.; writing—original draft preparation: P.B., N.S., and E.M.; writing—review and editing: all authors; visualization: P.B.; supervision: S.K. and T.L.; project administration: S.K.; funding acquisition: S.K. and B.P.

Acknowledgments: We thank the technicians of the German Heart Center Berlin for the performance of high-quality CMR and cardiac CT examinations.

References

1. Caforio, A.L.P.; Adler, Y.; Agostini, C.; Allanore, Y.; Anastasakis, A.; Arad, M.; Böhm, M.; Charron, P.; Elliott, P.M.; Eriksson, U.; et al. Diagnosis and management of myocardial involvement in systemic immune-mediated diseases: A position statement of the European Society of Cardiology Working Group on Myocardial and Pericardial Disease. *Eur. Heart J.* **2017**, *38*, 2649–2662. [CrossRef] [PubMed]

2. Prasad, M.; Hermann, J.; Gabriel, S.E.; Weyand, C.M.; Mulvagh, S.; Mankad, R.; Oh, J.K.; Matteson, E.L.; Lerman, A. Cardiorheumatology: Cardiac involvement in systemic rheumatic disease. *Nat. Rev. Cardiol.* **2015**, *12*, 168–176. [CrossRef] [PubMed]

3. Pedrizzetti, G.; Lapinskas, T.; Tonti, G.; Stoiber, L.; Zaliunas, R.; Gebker, R.; Pieske, B.; Kelle, S. The Relationship Between EF and Strain Permits a More Accurate Assessment of LV Systolic Function. *JACC Cardiovasc. Imaging* **2019**, *3033*. [CrossRef] [PubMed]

4. Pagourelias, E.D.; Mirea, O.; Duchenne, J.; Van Cleemput, J.; Delforge, M.; Bogaert, J.; Kuznetsova, T.; Voigt, J.-U. Echo Parameters for Differential Diagnosis in Cardiac Amyloidosis: a head-to-head comparison of deformation and nondeformation parameters. *Circ. Cardiovasc. Imaging* **2017**, *10*, e005588. [CrossRef] [PubMed]

5. Guerra, F.; Stronati, G.; Fischietti, C.; Ferrarini, A.; Zuliani, L.; Pomponio, G.; Capucci, A.; Danieli, M.G.; Gabrielli, A. Global longitudinal strain measured by speckle tracking identifies subclinical heart involvement in patients with systemic sclerosis. *Eur. J. Prev. Cardiol.* **2018**, *25*, 1598–1606. [CrossRef] [PubMed]

6. Fine, N.M.; Crowson, C.S.; Lin, G.; Oh, J.K.; Villarraga, H.R.; Gabriel, S.E. Evaluation of myocardial function in patients with rheumatoid arthritis using strain imaging by speckle-tracking echocardiography. *Ann. Rheum Dis.* **2014**, *73*, 1833–1839. [CrossRef] [PubMed]

7. Cho, M.-J.; Lee, J.-W.; Lee, J.; Shin, Y.B. Evaluation of Early Left Ventricular Dysfunction in Patients with Duchenne Muscular Dystrophy Using Two-Dimensional Speckle Tracking Echocardiography and Tissue Doppler Imaging. *Pediatr. Cardiol.* **2018** *39*, 1614–1619. [CrossRef] [PubMed]

8.   Obokata, M.; Nagata, Y.; Wu, V.C.-C.; Kado, Y.; Kurabayashi, M.; Otsuji, Y.; Takeuchi, M. Direct comparison of cardiac magnetic resonance feature tracking and 2D/3D echocardiography speckle tracking for evaluation of global left ventricular strain. *Eur. Heart J. Cardiovasc. Imaging* **2016**, *17*, 525–532. [CrossRef]

9.   Mavrogeni, S.; Markousis-Mavrogenis, G.; Koutsogeorgopoulou, L.; Kolovou, G. Cardiovascular magnetic resonance imaging: Clinical implications in the evaluation of connective tissue diseases. *J. Inflamm. Res.* **2017**, *10*, 55–61. [CrossRef]

10. Scatteia, A.; Baritussio, A.; Bucciarelli-Ducci, C. Strain imaging using cardiac magnetic resonance. *Heart Fail. Rev.* **2017**, *22*, 465–476. [CrossRef]

11. Fukui, M.; Xu, J.; Abdelkarim, I.; Sharbaugh, M.S.; Thoma, F.W.; Althouse, A.D.; Pedrizzetti, G.; Cavalcante, J.L. Global longitudinal strain assessment by computed tomography in severe aortic stenosis patients—Feasibility using feature tracking analysis. *J. Cardiovasc. Comput. Tomogr.* **2019**, *13*, 157–162. [CrossRef] [PubMed]

12. Buss, S.J.; Schulz, F.; Mereles, D.; Hosch, W.; Galuschky, C.; Schummers, G.; Stapf, D.; Hofmann, N.; Giannitsis, E.; Hardt, S.E.; et al. Quantitative analysis of left ventricular strain using cardiac computed tomography. *Eur. J. Radiol.* **2014**, *83*, e123–e130. [CrossRef] [PubMed]

13. Baumgartner, H.; Falk, V.; Bax, J.J.; De Bonis, M.; Hamm, C.; Holm, P.J.; Lung, B.; Lancellotti, P.; Lansac, E.; Rodriguez Munoz, D.; et al. 2017 ESC/EACTS Guidelines for the management of valvular heart disease. *Eur. Heart J.* **2017**, *38*, 2739–2791. [CrossRef] [PubMed]

14. Morton, G.; Schuster, A.; Jogiya, R.; Kutty, S.; Beerbaum, P.; Nagel, E. Inter-study reproducibility of cardiovascular magnetic resonance myocardial feature tracking. *J. Cardiovasc. Magn. Reson.* **2012**, *14*, 43. [CrossRef] [PubMed]

15. Oppo, K.; Leen, E.; Angerson, W.J.; Cooke, T.G.; McArdle, C.S. Doppler perfusion index: An interobserver and intraobserver reproducibility study. *Radiology* **1998**, *208*, 453–457. [CrossRef] [PubMed]

16. Helle-Valle, T.M.; Yu, W.C.; Fernandes, V.R.S.; Rosen, B.D.; Lima, J.A.C. Usefulness of radial strain mapping by multidetector computer tomography to quantify regional myocardial function in patients with healed myocardial infarction. *Am. J. Cardiol.* **2010**, *106*, 483–491. [CrossRef] [PubMed]

17. Tanabe, Y.; Kido, T.; Kurata, A.; Sawada, S.; Suekuni, H.; Kido, T.; Yokoi, T.; Uetani, T.; Inoue, K.; Miyagawa, M.; et al. Three-dimensional maximum principal strain using cardiac computed tomography for identification of myocardial infarction. *Eur. Radiol.* **2017**, *27*, 1667–1675. [CrossRef] [PubMed]

18. Marwan, M.; Ammon, F.; Bittner, D.; Röther, J.; Mekkhala, N.; Hell, M.; Schuhbaeck, A.; Gitsioudis, G.; Feryrer, R.; Schlundt, C.; et al. CT-derived left ventricular global strain in aortic valve stenosis patients: A comparative analysis pre and post transcatheter aortic valve implantation. *J. Cardiovasc. Comput. Tomogr.* **2018**, *12*, 240–244. [CrossRef] [PubMed]

19. Ammon, F.; Bittner, D.; Hell, M.; Mansour, H.; Achenbach, S.; Arnold, M.; Marwan, M. CT-derived left ventricular global strain: A head-to-head comparison with speckle tracking echocardiography. *Int. J. Cardiovasc. Imaging* **2019**, *35*, 1701–1707. [CrossRef] [PubMed]

20. Rösner, A.; Barbosa, D.; Aarsæther, E.; Kjønås, D.; Schirmer, H.; D'hooge, J. The influence of frame rate on two-dimensional speckle-tracking strain measurements: A study on silico-simulated models and images recorded in patients. *Eur. Heart J. Cardiovasc. Imaging* **2015**, *16*, 1137–1147. [CrossRef] [PubMed]

21. Schulz-Menger, J.; Bluemke, D.A.; Bremerich, J.; Flamm, S.D.; Fogel, M.A.; Friedrich, M.G.; Kim, R.J.; von Knobelsdorff-Brenkenhoff, F.; Kramer, C.M.; Pennell, D.J.; et al. Standardized image interpretation and post processing in cardiovascular magnetic resonance: Society for Cardiovascular Magnetic Resonance (SCMR) Board of Trustees Task Force on Standardized Post Processing. *J. Cardiovasc. Magn. Reson.* **2013**, *15*, 35. [CrossRef] [PubMed]

22. Greupner, J.; Zimmermann, E.; Grohmann, A.; Dübel, H.-P.; Althoff, T.; Borges, A.C.; Rutsch, W.; Schlattmann, P.; Hamm, B.; Dewey, M. Head-to-Head Comparison of Left Ventricular Function Assessment with 64-Row Computed Tomography, Biplane Left Cineventriculography, and Both 2- and 3-Dimensional Transthoracic Echocardiography. *J. Am. Coll. Cardiol.* **2012**, *59*, 1897–1907. [CrossRef] [PubMed]

23. Wu, Y.-W.; Tadamura, E.; Yamamuro, M.; Kanao, S.; Okayama, S.; Ozasa, N.; Toma, M.; Kimura, T.; Komeda, M.; Togashi, K. Estimation of global and regional cardiac function using 64-slice computed

tomography: A comparison study with echocardiography, gated-SPECT and cardiovascular magnetic resonance. *Int. J. Cardiol.* **2008**, *128*, 69–76. [CrossRef] [PubMed]

24. Sarwar, A.; Shapiro, M.D.; Nasir, K.; Nieman, K.; Nomura, C.H.; Brady, T.J.; Cury, R.C. Evaluating global and regional left ventricular function in patients with reperfused acute myocardial infarction by 64-slice multidetector CT: A comparison to magnetic resonance imaging. *J. Cardiovasc. Comput. Tomogr.* **2009**, *3*, 170–177. [CrossRef] [PubMed]

25. Cao, J.J.; Ngai, N.; Duncanson, L.; Cheng, J.; Gliganic, K.; Chen, Q. A comparison of both DENSE and feature tracking techniques with tagging for the cardiovascular magnetic resonance assessment of myocardial strain. *J. Cardiovasc. Magn. Reson.* **2018**, *20*, 26. [CrossRef] [PubMed]

10

Hybrid Coronary Percutaneous Treatment with Metallic Stents and Everolimus-Eluting Bioresorbable Vascular Scaffolds: 2-Years Results from the GABI-R Registry

Tommaso Gori [1,2,*], Stephan Achenbach [3], Thomas Riemer [4], Julinda Mehilli [5,6], Holger M. Nef [7], Christoph Naber [8], Gert Richardt [9], Jochen Wöhrle [10], Ralf Zahn [11], Till Neumann [12], Johannes Kastner [13], Axel Schmermund [14], Christian Hamm [7,15] and Thomas Münzel [1,2]
for the GABI-R Study Group

[1]   Zentrum für Kardiologie, University Medical Center, Johannes Gutenberg University Mainz, 55131 Mainz, Germany; tmuenzel@uni-mainz.de
[2]   German Centre for Cardiovascular Research, partner site Rhine Main, 55131 Mainz, Germany
[3]   Department of Cardiology, Friedrich-Alexander University Erlangen-Nürnberg, 91054 Erlangen, Germany; achenbach@uni-erlangen.de
[4]   IHF GmbH-Institut für Herzinfarktforschung, 67063 Ludwigshafen, Germany; riemer@ihf.de
[5]   Department of Cardiology, Munich University Clinic, LMU, 80539 Munich, Germany; mehilli@lmu.de
[6]   German Centre for Cardiovascular Research, partner site Munich Heart Alliance, 80539 Munich, Germany
[7]   Department of Cardiology, University of Giessen, Medizinische Klinik I, 35392 Giessen, Germany; h.nef@me.com (H.M.N.); hamm@neuheim.de (C.H.)
[8]   Klinik für Kardiologie und Angiologie, Elisabeth-Krankenhaus, 45138 Essen, Germany; naber@contilia.de
[9]   Herzzentrum, Segeberger Kliniken GmbH, 23795 Bad Segeberg, Germany; richrdt@segeberg.de
[10] Department of Internal Medicine II, University of Ulm, 89081 Ulm, Germany; woehrle@ulm.de
[11] Abteilung für Kardiologie, Herzzentrum Ludwigshafen, 67063 Ludwigshafen, Germany; zahn@klinikum.de
[12] Department of Cardiology, University of Essen, 45138 Essen, Germany; neumann@uniwien.at
[13] Department of Cardiology, University of Vienna Medical School, 1090 Wien, Austria; kastner@viennw.at
[14] Bethanien Hospital, 60389 Frankfurt, Germany; schmermund@ccb.de
[15] Department of Cardiology, Kerckhoff Heart and Thorax Center, 61231 Bad Nauheim, Germany
*   Correspondence: tomgori@hotmail.com

Abstract: The limitations of the first-generation everolimus-eluting coronary bioresorbable vascular scaffolds (BVS) have been demonstrated in several randomized controlled trials. Little data are available regarding the outcomes of patients receiving hybrid stenting with both BVS and drug-eluting stents (DES). Of 3144 patients prospectively enrolled in the GABI-Registry, 435 (age 62 ± 10, 19% females, 970 lesions) received at least one BVS and one metal stent (hybrid group). These patients were compared with the remaining 2709 (3308 lesions) who received BVS-only. Patients who had received hybrid stenting had more frequently a history of cardiovascular disease and revascularization ($p < 0.05$), had less frequently single-vessel disease ($p < 0.0001$), and the lesions treated in these patients were longer ($p < 0.0001$) and more frequently complex. Accordingly, the incidence of periprocedural myocardial infarction ($p < 0.05$) and that of cardiovascular death, target vessel and lesion failure and any PCI at 24 months was lower in the BVS-only group (all $p < 0.05$). The 24-months rate of definite and probable scaffold thrombosis was 2.7% in the hybrid group and 2.8% in the BVS-only group, that of stent thrombosis in the hybrid group was 1.86%. In multivariable analysis, only implantation in bifurcation lesions emerged as a predictor of device thrombosis, while the device type was not associated with this outcome ($p = 0.21$). The higher incidence of events in patients receiving hybrid stenting reflects the higher complexity of the lesions in these patients; in patients treated with a hybrid strategy, the type of device implanted did not influence patients´ outcomes.

Keywords: coronary artery disease; drug eluting stents; stent bioresorbable

1. Introduction

A number of randomized controlled trials comparing the outcomes of drug eluting stents compared to first-generation everolimus-eluting coronary bioresorbable vascular scaffolds (BVS) have shown the limitations of this novel type of devices [1–4]. When compared with drug eluting stents (DES), the mechanical limitations of BVS, including thicker and wider struts, lower radial strength, and limited expansion capabilities [5,6] represent important limitations for the treatment of complex lesions, including ostial or calcific ones, bifurcations, and lesions in small vessels. Supporting this concept, a number of post-hoc analyses have shown that this type of lesions represents predictors for BVS failure [7–9] unless a dedicated implantation technique is used [10,11]. Additionally, lesions in the left main, in by-pass grafts, and restenotic lesions have been excluded from the CE certification from the very beginning.

Based on these considerations, some authors have advocated for the use of a hybrid approach, which consists of limiting the use of BVS to settings in which the use of BVS is allowed (or considered to be safe) [12]. While this strategy is in conflict with the concept of "vascular regeneration" which represents the foundation of the use of BVS, it might still have the theoretical advantage that vessels (e.g., the proximal segments) in which long-term complications are clinically more relevant, would be "stent-free" after device resorption. Independently of the clinical rationale supporting the use of hybrid stenting, this setting however allows a direct head-to-head comparison of the outcomes of the device types independently of patients´ characteristics and clinical presentation.

The multicenter German-Austrian ABSORB Registry (GABI-R) was designed to monitor the usage of BVS in everyday practice. Details on this international registry have been published elsewhere [13]. In the current analysis, we set out to assess the incidence of clinical events in patients receiving hybrid percutaneous coronary interventions.

2. Methods

Between November 2013 and January 2016, consecutive patients undergoing implantation of at least one BVS (Absorb; Abbott Vascular, Santa Clara, CA, USA) were enrolled in a prospective single-arm registry in 92 GABI-R centers. Details on the methods for patients' inclusion and follow-up in this observational registry have been previously published [13–15]. The study was conducted in accordance with the provisions of the Declaration of Helsinki and with the International Conference on Harmonization Good Clinical Practices, the protocol was approved by each local ethics committee (first Vote: Ethic committee of the Justus Liebig Universität Giessen 190/13) and all patients provided written, informed consent. Clinicaltrial.gov NCT02066623

2.1. Objective of the Study

The objective of this study was to investigate the outcome of patients receiving hybrid stenting with at least one drug eluting stent and one bioresorbable scaffold.

2.2. Procedures

Lesion preparation, BVS implantation, postdilation and use of intracoronary imaging, as well as medical therapy, were left to the operator's discretion. The protocol recommended use of pre- and postdilation. High-pressure dilation was defined as dilation with ≥14ATM. Antiplatelet therapy consisted of aspirin (loading dose 250–500 mg and maintenance dose 100 mg/day) and clopidogrel (loading dose at least 300 mg and maintenance dose 75 mg/day), prasugrel (loading dose 60 mg and maintenance dose 10 mg), or ticagrelor (loading dose 180 mg and maintenance dose 90 mg bid). Dual antiplatelet therapy was recommended for at least 12 months.

2.3. Definitions

For the purpose of the present analysis, hybrid stenting was defined as implantation of at least one Absorb BVS and one metallic stent (BMS or DES) in the same patient. The primary endpoint of the present study was the incidence of definite/probable device thrombosis in lesions/patients treated with BVS compared to metallic stents.

Procedural success was defined as visually estimated residual stenosis <30% with thrombolysis in myocardial infarction flow grade III. Other definitions were based on the Academic Research Consortium (ARC) criteria [16]. Scaffold thrombosis was defined as definite or probable. Cardiac death was defined as death from immediate cardiac causes or complications related to the procedure as well as any death in which a cardiac cause could not be excluded. Myocardial infarction (MI) was defined according to the World Health Organization extended definition. Target lesion failure (TLF) was defined as a composite of cardiac death, target vessel MI, and clinically-driven target lesion revascularization (TLR). Target vessel failure (TVF) was defined as a composite of cardiac death, target-vessel MI, and clinically driven target vessel revascularization (TVR).

2.4. Data Management and Outcomes of Interest

Data in the GABI-R were collected electronically via an internet-based application and centralized by the IHF GmbH-Institut für Herzinfarktforschung (Ludwigshafen, Germany). Patients were contacted by telephone at 30 days, six months and two years using standardized questionnaires. Follow-up, source verification, quality controls were performed centrally. All events were adjudicated and classified by an independent event adjudication committee.

2.5. Statistical Analysis

Data are presented as mean ± standard deviation, absolute frequencies and percentages, or median (lower, upper quartile) as appropriate. Data are presented per patient and per lesion. Odds-ratios (95% confidence limits) are presented to characterize the differences in event frequencies among groups. The incidence of events in the periprocedural interval and at each of the follow-up times was tested with Pearson's Chi-squared test. Concerning device thrombosis, testing for differences on patient level had to face a highly unbalanced design: There was no reference group for DES/BMS-only treatment. Thus, we implemented a loglinear model for an incomplete contingency table and three factors: BVS thrombosis, stent thrombosis, and hybrid treatment, accounting for interactions between the treatment and device type. To compare times to event (= device thrombosis) and assess the impact of the device type and hybrid stenting on outcomes, a proportional-hazard model ("Cox regression") on stent level was implemented. Intra-subject correlations were considered by using a robust sandwich estimate aggregating stent residuals to subject level. This multiple regression model included the device type as a main factor and additional pre-defined predictor variables that have been previously shown to be associated with scaffold/stent thrombosis in the GABI-R: Total stent length, lesion type, bifurcation lesion, and time of implantation (before or after January 2015). Missing values were imputed either by random drawing from the standardized empirical distribution (in case of missing times-to-event), by modal values (binary) or by median values (metrical variables). A two-tailed p value <0.05 was considered to indicate statistical significance. Statistical analyses were performed using the SAS® software, version 9.4 for Windows. Copyright © 2002–2012 SAS Institute Inc. SAS and all other SAS Institute Inc. product or service names are registered trademarks or trademarks of SAS Institute Inc., Cary, NC, USA.

3. Results

3.1. Patient Characteristics

CONSORT flow diagrams are presented in Figure 1 (left and right panel). Of 3144 (4278 lesions) patients included in the GABI-R registry who received at least one BVS and whose two-years vital status was known, 2709 (3308 lesions) were treated with scaffolds only (BVS-only group) while 435 (970 lesions) were treated with at least one additional metallic stent (hybrid group).

Patient characteristics are presented in Table 1. Patients in the hybrid group consistently showed characteristics compatible with a higher complexity: Glomerular filtration rate was lower ($p < 0.05$), the prevalence of prior PCI ($p < 0.01$), myocardial infarction ($p < 0.01$), multivessel disease ($p < 0.0001$), male sex ($p < 0.05$) were all higher in the hybrid group and there was a trend towards older age and higher diabetes prevalence in this group (both = 0.06). In line with this, procedure duration, contrast use, radiation time, and the number of lesions treated per patient were larger in the hybrid group (all $p < 0.0001$). DAPT with prasugrel was used more commonly in the hybrid group ($p < 0.05$). The prevalence of smoking was higher in the BVS-only group ($p < 0.05$).

Table 1. Baseline characteristics of the cohort.

	Total (Hybrid + BVS-Only) $n = 3144$	Hybrid Group $n = 435$	BVS Only $n = 2709$	p Value
Female gender	22.9% (721/3144)	19.1% (83/435)	23.6% (638/2709)	<0.05
Age (years, rounded)	60.87 ± 11.02	61.91 ± 10.36,	60.7 ± 11.11	0.06
Diabetes mellitus	20.9% (651/3117)	24.2% (105/433)	20.3% (546/2684)	0.06
Current smoker	34.9% (1039/2978)	30.4% (128/421)	35.6 % (911/2557)	<0.05
Arterial hypertension	73.4% (2274/3100)	75.3% (324/430)	73% (1950/2670)	0.31
Hypercholesterolemia	56.5% (1702/3010)	59.6% (243/408)	56.1% (1459/2602)	0.19
Glomerular filtration rate	79.39 ± 23.68, $n = 1590$	75.33 ± 22.55, $n = 165$	79.86 ± 23.77, $n = 1425$	<0.05
History of myocardial infarction	22.2% (687/3094)	27.4% (117/427)	21.4% (570/2667)	<0.01
History of PCI	33.9% (1044/3079)	39.6% (169/427)	33% (875/2652)	<0.01
History of aorto-coronary bypass surgery	2.5% (79/3131)	3% (13/433)	2.4% (66/2698)	0.49
History of CAD	41.1% (1137/2768)	44% (178/405)	40.6% (959/2363)	0.20
History of stroke	2.7% (85/3143)	3% (13/435)	2.7% (72/2708)	0.69
Acute coronary syndrome at presentation	51.4% (1617/3143)	47.8% (208/435)	52% (1409/2708)	0.10
Stable angina pectoris	33.5% (1053/3143)	33.1% (144/435)	33.6% (909/2708)	0.85
Left ventricular ejection fraction	56.09 ± 10.5, $n = 1930$	54.84 ± 10.15, $n = 282$	56.31 ± 10.55, $n = 1648$	<0.05
1-vessel CAD	41.9% (1317/3144)	20% (87/435)	45.4% (1230/2709)	<0.0001
2-vessels CAD	31% (974/3144)	35.6% (155/435)	30.2% (819/2709)	<0.05
3-vessel CAD	27.1% (852/3144)	44.4% (193/435)	24.3% (659/2709)	<0.0001

Values are mean ± SD or % (absolute number/number of available records); CAD = coronary artery disease; PCI = percutaneous coronary intervention, CBR = clinical BVS restenosis.

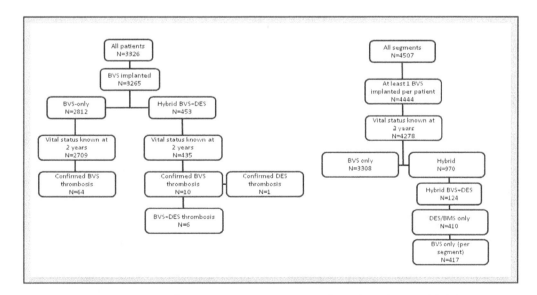

Figure 1. Study flow per patient (**left** panel) and per lesion (**right**).

Lesion characteristics are presented in Table 2. A total of 4962 BVS/Stents (4349 BVS, 631 in the hybrid group and 3718 in the BVS-only group, and 613 stents, all in the hybrid group) were implanted.

The large majority of metallic stents were DES (total of DES used: 610), and only three BMS were used. Interventions in the hybrid group were more frequent in the LAD, those in the BVS-only group were more frequent in the RCA ($p < 0.0001$ and $p < 0.05$). Compatible with the above differences between groups, all parameters expressing lesion complexity were more frequent in the hybrid group: The prevalence of B2 ($p < 0.05$), C1 ($p < 0.0001$), C2 ($p < 0.05$) lesions, bifurcation lesions ($p < 0.0001$), chronic total occlusions ($p < 0.0001$), lesions with severe tortuosity ($p < 0.05$), presence of calcium ($p < 0.05$), and lesion length ($p < 0.0001$) were higher in the hybrid group than in the BVS only group. Predilatation was performed in 93.5% of BVS-only treated patients and 85.7% of patients treated with hybrid-PCI ($p < 0.0001$). The use of high-pressure inflations, scoring balloons, rotablator, was more frequent in the hybrid group ($p < 0.001$). In contrast, postdilation was performed more frequently (73.6% compared to 68.4% in BVS-only patients.

Table 2. Angiographic and procedural characteristics.

	Total (Hybrid + BVS-Only)	Hybrid Group	BVS Only	p Value
Procedure duration, minutes	58.90 ± 28.91, $n = 3141$	77.83 ± 35.96, $n = 435$	55.85 ± 26.38, $n = 2706$	<0.0001
Radiation time, minutes	11.84 ± 8.22, $n = 3143$	18.05 ± 10.64, $n = 435$	10.84 ± 7.28, $n = 2708$	<0.0001
Amount of contrast medium, mL	174.76 ± 74.65, $n = 3140$	223.40 ± 91.21, $n = 435$	166.94 ± 68.50, $n = 2705$	<0.0001
IVUS	3% (94/3142)	2.8% (12/435)	3% (82/2707)	0.76
OCT	4.5% (141/3142)	4.6% (20/435)	4.5% (121/2707)	0.90
Per lesion				
Treated segments	4278	970	3308	
Lesions treated with BRS only	87.3% (3670/4204)	43.8% (417/951)	100% (3253/3253)	
Lesions treated with stents only	9.8% (410/4204)	43.1% (410/951)	0% (0/3253)	
Intervention in LAD	74.7% (1582/2118)	84.7% (287/339)	72.8% (1295/1779)	<0.0001
Intervention in LCX	59.6% (813/1363)	63.8% (153/240)	58.8% (660/1123)	0.15
Intervention in RCA	68.4% (1051/1537)	62.8% (155/247)	69.5% (896/1290)	<0.05
Graft	23.8% (5/21)	0% (0/1)	25% (5/20)	0.57
Lesion type				
A	26.5% (1133/4270)	19.4% (187/964)	28.6% (946/3306)	<0.0001
B1	37% (1579/4270)	36.1% (348/964)	37.2% (1231/3306)	0.52
B2	19.6% (836/4270)	21.9% (211/964)	18.9% (625/3306)	<0.05
C1	12.6% (539/4270)	17% (164/964)	11.3% (375/3306)	<0.0001
C2	4.3% (183/4270)	5.6% (54/964)	3.9% (129/3306)	<0.05
De novo lesion	94.2% (4025/4272)	92.9% (897/966)	94.6% (3128/3306)	<0.05
Ostial lesion	0.8% (36/4272)	0.5% (5/966)	0.9% (31/3306)	0.21
Bifurcation lesion	2.9% (123/4272)	5.5% (53/966)	2.1% (70/3306)	<0.0001
100% stenosis	5.6% (241/4272)	5.7% (55/966)	5.6% (186/3306)	0.94
Chronic total occlusion	37.3% (90/241)	63.6% (35/55)	29.6% (55/186)	<0.0001
Severe tortuosity	1.2% (52/4263)	1.9% (18/961)	1% (34/3302)	<0.05
No calcification	35.9% (1533/4270)	33.2% (320/964)	36.7% (1213/3306)	<0.05
% Stenosis	86.30 ± 11.73, $n = 4275$	84.92 ± 11.93, $n = 968$	86.71 ± 11.65, $n = 3307$	<0.0001
Imaging	3.2% (136/4275)	1.8% (17/968)	3.6% (119/3307)	<0.01
FFR	5.2% (223/4262)	6.7% (64/961)	4.8% (159/3301)	<0.05
RVD	2.95 ± 0.63, $n = 93$	3.15 ± 0.43, $n = 11$	2.92 ± 0.64, $n = 82$	0.26
Lesion length	17.12 ± 9.30, $n = 4258$	18.84 ± 10.51, $n = 956$	16.62 ± 8.85, $n = 3302$	<0.0001
Lesion length >34 mm	5.6% (238/4258)	8.4% (80/956)	4.8% (158/3302)	<0.0001
Any lesion preparation	91.7% (3921/4274)	85.7% (830/968)	93.5% (3091/3306)	<0.0001
Pre-dilatation	100% (3920/3921)	100% (830/830)	100% (3090/3091)	0.60
High pressure balloon	43% (1680/3908)	49.3% (408/828)	41.3% (1272/3080)	<0.0001
Non-compliant balloon	73% (1215/1665)	85.3% (348/408)	69% (867/1257)	<0.0001
Use of scoring balloon	3% (116/3921)	5.4% (45/830)	2.3% (71/3091)	<0.0001
Rotablation	0.2% (6/3921)	0.6% (5/830)	0% (1/3091)	<0.001
Stent/BVS size, mm	3.07 ± 0.59, $n = 4960$	3.03 ± 0.45, $n = 1243$	3.08 ± 0.63, $n = 3717$	<0.001
Postdilatation performed	72.4% (3093/4271)	68.4% (660/965)	73.6% (2433/3306)	<0.01
High-pressure Postdilation	89.5% (2766/3090)	86.9% (573/659)	90.2% (2193/2431)	<0.05
PSP-technique	6.4% (244/3794)	12.6% (68/541)	5.4% (176/3253)	<0.0001
Procedural success	99% (4229/4273)	98.7% (954/967)	99.1% (3275/3306)	0.27
Glycoprotein IIb/IIIa inhibitors	8% (252/3143)	6.7% (29/435)	8.2% (223/2708)	0.26
Medical therapy at discharge				
Aspirin	97.3% (3056/3141)	95.9% (417/435)	97.5% (2639/2706)	<0.05
P2Y12-receptor inhibitorsClopidogrel	44% (1351/3068)	41.2% (175/425)	44.5% (1176/2643)	0.2
Prasugrel	34.1% (1045/3068)	38.6% (164/425)	33.3% (881/2643)	<0.05
Ticagrelor	21.9% (672/3068)	20.2% (86/425)	22.2% (586/2643)	0.37

Values are mean ± SD, median (quartiles) or % (absolute number/number of available records); BVS = bioresorbable vascular scaffold; CBR = clinical BVS restenosis; DES = drug eluting stent; PCI = percutaneous coronary intervention.

Lesion and procedural characteristics in the hybrid group are presented in Table 3. Of the 970 lesions in patients in the hybrid group, 417 (43.8%) had been treated with BVS only, 410 (43.1%) with DES/BMS only and there was a total of 124 lesions treated with overlapping hybrid strategy (2.9% of the total, 12.8% of the lesions treated in patients who received hybrid revascularization). An additional 19 were not classified in the database. When lesions treated with BVS-only were compared to lesions treated with DES/BMS only, BVS-only lesions were longer, more frequently type C2 (both $p < 0.05$), and there was a trend towards more frequent chronic total occlusions ($p = 0.06$). Only the prevalence of bifurcation lesions was higher in the DES/BMS-treated lesions ($p < 0.0001$). There was a total of 25 Medina 1,1,1 lesions, and 2 Medina 0,1,1 lesions in the hybrid group. There were only three cases of hybrid bifurcation stenting (metallic stent + BVS in the same bifurcation lesion). In terms of procedural parameters, larger predilation balloons, imaging and postdilation were used more frequently in BVS-treated lesions ($p < 0.01$, $p < 0.05$ and $p < 0.0001$). Procedural success was 99% in both groups.

Table 3. Lesion-level analysis, bioresorbable vascular scaffold (BVS)-treated lesions compared to lesions treated with metallic stents in the hybrid group.

	Total	BVS Only	DES/BMS Stent Only	p Value	OR (95%-CI)
Number of lesions	827	417	410		
Stenosis (%) before PCI	84.42 ± 11.94, $n = 827$	84.47 ± 11.36, $n = 417$	84.37 ± 12.51, $n = 410$	0.69	
RVD (mm)	2.96 ± 0.29, $n = 6$	2.96 ± 0.24, $n = 3$	2.95 ± 0.39, $n = 3$	1	
Lesion length (mm)	18.01 ± 9.9, $n = 815$	18.6 ± 9.66, $n = 411$	17.41 ± 10.1, $n = 404$	<0.05	
Lesion length >34 mm	6.5 % (53/815)	6.8% (28/411)	6.2% (25/404)	0.72	1.11 (0.63–1.94)
Morphology					
A	20.4% (168/823)	21.4% (89/416)	19.4% (79/407)	0.48	1.13 (0.80–1.59)
B1	36.2% (298/823)	36.8% (153/416)	35.6% (145/407)	0.73	1.05 (0.79–1.40)
B2	22.6% (186/823)	20% (83/416)	25.3% (103/407)	0.07	0.74 (0.53–1.02)
C1	15.6% (128/823)	15.1% (63/416)	16% (65/407)	0.74	0.94 (0.64–1.37)
C2	5.2% (43/823)	6.7% (28/416)	3.7% (15/407)	<0.05	1.89 (0.99–3.59)
De novo vessel	93% (767/825)	93.8% (391/417)	92.2% (376/408)	0.37	1.28 (0.75–2.19)
In-stent re-stenosis	1% (8/825)	0.5 % (2/417)	1.5% (6/408)	0.15	0.32 (0.06–1.61)
Bifurcation	5.9% (49/825)	2.4% (10/417)	9.6% (39/408)	<0.0001	0.23 (0.11–0.47)
Complete occlusion	5.3% (44/825)	6.2% (26/417)	4.4% (18/408)	0.24	1.44 (0.78–2.67)
CTO	61.4% (27/44)	73.1% (19/26)	44.4% (8/18)	0.06	3.39 (0.95–12.09)
Ostial lesion	0.6% (5/825)	0.2% (1/417)	1% (4/408)	0.17	0.24 (0.03–2.18)
Severe tortuosity	2% (16/820)	1.2% (5/416)	2.7% (11/404)	0.12	0.43 (0.15–1.26)
No calcification	33.7% (277/823)	36.3% (151/416)	31% (126/407)	0.11	1.27 (0.95–1.7)
Mild	43.7% (360/823)	44.2% (184/416)	43.2% (176/407)	0.78	1.04 (0.79–1.37)
Moderate	18.2% (150/823)	15.9% (66/416)	20.6% (84/407)	0.08	0.73 (0.51–1.04)
Severe	4.4% (36/823)	3.6% (15/416)	5.2% (21/407)	0.28	0.69 (0.35–1.35)

Table 3. *Cont.*

	Total	BVS Only	DES/BMS Stent Only	*p* Value	OR (95%-CI)
		Procedural Characteristics			
Pre-dilatation	100% (693/693)	100% (396/396)	100% (297/297)	n.d.	
High pressure balloon	51.1% (353/691)	52.3% (207/396)	49.5% (146/295)	0.47	1.12 (0.83–1.51)
Maximum balloon diameter (mm)	2.75 ± 0.46, n = 689	2.79 ± 0.41, n = 395	2.69 ± 0.5, n = 294	<0.01	
Scoring balloon	5.8% (40/693)	6.8% (27/396)	4.4 % (13/297)	0.17	1.6 (0.81–3.15)
Rotablation	0.6% (4/693)	0.5% (2/396)	0.7% (2/297)	0.77	0.75 (0.10–5.35)
Post-dilatation	66.8% (551/825)	85.5% (355/415)	47.8% (196/410)	<0.0001	
High pressure balloon	86.5% (476/550)	89.9% (319/355)	80.5% (157/195)	<0.01	
Intravasc. imaging (IVUS/OCT/QCA) after PCI	1.6% (13/827)	2.6% (11/417)	0.5% (2/410)	<0.05	
Procedural success	99% (819/827)	99% (413/417)	99% (406/410)	0.98	

Values are mean ± SD or % (absolute number/number of available records).

3.2. Clinical Outcomes

The incidence of periprocedural myocardial infarction ($p < 0.05$, OR 4.2(1.2–14.9)) and vessel perforation ($p < 0.001$, OR 4.9(1.8–13.2)) was higher in the hybrid group. Otherwise, there was no difference in the incidence of periprocedural events.

At 30 days (Table 4), the incidence of cardiovascular death, target vessel and target lesion failure were higher in the hybrid group. Similarly, at 24-month follow-up (follow up available in 98.4% of the patients), the incidence of cardiovascular death ($p < 0.05$, OR 2.3(1.0–5.2)), target vessel failure ($p < 0.01$, OR 1.7(1.2–2.3)) and target lesion failure ($p < 0.05$, OR 1.6(1.1–2.3)), and that of any PCI ($p < 0.05$, OR 1.4(1.1–1.8)), were higher in the hybrid group.

There was no significant difference ($p = 0.13$) in the incidence of target lesion revascularization (estimates and confidence limits presented in Figure 2).

A total of 17 definite/probable stent thromboses occurred in the hybrid group during the 24-months follow-up: In six cases, they affected both (at least) a DES and a BVS in the same patient; in four cases, they only affected a BVS, and in one case only one DES.

Figure 3A,B show the two-years incidence, as well as estimates and confidence limits for the incidence of stent and BVS thrombosis in both the hybrid and BVS-only group. Before testing for differences, effects of the device type and hybrid treatment had to be separated and adjusted for possible interactions. Thereafter, with regard to treatment strategy, only a trend towards a higher incidence of BVS thrombosis remained in the BVS-only group ($p = 0.07$). With regards to the device type, BVS and stent thrombosis rates did not differ significantly, neither within the hybrid group ($p = 0.22$), between hybrid and BVS-only group ($p = 0.31$), nor pooled over all treatments ($p = 0.07$).

In the multivariable analysis, only the implantation in bifurcation lesions emerged as an independent predictor of device thrombosis (Table 5). In separate analyses neither acute coronary syndrome at index nor the implantatation technique used modified this association ($p = 0.241$ and $p = 0.637$, respectively).

Table 4. Clinical Outcomes.

	Total (*n* = 3144)	Hybrid Stenting (*n* = 435)	BVS Only (*n* = 2709)	*p* Value	OR (95%-CI)
Periprocedural complications					
Death	0% (0/3143)	0% (0/435)	0% (0/2708)	n.d.	-
MI	0.3% (10/3143)	0.9% (4/435)	0.2% (6/2708)	<0.05	4.18 (1.17–14.87)
CABG - emergency operation	0% (0/3143)	0% (0/435)	0% (0/2708)	n.d.	-
Coronary thrombosis	0.4% (12/3143)	0.9% (4/435)	0.3% (8/2708)	0.05	3.13 (0.94–10.45)
Coronary perforation	0.5% (16/3140)	1.6% (7/435)	0.3% (9/2705)	<0.001	4.9 (1.82–13.22)
30-days follow-up					
All-cause mortality	0.51% (16/3144)	1.15% (5/435)	0.41% (11/2709)	<0.05	2.85 (0.99–8.25)
Cardiovascular mortality	0.32% (10/3144)	0.92% (4/435)	0.22% (6/2709)	< 0.05	4.18 (1.18–14.88)
Scaffold thrombosis Definite	0.86% (27/3144)	1.15% (5/435)	0.81% (22/2709)	0.48	1.42 (0.53–3.77)
- Probable	0.35% (11/3144)	0.69% (3/435)	0.3% (8/2709)	0.20	2.34 (0.62–8.87)
Stent thrombosis Definite	0.23% (1/435)	0.23% (1/435)		-	-
- Probable	0.69% (3/435)	0.69% (3/435)		-	-
Any myocardial infarction	1.43% (45/3144)	1.84% (8/435)	1.37% (37/2709)	0.44	1.35 (0.63–2.93)
Target vessel related MI	1.18% (37/3144)	1.61% (7/435)	1.11% (30/2709)	0.37	1.46 (0.64–3.35)
Target lesion revascularization	1.08% (34/3144)	1.38% (6/435)	1.03% (28/2709)	0.52	1.34 (0.55–3.25)
Target lesion failure	1.49% (47/3144)	2.76% (12/435)	1.29% (35/2709)	<0.05	2.17 (1.12–4.21)
Target vessel failure	1.72% (54/3144)	2.99% (13/435)	1.51% (41/2709)	<0.05	2 (1.07–3.77)
24-months follow-up					
Follow-up available	98.4% (3094/3144)	97.2% (423/435)	98.6% (2671/2709)		
All-cause mortality	3.06% (96/3135)	4.37% (19/435)	2.85% (77/2700)	0.09	1.56 (0.93–2.6)
Cardiovascular mortality	0.96% (30/3135)	1.84% (8/435)	0.81% (22/2700)	<0.05	2.28 (1.01–5.16)
Scaffold thrombosis Definite	2% (54/2694)	1.33% (5/375)	2.11% (49/2319)	0.32	0.63 (0.25–1.58)
- Probable	0.78% (21/2688)	1.33% (5/377)	0.69% (16/2311)	0.19	1.93 (0.7–5.29)
Stent thrombosis Definite	0.53% (2/374)	0.53% (2/374)		-	-
- Probable	1.33% (5/377)	1.33% (5/377)		-	-
Any myocardial infarction	5.07% (137/2703)	5.31% (20/377)	5.03% (117/2326)	0.82	1.06 (0.65–1.72)
Target vessel related MI	3.37% (91/2700)	3.19% (12/376)	3.4% (79/2324)	0.84	0.94 (0.51–1.74)
Target lesion revascularization	6% (162/2698)	7.71% (29/376)	5.73% (133/2322)	0.13	1.38 (0.91–2.09)
Target lesion failure	7.19% (195/2711)	10.24% (39/381)	6.7% (156/2330)	<0.05	1.59 (1.1–2.3)
Target vessel failure	10.21% (277/2714)	14.7% (56/381)	9.47% (221/2333)	<0.01	1.65 (1.2–2.26)
Any PCI	18.52% (505/2727)	23.02% (87/378)	17.79% (418/2349)	<0.05	1.38 (1.06–1.79)

Values are mean ± SD or % (absolute number/number of available records); BRS = bioresorbable vascular scaffold; CI = confidence interval; PCI = percutaneous coronary intervention; OR = Odds ratio.

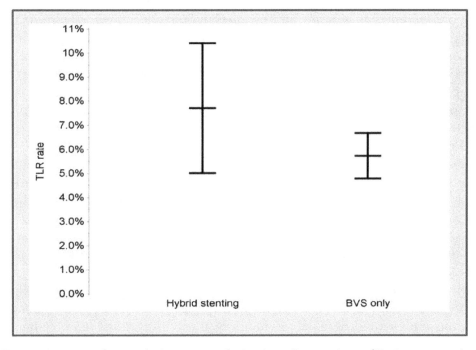

Figure 2. Two-years rates of target lesion revascularization. Comparison of Patients treated with hybrid vs. BVS-only strategy.

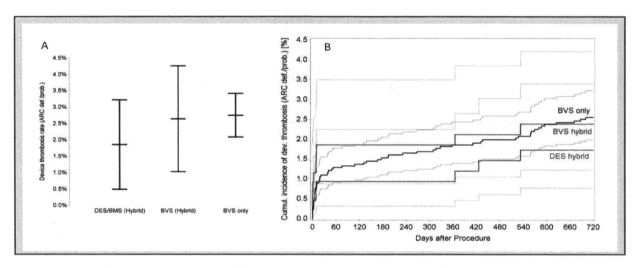

Figure 3. (**A**) Two-years incidence of device thrombosis. There was no difference among lesions treated with BVS only, metal stents only, or hybrid strategies; (**B**) cumulative incidence curves showing an overlap of the confidence intervals.

Table 5. Multivariate analysis of the predictors of definite/probable device thrombosis.

Analysis of Maximum Likelihood Estimates					
Parameter	Parameter Estimate	Standard Error	Chi-Square	Pr > ChiSq	Hazard Ratio
Device type	0.44883	0.36030	1.5518	0.2129	1.566
Total stent length	0.21102	0.16178	1.7015	0.1921	1.235
Lesion type B2/C	−0.32342	0.26101	1.5354	0.2153	0.724
Implantation after Jan. 2015	−0.33539	0.23905	1.9683	0.1606	0.715
Bifurcation	1.04114	0.48421	4.6233	0.0315	2.832

4. Discussion

The GABI-R is a large international registry on the use of BVS. In the present analysis, we investigate the characteristics and outcomes of patients who received hybrid stenting (i.e., at least one BVS and at least one metallic stent). The major findings of the current analysis include: (i) Patients treated with hybrid stent/scaffold therapy had a more complex presentation and worse outcomes than those treated with BVS alone; (ii) During a two-years follow-up, the incidence of adverse events at the level of the lesions treated with BVS was not worse than that of the lesions treated with metallic stents.

The concept of a vascular scaffold that provides temporary mechanical support and is resorbed during follow-up to avoid a permanent unnecessary foreign body remains an attractive concept for percutaneous coronary intervention. Although initial randomized trials reported non-inferiority as compared to metallic drug-eluting stents [17,18], with signals that these devices might also be used in more complex lesion [19–22], more recent trials have consistently demonstrated a higher incidence of adverse events both early and late after implantation [3,4,23]. Mechanistic evidence shows that these increased rates might depend on the technique used at the time of implantation, inadequate selection of lesions, and, importantly, on the mechanical limitations of the devices, including increased strut thickness, reduced expansion limits, reduced radial resistance [6,8]. Further, particular settings, such as chronic total occlusions, acute coronary syndromes, treatment of ostial lesions and a lack of care at the time of implantation have all been associated with increased events, including thrombosis and restenosis [3,24–28]. Based on these notions, the general recommendation is that patients who have been treated with BVS should prolong their dual antiplatelet therapy until complete resorption of the device. This recommendation is likely to be particularly important in patients treated for complex lesions, such as those presented here. Knowledge of these limitations lead to the hypothesis that, by avoiding implantation in the presence of adverse lesion characteristics (e.g., long lesions with proximal or distal reference vessel diameters unsuitable for BVSs, very calcific or bifurcation lesions) may represent an adequate compromise between the benefit of the BVS and the risk of adverse events.

Interestingly, this setting also allows within-patients comparison of the outcomes, i.e., removes the confounding influence of differences in patient-related risk factors among groups.

Beyond any consideration on the safety of the devices implanted, it might be hypothesized that the use of BVS might be more advantageous in long and proximal segments, which might thereafter regain the possibility to adjust their diameter in response to biochemical and physical stimuli. Calcific lesions, in contrast, might have theoretically less potential for regeneration. Thrombotic lesions might also represent a setting for BVS, allowing "plaque stabilization" as previously reported [29]. The use of BVS in CTO lesions has also been reported, but no data are available regarding the capacity of these lesions to regenerate [30]. In the present database, lesions treated with BVS-only were indeed longer and more frequently of type C (thrombotic). There was a trend towards less calcific lesions being treated with BVS-only, but this difference remains speculative. Finally, in theory there is also a rationale for the use of BVS in ostial or bifurcation lesions to limit (in time) the risks associated with malapposed struts, but the evidence on their (lack of) safety in these settings clearly discouraged their use [31]. Based on the instructions for use, in the present database, bifurcation lesions were almost exclusively treated with metallic stents.

Reports on the short-term outcomes of this so-called hybrid stenting strategy (the use of both metallic stents and BVS in the same patient or lesion) have been previously published [32–35]. Collectively, these studies reported that the use of a hybrid approach might be an acceptable compromise to overcome the limitations of BVS. In the present study, we report data from a larger database with longer follow-up. In our study, the incidence of events was similar between BVS and metallic stents, while treatment of complex patients and lesions (particularly bifurcation lesions) remained an independent predictor of events. These findings confirm the hypothesis that a hybrid approach, in which more complex settings are treated with DES, might be a feasible option, although its rationale needs to be validated. While polymeric devices of the first generation (Absorb, Abbott vascular) have been removed from the market following the evidence of increased adverse events, the present results might also apply to other similar devices for which data from large databases are not available. Further, they provide a perspective for novel devices of this type.

5. Limitations

The GABI-R was a prospective registry designed to provide information on the real-life use of BVS and is therefore affected by the limitations of this type of study design. Centralized data monitoring, quality assessment, and follow-up were however performed to limit these issues. With regards to the present analysis, hybrid treatment of lesions complicates the adjudications of the events to one or the other device type. For this reason, the comparison of the incidence of device thrombosis was limited to lesions treated with only one type of device. Despite the size of the database, conclusions on very rare subsets (e.g., bifurcation lesions treated with hybrid strategy) were not possible. As well, data on the antiplatelet regimen at the time of the event are missing. The present data should not be directly extrapolated to second-generation BVS. However, they provide an insight that a prudent strategy of hybrid stenting might allow combining the benefit of bioresorbable devices with the safety of standard metallic stents also in more complex settings. The impact of a correct implantation technique has been demonstrated in a number of papers, including those from our group [8,18,24,25,27,28]. Unfortunately, the absence of a central quantitative coronary analysis in the present database does not allow clear conclusions to this regard. Finally, the comparison of the outcomes within hybrid patients removes patient-related confounders but not lesion-related confounders, which would be better addressed in trials with a randomization at lesion level.

6. Conclusions

We report on the outcome of patients undergoing BVS and DES implantation, a particularly complex subset among patients treated with BVS. In this database, which is one of the largest ones worldwide on the use of BVS, the type of device implanted did not influence patients' outcomes.

Hybrid stenting is a negotiation between the concept of "full vascular regeneration" and the mechanical limitations of these novel devices. Whether the use of metallic stents, although limited as compared to a full-metal strategy, compromises the benefits of BVS remains however to be discussed. Whether the use of a hybrid strategy with newer (and safer) scaffolds will present any advantage as compared to a full-DES strategy, will need to be studied in the future.

Author Contributions: Conceptualization, H.N. and T.G.; Methodology, T.G. and H.N.; Formal Analysis, T.G.; Writing—Original Draft Preparation, T.G.; Supervision, H.N.; Revision for intellectual content: S.A., T.R., J.M., C.N., G.R., J.W., R.Z., T.N., J.K., A.S., C.H., T.M.

References

1.   Kereiakes, D.J.; Ellis, S.G.; Metzger, C.; Caputo, R.P.; Rizik, D.G.; Teirstein, P.S.; Litt, M.R.; Kini, A.; Kabour, A.; Marx, S.O.; et al. 3-Year Clinical Outcomes With Everolimus-Eluting Bioresorbable Coronary Scaffolds: The ABSORB III Trial. *J. Am. Coll. Cardiol.* **2017**, *70*, 2852–2862. [CrossRef]

2.   Mahmoud, A.N.; Barakat, A.F.; Elgendy, A.Y.; Schneibel, E.; Mentias, A.; Abuzaid, A.; Elgendy, I.Y. Long-Term Efficacy and Safety of Everolimus-Eluting Bioresorbable Vascular Scaffolds Versus Everolimus-Eluting Metallic Stents: A Meta-Analysis of Randomized Trials. *Circ. Cardiovasc. Interv.* **2017**, *10*, e005286. [CrossRef] [PubMed]

3.   Polimeni, A.; Anadol, R.; Munzel, T.; Indolfi, C.; De Rosa, S.; Gori, T. Long-term outcome of bioresorbable vascular scaffolds for the treatment of coronary artery disease: a meta-analysis of RCTs. *BMC Cardiovasc. Disord.* **2017**, *17*, 147. [CrossRef] [PubMed]

4.   Wykrzykowska, J.J.; Kraak, R.P.; Hofma, S.H.; van der Schaaf, R.J.; Arkenbout, E.K.; Ijsselmuiden, A.J.; Elias, J.; van Dongen, I.M.; Tijssen, R.Y.G.; Koch, K.T.; et al. Bioresorbable Scaffolds versus Metallic Stents in Routine PCI. *N. Engl. J. Med.* **2017**, *376*, 2319–2328. [CrossRef]

5.   Foin, N.; Lee, R.; Mattesini, A.; Caiazzo, G.; Fabris, E.; Kilic, I.D.; Chan, J.N.; Huang, Y.; Venkatraman, S.S.; Di Mario, C.; et al. Bioabsorbable vascular scaffold overexpansion: insights from in vitro post-expansion experiments. *EuroIntervention* **2016**, *11*, 1389–1399. [CrossRef] [PubMed]

6.   Ormiston, J.A.; Webber, B.; Ubod, B.; Darremont, O.; Webster, M.W. An independent bench comparison of two bioresorbable drug-eluting coronary scaffolds (Absorb and DESolve) with a durable metallic drug-eluting stent (ML8/Xpedition). *EuroIntervention* **2015**, *11*, 60–67. [CrossRef]

7.   Anadol, R.; Lorenz, L.; Weissner, M.; Ullrich, H.; Polimeni, A.; Münzel, T.; Gori, T. Characteristics and outcome of patients with complex coronary lesions treated with bioresorbable scaffolds Three years follow-up in a cohort of consecutive patients. *EuroIntervention* **2018**, *14*, e1011–e1019. [CrossRef]

8.   Ellis, S.G.; Gori, T.; Serruys, P.W.; Nef, H.; Steffenino, G.; Brugaletta, S.; Munzel, T.; Feliz, C.; Schmidt, G.; Sabaté, M. Clinical, Angiographic, and Procedural Correlates of Very Late Absorb Scaffold Thrombosis: Multistudy Registry Results. *JACC. Cardiovasc. Interv.* **2018**, *11*, 638–644. [CrossRef] [PubMed]

9.   Wohrle, J.; Nef, H.M.; Naber, C.; Achenbach, S.; Riemer, T.; Mehilli, J.; Münzel, T.; Schneider, S.; Markovic, S.; Seeger, J.; et al. Predictors of early scaffold thrombosis: results from the multicenter prospective German-Austrian ABSORB RegIstRy. *Coron. Artery Dis.* **2018**, *29*, 389–396. [CrossRef]

10.   Regazzoli, D.; Latib, A.; Ezhumalai, B.; Tanaka, A.; Leone, P.P.; Khan, S.; Kumar, V.; Rastogi, V.; Ancona, M.B.; Mangieri, A.; et al. Long-term follow-up of BVS from a prospective multicenter registry: Impact of a dedicated implantation technique on clinical outcomes. *Int. J. Cardiol.* **2018**, *270*, 113–117. [CrossRef] [PubMed]

11.   Anadol, R.; Gori, T. The mechanisms of late scaffold thrombosis. *Clin. Hemorheol. Microcirc.* **2017**, *67*, 343–346. [CrossRef] [PubMed]

12.   Tanaka, A.; Jabbour, R.J.; Mitomo, S.; Latib, A.; Colombo, A. Hybrid Percutaneous Coronary Intervention With Bioresorbable Vascular Scaffolds in Combination With Drug-Eluting Stents or Drug-Coated Balloons for Complex Coronary Lesions. *JACC. Cardiovasc. Interv.* **2017**, *10*, 539–547. [CrossRef]

13.   Nef, H.; Wiebe, J.; Achenbach, S.; Münzel, T.; Naber, C.; Richardt, G.; Mehilli, J.; Wöhrle, J.; Neumann, T.; Biermann, J.; et al. Evaluation of the short- and long-term safety and therapy outcomes of the

everolimus-eluting bioresorbable vascular scaffold system in patients with coronary artery stenosis: Rationale and design of the German-Austrian ABSORB RegIstRy (GABI-R). *Cardiovasc. Revasc. Med.* **2016**, *17*, 34–37. [CrossRef] [PubMed]

14. Nef, H.M.; Wiebe, J.; Kastner, J.; Mehilli, J.; Muenzel, T.; Naber, C.; Neumann, T.; Richardt, G.; Schmermund, A.; Woehrle, J.; et al. Everolimus-eluting bioresorbable scaffolds in patients with coronary artery disease: Results from the German-Austrian ABSORB RegIstRy (GABI-R). *EuroIntervention* **2017**, *13*, 1311–1318. [CrossRef]

15. Mehilli, J.; Achenbach, S.; Woehrle, J.; Baquet, M.; Riemer, T.; Muenzel, T.; Nef, H.; Naber, C.; Richardt, G.; Zahn, R.; et al. Clinical restenosis and its predictors after implantation of everolimus-eluting bioresorbable vascular scaffolds: results from GABI-R. *EuroIntervention* **2017**, *13*, 1319–1326. [CrossRef]

16. Cutlip, D.E.; Windecker, S.; Mehran, R.; Boam, A.; Cohen, D.J.; van Es, G.A.; Steg, P.G.; Morel, M.A.; Mauri, L.; Vranckx, P.; et al. Clinical end points in coronary stent trials: a case for standardized definitions. *Circulation* **2007**, *115*, 2344–2351. [CrossRef]

17. Kimura, T.; Kozuma, K.; Tanabe, K.; Nakamura, S.; Yamane, M.; Muramatsu, T.; Saito, S.; Yajima, J.; Hagiwara, N.; Mitsudo, K.; et al. A randomized trial evaluating everolimus-eluting Absorb bioresorbable scaffolds vs. everolimus-eluting metallic stents in patients with coronary artery disease: ABSORB Japan. *Eur. Heart J.* **2015**, *36*, 3332–3342. [CrossRef]

18. Stone, G.W.; Gao, R.; Kimura, T.; Kereiakes, D.J.; Ellis, S.G.; Onuma, Y.; Cheong, W.F.; Jones-McMeans, J.; Su, X.; Zhang, Z.; et al. 1-year outcomes with the Absorb bioresorbable scaffold in patients with coronary artery disease: a patient-level, pooled meta-analysis. *Lancet* **2016**, *387*, 387–1277. [CrossRef]

19. De Ribamar Costa, J.; Abizaid, A.; Bartorelli, A.L.; Whitbourn, R.; Jepson, N.; Perin, M.; Steinwender, C.; Stuteville, M.; Ediebah, D.; Sudhir, K.; et al. One-year clinical outcomes of patients treated with everolimus-eluting bioresorbable vascular scaffolds versus everolimus-eluting metallic stents: a propensity score comparison of patients enrolled in the ABSORB EXTEND and SPIRIT trials. *EuroIntervention* **2016**, *12*, 1255–1262. [CrossRef] [PubMed]

20. La Manna, A.; Chisari, A.; Giacchi, G.; Capodanno, D.; Longo, G.; Di Silvestro, M.; Capranzano, P.; Tamburino, C. Everolimus-eluting bioresorbable vascular scaffolds versus second generation drug-eluting stents for percutaneous treatment of chronic total coronary occlusions: Technical and procedural outcomes from the GHOST-CTO registry. *Catheter Cardiovasc. Interv.* **2016**, *88*, E155–E163. [CrossRef]

21. Tamburino, C.; Capranzano, P.; Gori, T.; Latib, A.; Lesiak, M.; Nef, H.; Caramanno, G.; Naber, C.; Mehilli, J.; Di Mario, C.; et al. 1-Year Outcomes of Everolimus-Eluting Bioresorbable Scaffolds Versus Everolimus-Eluting Stents: A Propensity-Matched Comparison of the GHOST-EU and XIENCE V USA Registries. *JACC. Cardiovasc. Interv.* **2016**, *9*, 9–440. [CrossRef]

22. Lesiak, M.; Zawada-Iwanczyk, S.; Lanocha, M.; Klotzka, A.; Lesiak, M. Bioresorbable scaffolds for complex coronary interventions. *Minerva Cardioangiol.* **2018**, *66*, 477–488. [PubMed]

23. Sorrentino, S.; Giustino, G.; Mehran, R.; Kini, A.S.; Sharma, S.K.; Faggioni, M.; Farhan, S.; Vogel, B.; Indolfi, C.; Dangas, G.D. Everolimus-Eluting Bioresorbable Scaffolds Versus Everolimus-Eluting Metallic Stents. *J. Am. Coll. Cardiol.* **2017**, *69*, 3055–3066. [CrossRef]

24. Dimitriadis, Z.; Polimeni, A.; Anadol, R.; Geyer, M.; Weissner, M.; Ullrich, H.; Münzel, T.; Gori, T. Procedural Predictors for Bioresorbable Vascular Scaffold Thrombosis: Analysis of the Individual Components of the "PSP" Technique. *J. Clin. Med.* **2019**, *8*, 93. [CrossRef] [PubMed]

25. Gori, T.; Polimeni, A.; Indolfi, C.; Räber, L.; Adriaenssens, T.; Münzel, T. Predictors of stent thrombosis and their implications for clinical practice. *Nat. Rev. Cardiol.* **2019**, *16*, 243–256. [CrossRef]

26. Polimeni, A.; Anadol, R.; Münzel, T.; De Rosa, S.; Indolfi, C.; Gori, T. Predictors of bioresorbable scaffold failure in STEMI patients at 3years follow-up. *I. J. Cardiol.* **2018**, *268*, 68–74.

27. Polimeni, A.; Weissner, M.; Schochlow, K.; Ullrich, H.; Indolfi, C.; Dijkstra, J.; Anadol, R.; Münzel, T.; Gori, T. Incidence, Clinical Presentation, and Predictors of Clinical Restenosis in Coronary Bioresorbable Scaffolds. *JACC. Cardiovasc. Interv.* **2017**, *10*, 1819–1827. [CrossRef]

28. Sorrentino, S.; De Rosa, S.; Ambrosio, G.; Mongiardo, A.; Spaccarotella, C.; Polimeni, A.; Sabatino, J.; Torella, D.; Caiazzo, G.; Indolfi, C. The duration of balloon inflation affects the luminal diameter of coronary segments after bioresorbable vascular scaffolds deployment. *BMC Cardiovasc. Disord.* **2015**, *15*, 169. [CrossRef] [PubMed]

29. Brugaletta, S.; Gomez-Lara, J.; Garcia-Garcia, H.M.; Heo, J.H.; Farooq, V.; van Geuns, R.J.; Chevalier, B.; Windecker, S.; McClean, D.; Thuesen, L. Analysis of 1 year virtual histology changes in coronary plaque located behind the struts of the everolimus eluting bioresorbable vascular scaffold. *Int. J. Cardiovasc. Imaging* **2012**, *28*, 1307–1314. [CrossRef] [PubMed]

30. Polimeni, A.; Anadol, R.; Münzel, T.; Geyer, M.; De Rosa, S.; Indolfi, C.; Gori, T. Bioresorbable vascular scaffolds for percutaneous treatment of chronic total coronary occlusions: a meta-analysis. *BMC Cardiovasc. Disord.* **2019**, *19*, 59. [CrossRef]

31. Gori, T.; Wiebe, J.; Capodanno, D.; Latib, A.; Lesiak, M.; Pyxaras, S.A.; Mehilli, J.; Caramanno, G.; Di Mario, C.; Brugaletta, S.; et al. Early and midterm outcomes of bioresorbable vascular scaffolds for ostial coronary lesions: insights from the GHOST-EU registry. *EuroIntervention* **2016**, *12*, e550–556. [CrossRef] [PubMed]

32. Gil, R.J.; Bil, J.; Pawłowski, T.; Yuldashev, N.; Kołakowski, L.; Jańczak, J.; Jabłoński, W.; Paliński, P. The use of bioresorbable vascular scaffold Absorb BVS(R) in patients with stable coronary artery disease: one-year results with special focus on the hybrid bioresorbable vascular scaffolds and drug eluting stents treatment. *Kardiol. Pol.* **2016**, *74*, 627–633. [CrossRef] [PubMed]

33. Rigatelli, G.; Avvocata, F.D.; Ronco, F.; Giordan, M.; Roncon, L.; Caprioglio, F.; Grassi, G.; Faggian, G.; Cardaioli, P. Edge-to-Edge Technique to Minimize Ovelapping of Multiple Bioresorbable Scaffolds Plus Drug Eluting Stents in Revascularization of Long Diffuse Left Anterior Descending Coronary Artery Disease. *J. Interv. Cardiol.* **2016**, *29*, 275–284. [CrossRef] [PubMed]

34. Karbassi, A.; Kassaian, S.E.; Poorhosseini, H.; Salarifar, M.; Jalali, A.; Nematipour, E.; Kazazi, E.H.; Alidoosti, M.; Hajizeinali, A.M.; Tokaldani, M.L. Selective versus exclusive use of drug-eluting stents in treating multivessel coronary artery disease: a real-world cohort study. *Tex. Heart Inst. J.* **2014**, *41*, 477–483. [CrossRef]

35. Naganuma, T.; Latib, A.; Ielasi, A.; Panoulas, V.F.; Sato, K.; Miyazaki, T.; Colombo, A. No more metallic cages: an attractive hybrid strategy with bioresorbable vascular scaffold and drug-eluting balloon for diffuse or tandem lesions in the same vessel. *Int. J.Cardiol.* **2014**, *172*, 618–619. [CrossRef] [PubMed]

11

Ischemic Heart Disease during Acute Exacerbations of COPD

Rosa Malo de Molina [1],*, **Silvia Aguado** [1], **Carlos Arellano** [2]⑩, **Manuel Valle** [1] and **Piedad Ussetti** [1]

[1] Department of Pulmonary Medicine, University Hospital Puerta de Hierro, Majadahonda, 28040 Madrid, Spain; s.aguado.ibanez@gmail.com (S.A.); rycmvalle@hotmail.com (M.V.); pied2152@separ.es (P.U.)

[2] Department of Cardiology, University Hospital Puerta de Hierro, Majadahonda, 28040 Madrid, Spain; arellano.serrano@gmail.com

* Correspondence: rmm02004@yahoo.es

Abstract: Patients with chronic obstructive pulmonary disease (COPD) have a higher risk of acute cardiovascular events, and around 30% die from cardiovascular diseases. Recent data suggest an increased risk of myocardial infarction in the following days of a severe exacerbation of COPD. Disruption in the balance during the exacerbation with tachycardia, increased inflammation and systemic oxidative stress as well as some other factors may confer an increased risk of subsequent cardiovascular events. A number of investigations may be useful to an early diagnosis, including electrocardiography, imaging techniques and blood test for biomarkers. Some drugs that have changed prognosis in the cardiovascular setting such as cardioselective beta-blockers may be underused in patients with COPD despite its demonstrated benefits. This review focuses on several aspects of exacerbation of COPD and cardiovascular events including epidemiology, possible mechanism, diagnosis and treatment.

Keywords: chronic obstructive pulmonary disease; cardiovascular; myocardial infarction; exacerbation; treatment; beta-blockers

1. Introduction

Patients with chronic obstructive pulmonary disease (COPD) often develop cardiovascular comorbidities [1]. In addition, they have a higher risk of acute cardiovascular events, and around 30% die from cardiovascular diseases (CVD) [2,3].

Focusing on ischemic heart disease, a recent meta-analysis showed that patients with COPD had a consistent risks of coronary heart disease (meta-odd ratio (OR) 186, 95% confidence interval (CI) 151–230; $p < 0.0001$), myocardial infarction (271, 169–435; $p < 0.0001$), and angina pectoris (816, 308–2159; $p < 0.0001$) [4].

Indeed, COPD patients with acute ischemic heart diseases (IHD) may have worse outcomes. The three-year follow-up of 4284 patients who received hospital treatment for coronary heart disease reported mortality rates of 21% for patients diagnosed with COPD versus 9% in those without COPD ($p \leq 0.001$) [5].

COPD patients who develop ST-segment elevation myocardial infarction (STEMI) at three-year follow-up had higher mortality than non-COPD patients in a web-based Italian registry of 11,118 consecutive patients with STEMI.

Remarkably, hospital readmissions for COPD emerged as a strong independent risk factor for recurrence of MI (HR, 2.1; 95% CI, 1.4–3.3) [6].

It is likely that part of this increased risk of IHD comes from shared risk factors, such as smoking or sedentary behavior, but also the increased cardiac stress associated with acute exacerbations that COPD patients suffer may play an important role [2].

In this line of research, recent data from the UK suggest a 2.58-fold increased risk of myocardial infarction (MI) in the following 91 days of a severe acute exacerbation of COPD (AECOPD) [7]. Notably, the cross-sectional nature of the evidence confers difficulties in assessing the directions of the association: whether myocardial infarction contributes to AECOPD or vice versa. Although the prevalence of myocardial infarction following hospitalization for AECOPD has been broadly described, no data related to the prevalence of COPD exacerbations during acute coronary events have been published to date.

The purpose of this review is to summarize current knowledge relating to epidemiology, diagnosis and treatment of ischemic heart disease in people with AECOPD and the mechanisms that may underlie its coexistence.

A search was conducted in MEDLINE (via PubMed) for observational studies published between January 1990 and August 2018 reporting ischemic heart disease including coronary heart disease, myocardial infarction, and angina pectoris in patients with acute exacerbations of COPD.

2. Epidemiology

Myocardial infarction is frequently unrecognized in patients hospitalized for COPD exacerbation. Five main articles analyzed the association between AECOPD and acute coronary events (Table 1). Brekke and coauthors retrospectively analyzed the electrocardiogram (ECG) from the day of admission of 897 patients with at least one AECOPD hospitalization. Of the 229 (25%) patients with ECG signs of previous infarction, only 30% (CI 24–36%, $n = 68$) had a recognized history of MI [8]. Unfortunately, they used a Cardiac Infarction Injury Score (CIIS) which does not include ST-segment changes in the algorithm and only 84% of COPD patients included had a spirometry in their medical record [8].

Donalson et al., using UK administrative data from 25,857 patients with COPD, reported an incidence rate of MI of 1.1 per 100 patient-years with a 2.27-fold (95% CI 1.1–4.7; $p = 0.03$) increased risk of MI 1–5 days after exacerbation (defined by prescription of both steroids and antibiotics) [9].

They analyzed aself-controlled case series of COPD, avoiding the need for multivariate analysis to adjust for confounders such as socioeconomic background or family history. However, the study has some limitations due to its retrospective nature. The study used administrative codes for COPD and MI and only some COPD patient had spirometry data recorded. Indeed, the date of the exacerbation onset could not be determined precisely only by the date of consultation and this may overestimate the time window for an acute coronary event.

Some of the limitations were solved by a prospective case series study looking at the incidence of MI in patients hospitalized with an acute exacerbation of COPD ($n =242$) in four hospitals. In total, 124 COPD patients (51%; 95% CI 48–58%) developed chest pain during the exacerbation, and 24 (10%) had raised troponin (Tn), among whom 20 (8.3%; 95% CI 5.1–12.5%) had chest pain and/or serial ECG changes, fulfilling the 2007 Universal Definition of Myocardial Infarction [10].

One in 12 patients had raised Tn along with serial ECG changes and/or chest pain and therefore a myocardial infarction diagnosis [10]. Patients with chest pain at admission were excluded.

From our point of view, patients whose primary presenting complaint was chest pain and have a diagnosis of AECOPD during hospital admission should also be evaluated, as being hospitalized by a MI does not exclude having symptoms concordant with an AECOPD before arrivingto hospital.

Table 1. Association between acute exacerbations of COPD and acute coronary events: epidemiological studies.

Author	Date	Size	Method	Outcome	Prevalence/Incidence/HR/IRR
Brekke et al. [8]	2008	897	Retrospective study from the Hospital data base	Cardiac Infarction Injury Score (CIIS) to assess the prevalence of prior MI in acute exacerbated COPD patients	229 (25%) patients with ECG signs of previous infarction, only 30% (95% CI 24–36%) had a previous recognized history of MI.
Donaldson et al. [9]	2010	25,857	Retrospective study using UK administrative data	Incidence rates of MI and stroke after exacerbation of COPD	Incidence rates of MI: 1.1 per 100 patient-years Risk of MI 1 to 5 days after AECOPD: IRR 2.27-fold (95% CI 1.1–4.7)
McAllister et al. [10]	2012	242	Prospective case series	Incidence of MI in patients hospitalized with an AECOPD	51% (95% CI 48–58%) develop chest pain; 8.3%; (95% CI 5.1–12.5%) had chest pain and/or serial ECG changes, fulfilling the 2007 Universal Definition of Myocardial Infarction
Kunisaki et al. [11]	2018	16,485	Secondary cohort analysis of the SUMMIT (Study to Understand Mortality and Morbidity) trial	Determine whether AECOPD events are associated with increased risk of subsequent cardiovascular disease	CVD events 30 days following AECOPD: HR 3.8; (95% CI 2.7–5.5) CVD events 30 days following AECOPD with hospitalization: HR 9.9; (95% CI 6.6–14.9).
Rothnie et al. [7]	2018	5696	Retrospective self-controlled case series using UK data database	Quantify the increased risks of MI and ischemic stroke risk associated with both moderate and severe AECOPD	Severe exacerbation-MI risk: IRR 2.58; (95%CI 2.26–2.95) Moderate exacerbation-MI risk: IRR 1.58; (95% CI 1.46–1.71)

AECOPD: Acute exacerbation of COPD; CI: confidence interval; COPD: chronic obstructive pulmonary disease; CVD: cardiovascular disease; ECG: electrocardiogram; HR: hazard ratio; IRR: incident rate ratio; MI: myocardial infarction.

Recent data from the SUMMIT trial (Study to Understand Mortality and MorbidITy), which investigated the effects of vilanterol and fluticasone furoate, by means of a secondary prospective cohort analysis of COPD patients with cardiovascular disease or cardiovascular risk, proved that exacerbations conferred an increased risk of subsequent CVD events, especially in hospitalized patients and within the first 30 days post-exacerbation. CVD events were a composite outcome of cardiovascular death, myocardial infarction, stroke, unstable angina, and transient ischemic attack. Among 16,485 participants in SUMMIT, 4704 participants had at least one AECOPD, 688 had at least one CVD event and 173 myocardial infarction. The 30-day hazard ratio (HR) for CV events following hospitalized AECOPD was more than two-fold higher than non-hospitalized COPD exacerbations [11].

Analysis restricted to only myocardial infarction events showed similar results, with a substantially increased risk of myocardial infarction in the first 30 days following AECOPD, a lower, but still significant, risk between 31days and 1 year, and no significant increased risk beyond 1 year. These data do not apply to COPD patients without CVD or CVD risk factor or those with severe airflow limitation (forced expiratory volume in 1 second or FEV 1 < 50%) [11].

Lately, in a within-individual analysis of 5696 COPD patients, from the UK Clinical Practice Research Datalink with linked Hospital Episodes Statistics data, Rothnie et al., investigated the rates of myocardial infarction and ischemic stroke following acute exacerbation compared to stable time [7]. They included 2850 COPD patients with a first myocardial infarction and at least one acute exacerbation, defined by a using prescription of antibiotics and oral steroids. Compared to stable periods, the 91 days following the onset of acute exacerbation were associated with a 65% increased risk of myocardial infarction (IRR 1.65, 95% CI 1.50–1.81). The increased myocardial infarction risk peaked in the first threedays post-AECOPD. The risk gradually fell back to a stable period level after 28 days for myocardial infarction.

The strength of this study was the sample size and also the analysisof previous cardiovascular medications, COPD medication, severity of airflow limitation and severity of AECOPD defined by those requiring hospitalization. However, the results in term of covariables were somewhat surprising as there was no modification of the associations between acute exacerbation and myocardial infarction by other previous cardiovascular diseases, cardiovascular drugs, COPD medicines, influenza vaccine in the baseline period, or by age or sex.

However, it is worth noting that those patients in whom primary prevention with these medicines was completely effective would not have been included in the study due to the case nature of the design.

More expected was the stronger association of acute exacerbation with myocardial infarction for those with severe airflow limitationas compared to mild-to-moderate (global initiative for chronic obstructive lung disease (GOLD) grade 1–2 IRR 1.69, (95% CI 1.45–1.98); GOLD grade 3–4 IRR 1.98, (95% CI 1.61–2.05); $p = 0.007$). With the evidence that we have now, mostly cross-sectional, it is not possible to assess the directions of the association (i.e., whether cardiovascular disease contributes to COPD or vice versa).

3. Possible Mechanisms of Ischemic Heart Diseases during Acute Exacerbations of COPD.

In this section, we briefly explore some of the mechanisms that are believed to underlie the association between AECOPD and IHD (Figure 1).

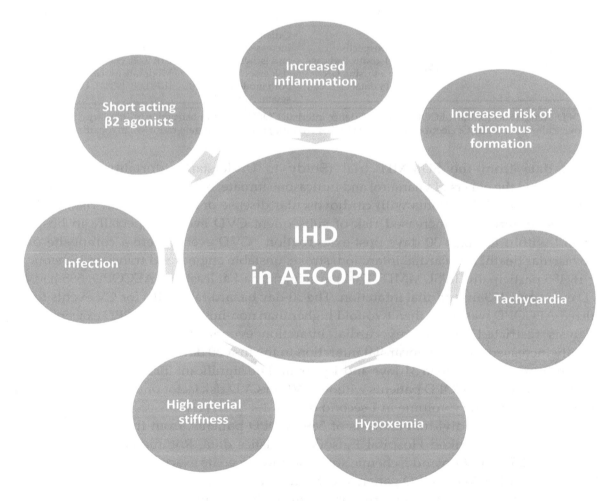

Figure 1. Potential factors contributing to acute ischemic heart disease in exacerbations of COPD. IHD: ischemic heart disease.

3.1. Infection as the Causal Mechanism of Acute Exacerbation of COPD (AECOPD)

Studies have shown that respiratory infection in the general population increases the likelihood of a MI. Meier et al. [12] reported a relative risk of 2.7 in healthy individuals during Days 1–5. Smeeth et al. [13], who investigated the relationship between lower respiratory tract infection (LRTI) and risks of myocardial infarction in 20,921 people from the general population, also reported a relative risk of 4.95 (95% CI 4.43–5.53) for myocardial infarction over Days 1–3 following LRTI. Clayton et al. [14] similarly reported in a case-controlled study an odds ratio of 2.10 with recent respiratory infection.

Whether this increased risk of MI in patients with AECOPD is restricted to those with infection as the causal mechanism of the exacerbation needs to be elucidated.

3.2. Increased Inflammation

Most COPD exacerbations are due to lower respiratory tract infections that are associated with an acute phase response with a rise in systemic inflammatory markers such as C reactive protein (CRP) [15].

This inflammatory state has been postulated as a causal mechanism of the increased risk of IHD during AECOPD.

Interestingly, systemic inflammatory mediators in stable COPD (such as CRP, fibrinogen, surfactant protein D, and neutrophils) have been associated with increased risk of CVD morbidity and mortality [16–18].

However, although previous studies suggested a potent independent association of CRP levels with cardiac events, the strength of this association has been shown to be weaker than previously reported in a recent large meta-analysis and in prospective studies [19].

Vanhaverbeke and colleagues, prospectively measured CRP in patients with a MI admitted to hospital. Median CRP levels were 1.89mg/L on admission with MI and peaked to 12.10 mg/L during hospitalization [20]. It seems that the inflammatory state was not the causal mechanism and the posterior inflammatory response is secondary to myocardial repair. Unfortunately, those were not COPD patients, but it would be interesting to perform a prospective measurement of this biomarker in a cohort of patients with AECOPD and MI and see if CRP may have different implications.

None of the observational studies mentioned in the epidemiology section of the review measured PCR. For this reason, to date, it is not possible to determine its potential contribution of inflammation in AECOPD to acute coronary events.

3.3. Increased Risk of Thrombus Formation

Platelet activation is present in stable COPD and increases during exacerbations [21]. Concentrations of other pro-atherothrombotic biomarkers, such as interleukins 6 and 8 and tumor necrosis factor α, and prothrombin fragments are also raised during exacerbations. These findings suggest that exacerbations of COPD lead to endothelial dysfunction and precipitate atherosclerotic plaque rupture and thrombosis [22].

Another possible explanation would be the increase in fibrinogen during AECOPD [23], biomarker that is directly thrombogenic [24].

3.4. Tachycardia

Hypoxemia and tachycardia associated with a COPD exacerbation can lead to adverse coronary artery events, especially in patients with pre-existing CHD or left ventricular dysfunction. The association between elevated heart rate and progression of coronary atherosclerosis has been shown in clinical studies. High minimum heart rate measured during a 24-h period in young men who survived a first myocardial infarction was associated with progression of both diffuse lesions and distinct stenos measured by angiography [25].

A positive association between a mean heart rate >80 bpm and the development of plaque disruption measured by coronary angiogram was found in an age- and sex-matched case-control study [26].

Indeed, some evidence shows that the mortality associated with increased troponin concentrationsin patients with COPD exacerbations might be linked to tachycardia [27]. This necessitates paying attention to cardiac frequency an adequately controlling it in case of AECOPD.

3.5. High Arterial Stiffness

Carotid-femoral aortic pulse wave velocity (aPWV) is a repeatable, validated gold standard noninvasive marker of cardiovascular risk and mortality, in apparently healthy and disease-specific populations. Increments of 1 ms^{-1} are associated with an increase in cardiovascular events and mortality of 12–18% depending on the risk profile of the population studied [28]. Higher arterial stiffness increases myocardial work against elevated systolic aortic pressures and reduces diastolic coronary artery blood flow, which in health is augmented by a slow reflected pulse wave arriving back at the coronary vasculature during diastole [29].

COPD exacerbations also provoke acute increases in arterial stiffness (assessed by aPWV) which then increases left ventricular afterload [30].

Arterial stiffness rose an average of 1.2 ms^{-1} (11.1%) from stable state to exacerbation ($n = 55$) and fell slowly during recovery in a prospective study of 98 COPD patients. In those with airway infection at exacerbation ($n = 24$), this rise was greater (1.4 ± 1.6 vs. 0.7 ± 1.3ms^{-1}; $p < 0.048$), prolonged, and related to sputum interleukin-6 (IL-6, rho < 0.753; $p = 0, 0.001$). In addition, the fact that exacerbation frequency status is independently associated with arterial stiffness raises the important possibility that acute exacerbations may accelerate this chronic ongoing cardiovascular process [30].

3.6. Short Acting β2 Agonists

High-dose of short acting β2 agonist inhaler therapy used to treat acute exacerbations of COPD might affect the β1 pathway and further aggravate tachycardia and sympathetic stress. These drugs are considered safe at standard doses in patients with stable COPD. However, the safety of these high doses during exacerbations has not been established in clinical trials. Although there is no evidence to confirm the hypothesis in patients with acute exacerbations of COPD at risk of ischemic heart diseases, high doses of β2 agonist may predispose to acute coronary events.

3.7. Hypoxemia

AECOPD may be associated with acute hypoxemia. It has been demonstrated that acute hypoxemia increases sympathetic nerve activity by stimulation of arterial chemoreceptors [31]. This sympathetic drive may link tachycardia and increases risk of ischemic coronary events [25,26].

4. Diagnosis

The diagnosis of heart disease in patients with COPD exacerbation is difficult, because many signs and symptoms are overlapping. The objective is to recognize acute coronary artery events in AECOPD as soon as possible. A delayed diagnosis of myocardial infarction in COPD patients has been demonstrated.In a UK database, 34,027 COPD patients with a first diagnosis of ST-elevation myocardial infarction (STEMI) were compared to 266,119 non-COPD patients. Patients with COPD who had a STEMI were more likely to have an initial diagnosis other than definite STEMI (OR 1.24, 95% CI 1.19–1.30) [32]. The following subsections discuss various diagnostic techniques.

4.1. Electrocardiogram

Acute exacerbated COPD patients should be evaluated for signs of acute ischemia in ECG (ST-segment depression or elevation), and previous MI (T-wave inversion, pathological Q-wave, loss of R, or left bundle branch block). In the 2007 Universal Definition statement, myocardial infarction was defined as a rise and/or fall of Tn concentration together with evidence of myocardial ischemia (at least one of the following: symptoms of ischemia; new ST-T changes; new left bundle branch block; or development of pathological Q waves in the ECG) [33].

McAllister and coauthors studied patients hospitalized with AECOPD and found that ECG was frequent abnormal: 12 (5%) had left bundle branch block, 34 (14%) T wave inversion, and 37 (15%) Q waves considered "diagnostic" in the Minnesota coding system. Only three patients developed Q waves during admission, but serial changes in T wave inversion/flattening and ST depression were common (65 (32%) and 19 (9%), respectively). Thirteen(6%) had serial changes in ST elevation. These changes in the T wave axis and dynamic ST segment depression on serial ECG, although common, were not associated with raised troponin [10]. These changes may reflect transient myocardial ischemia secondary to increased oxygen demand or reduced supply that is insufficient to induce MI.

Rothnie et al., in a self-controlled case-series of 5696 adults with COPD with a first myocardial infarction (n = 2850), investigated the rates of myocardial infarction following acute exacerbation compared to stable time, within individuals, and found that the association of acute exacerbation with myocardial infarction in the 91 days following acute exacerbation was higher for non-STEMIs (IRR 1.80, 95% CI 1.56–2.06) than for STEMIs (IRR 1.39, 95% CI 1.16–1.68) [7]. From a clinical point of view, these findings may help us to carefully look for these kinds of ECG alterations in AECOPD.

4.2. Echocardiogram

An echocardiogram may assess biventricular cardiac function and identify ischemic areas when IHD is suspected. However, it is often less useful in an exacerbating patient as a high proportion of tests are limited by poor acoustic window.

No data related to echocardiography findings in exacerbated COPD patients with acute ischemic heart disease have been published yet.

4.3. Cardiac Magnetic Resonance

Currently, the gold standard for assessing biventricular function, cardiac morphology and viability is Cardiac MRI, especially in patients with poor acoustic window on echocardiogram. However, this technique has important limitations: long duration, cost and claustrophobic nature of an MRI scanner. These limitations make this technique impractical in patients with COPD exacerbation [34].

4.4. Cardiac Computed Tomography (CT)

In patients with suspected coronary artery disease, multicenter studies using 64-slice CT have demonstrated sensitivities of 95–99% and specificities of 64–83% as well as negative predictive values of 97–99% for the identification of individuals with at least one coronary artery stenosis [35].

Dynamic cardiac CT can be used to assess biventricular function, pulmonary artery anatomy, coronary artery calcification, and pulmonary structure. In exacerbated COPD patient, this technique may also be a good diagnostic strategy.

Interestingly, low-dose ungated multidetector CT performed for lung evaluations is reliable to predict the presence of coronary artery calcification (CAC) and assessment of Agatston score. Correlations between gated and ungated CAC were excellent (r = 0.96) [36].

4.5. Biomarkers

Both troponin (Tn) and brain natriuretic peptide (BNP) are markers of myocardial stress, which can be easily measured and relatively cheap as a bedside test.

A rise of Tn concentration is a necessary condition to diagnose myocardial infarction [33]. However, although Tn measurements are specific for myocardial necrosis, they are not specific for ischemic injury because cardiac Tn can also be raised in heart failure, renal dysfunction, pulmonary embolism, pulmonary hypertension, tachyarrhythmias, and sepsis.

In most cases, during exacerbations, high sensitivity measurements show higher circulating cardiac Tn concentrations than the upper normal limit, particularly in patients with known ischemic heart disease [27,37,38].

In a meta-analysis of eight studies of patients with AECOPD, Cardiac Tn elevation ranged from 18% to 73%. They found that cardiac Tn elevation was significantly related to an increased risk for all-cause mortality (OR 1.69; 95% CI 1.25–2.29; I2 40%). This finding was independent to the follow-up length of studies ($\leq$6 months: OR 3.22, 95% CI 1.31–7.91; >6 months: OR 1.38,95% CI 1.02–1.86). When they compared the kind of troponin with the mortality prediction, Tn T seemed to be more helpful in predicting all-cause mortality as compared to Tn I (OR 1.54,95% CI 1.2–1.96 vs. OR 3.39, 95% CI 0.86–13.36, respectively) [37].

In a recent issue of Open Heart, Buhan et al. reviewed the role of cardiac biomarkers for predicting left ventricular dysfunction and cardiovascular mortality in acute exacerbations of COPD [39].

Of the ten included papers that measured Tn, seven analyzed mortality, and, in all of these, a significant association was found between elevated levels of Tn and increased mortality. Most of the studies were generally long term (more than 30 days after measurement), although various time points were used in the follow up (from in-hospital deaths to 50 months). In addition, increased levels of Tn at discharge was a predictor of readmission to hospital (HR = 2.89, 95% CI 1.13–7.36) [39]. In addition, not only the Tn level but also whether it rises, then falls or remains elevated during an AECOPD may also have prognostic value [40].

Brain natriuretic peptide is not useful to predict acute ischemic heart disease but may be important to assess left ventricular failure that may accompany MI in some exacerbated COPD patients. Another important reason to measure BNP or NT-proBNP in AECOPD is because its raise is associated to increased short term mortality. The measure of NT-proBNP during AECOPD then is justified as a prognosis marker and as a strategy to diagnose cardiac failure [39].

5. Treatment

Patients with AECOPD who develop MI should be treated as guidelines and no restriction should be made with cardiovascular medication. It has been shown that patients with COPD receive less guideline-recommended treatment for CVD, such as revascularization, than patients with CVD but without COPD [32].

We summarizesome data on cardiovascular treatment and AECOPD.

5.1. Acetylic Salicylic Acid (ASA)

In a prospective observationalstudy of 1343 patients with COPD who were admitted to hospital with acute exacerbation [35], thrombocytosis (>400 $\times$ 10^9 cells per mm^3) at admission was independently associated with increased in-hospital and one-year all-cause mortality, and antiplatelet therapy was associated with reduced one-year all-cause mortality after an acute exacerbation of COPD [41].

This has been verified in subsequent meta-analysis [42] in which all-cause mortality was significantly lower in COPD patients receiving antiplatelet treatment (OR 0.81,95%CI 0.75–0.88). This association was observed inboth stable COPD patients and those with acute exacerbation of COPD. Overall, the five studies included 11,117 COPD patients, 3069 with AECOPD. Antiplatelet therapy administration was common (47%, 95% CI 46–48%), ranging from 26% to 61%. A strength of the studies included was that IHD, present in 33% of COPD patients, was analyzed as a confounding factor by all the authors.

In this line, a recent retrospective cohort study using a large population-based data of 206,686 patients hospitalized for AECOPD, aspirin use was associated with lower rates of in-hospital mortality (1.0% vs. 1.4%; OR 0.60 (95% CI 0.50–0.72); p < 0.001), invasive mechanical ventilation use (1.7% vs. 2.6%; OR 0.64 (95% CI 0.55–0.73); p < 0.001), and shorter length-of-stay compared to non-users [43].

In a recent self-control case series, there was no modification of the increased risk of myocardial infarction in acute exacerbation compared to stable stateby previous aspirin use [7].

A randomized control trial (RCT) of COPD patients receiving either once daily 500 mg of ASA or placebo for 12 weeks in addition to their preexisting medication was stopped after an interim analysis was performed as the treatment had no effect on the lung function, measured as forced expiratory volume in 1 s (main outcome),dyspnea (measured by transition dyspnea index (TDI)) or quality of life (St. George's Respiratory Questionnaire (SGRQ)) [44].

From our point of view, a trial looking at whether antiplatelet therapy might be effective in AECOPD in terms of mortality or acute coronary events instead of lung function would add relevant evidence to adequately manage these patients.

5.2. β Blockers

An important matter is the use of β blockers, especially cardio-selective ones in COPD patients as secondary prevention [45]. Beta-blocker therapy has a proven survival benefit in patients with coronary artery disease. Unfortunately, COPD patients with comorbid cardiac disease are less likely to be prescribed β blockers as secondary prevention [46].

Data from the UK national registry of myocardial infarction (Myocardial Ischemia National Audit Project (MINAP) also reported that secondary prevention was less likely to be prescribed in patients with COPD and acute cardiac syndrome. These results were particularly evident for beta blockers (with an odds ratio of 0.25 (95% CI 0.24–0.25) for patients with non-ST elevation myocardial infarctions and 0.26 (95% CI 0.25–0.27) for those with ST-elevation myocardial infarction) [47].

This is probablydue to the ongoing fear of inducing bronchoconstriction. However, a Cochrane systematic review analyzed this issue and described that cardio-selective beta-blockers, given to patients with COPD in the identified studies, did not produce adverse respiratory effects [48].

Some non-randomized studies suggest that beta-blockers have also been associated with reduced exacerbation rates [49] and that mortality is lower in patients taking beta-blockers at the time of an exacerbation than in those who do not [50,51].

A meta-analysis of about fifteen original observational cohort studies revealed that beta-blockers treatment significantly decreased the risk of overall mortality (RR 0.72,95% CI 0.63–0.83) and exacerbation of COPD (RR 0.63,95% CI 0.57–0.71). Indeed, the risk for mortality was more significantly decreased in COPD patient with coronary artery disease (RR 0.64,95% CI 0.54–0.76) [52].

From a clinical stand point, an acute exacerbation of COPD may be a good opportunity to check for a correct diagnosis and treatment of a possible unrecognized CHD.

5.3. Statins

Other drugs that have changed prognosis in the cardiovascular setting are statins. The results of retrospective studies suggest that mortality may be lower in patients with COPD who take these drugs than in those who do not [53,54]. One randomized study using simvastatin versus placebo in the prevention of COPD exacerbations did not finddifferences in exacerbation rates, time to first exacerbation, serious adverse events, and mortality [55]. However, this study had a follow up of (±SD) of 641 ± 354 days and we donot know if longer duration of treatment would change the results. Indeed, patients with cardiovascular diseases who may have more impact on treatment were excluded.

Data on previous COPD treatment and acute ischemic heart disease are as follows:

Bronchodilators, principally long-acting muscarinic antagonists (LAMAs) and long-acting beta agonists (LABAs) have long been the mainstay pharmacological treatment of COPD, despite some observational evidence that their use may worsen existing underlying CVD or even increase the risk of developing CVD including cardiac ischemia [56].

However, accumulated evidence from previous clinical trials suggests that inhaled COPD therapies do not pose a significant CVD risk, at least in people free from cardiovascular comorbidities [56].

Lately, some randomized clinical trials on COPD medication including patients with history of heart disease showed more evidence of the cardiovascular safety of LAMA, LABA and inhaled corticosteroids (ICS) [57,58].

In a nested case-control study of more than 280,000 patients with COPD, new use of LABAs or LAMAs was associated with an approximate 1.5-fold increased cardiovascular risk within 30 days of initiation therapy. Although these findings need to be replicated, the results may be explained by the fact that worsening of COPD may have prompted the use of LABAs or LAMAs instead of adequately treat a possible exacerbation of COPD and its increased cardiovascular associated risk [59].

It makes sense that adequately prescribed COPD medications that reduce the risk of AECOPD consequently reduce also its associated increased risk of MI, but this needs to be prospectively verified.

6. Conclusions

An early recognition and treatment of ischemic heart diseases in acute exacerbations of COPD may determine prognosis.For this reason, diagnostic techniques for acute IHDshould be accessible for patients with COPD exacerbations. Understanding the complexity of the different possible mechanisms that may contribute to the increased risk of myocardial infarctionin COPD exacerbation, itis important to better delineate possible therapeutic targets in a susceptible population. Cardiac dysfunction during exacerbation represents a research challenge not only in terms of etiology but also concerning treatment strategies.

References

1.   Mullerova, H.; Agusti, A.; Erqou, S.; Mapel, D.W. Cardiovascular comorbidity in COPD: Systematic literature review. *Chest* **2013**, *144*, 1163–1178. [CrossRef] [PubMed]

2.   Sin, D.D.; Anthonisen, N.R.; Soriano, J.B.; Agusti, A.G. Mortality in COPD: Role of comorbidities. *Eur. Respir. J.* **2006**, *28*, 1245–1257. [CrossRef] [PubMed]

3.   Wise, R.A.; McGarvey, L.P.; John, M.; Anderson, J.A.; Zvarich, M.T. Reliability of cause-specific mortality adjudication in a COPD clinical trial. In Proceedings of the American Thoracic Society Annual Meeting, San Diego, CA, USA, 19–24 May 2006; p. A120.

4.   Chen, W.; Thomas, J.; Sadatsafavi, M.; Fitz Gerald, J.M. Risk of cardiovascular comorbidity in patients with chronic obstructive pulmonary disease: A systematic review and meta-analysis. *Lancet Respir. Med.* **2015**, *3*, 631–639. [CrossRef]

5.   Berger, J.S.; Sanborn, T.A.; Sherman, W.; Brown, D.L. Effect of chronic obstructive pulmonary disease on survival of patients with coronary heart disease having percutaneous coronary intervention. *Am. J. Cardiol.* **2004**, *94*, 649–651. [CrossRef] [PubMed]

6.   Campo, G.; Guastaroba, P.; Marzocchi, A.; Santarelli, A.; Varani, E.; Vignali, L.; Sangiorgio, P.; Tondi, S.; Serenelli, C.; De Palma, R.; et al. Impact of COPD on Long-term Outcome After ST-Segment Elevation Myocardial Infarction Receiving Primary Percutaneous Coronary Intervention. *Chest* **2013**, *144*, 750–757. [CrossRef] [PubMed]

7.   Rothnie, K.J.; Connell, O.; Müllerová, H.; Smeeth, L.; Pearce, N.; Douglas, I.; Quint, J.K. Myocardial Infarction and Ischaemic Stroke Following Exacerbations of Chronic Obstructive Pulmonary Disease. *Ann. Am. Thorac. Soc.* **2018**, *15*, 935–946. [CrossRef] [PubMed]

8.   Brekke, P.H.; Omland, T.; Smith, P.; Soyseth, V. Underdiagnosis of myocardial infarctionin COPD—Cardiac infarction injury score (CIIS) in patients hospitalised for COPD exacerbation. *Respir. Med.* **2008**, *102*, 1243–1247. [CrossRef] [PubMed]

9.   Donaldson, G.C.; Hurst, J.R.; Smith, C.J.; Hubbard, R.B.; Wedzicha, J.A. Increased Risk of Myocardial Infarction and Stroke Following Exacerbation of COPD. *Chest* **2010**, *137*, 1091–1097. [CrossRef] [PubMed]

10. McAllister, D.A.; Maclay, J.D.; Mills, N.L.; Leitch, A.; Reid, P.; Carruthers, R.; MacNee, W. Diagnosis of myocardial infarction following hospitalization for exacerbation of COPD. *Eur. Respir. J.* **2012**, *39*, 1097–1103. [CrossRef] [PubMed]

11. Kunisaki, K.M.; Dransfield, M.T.; Anderson, J.A.; Niewoehner, D.E. Exacerbations of Chronic Obstructive Pulmonary Disease and Cardiac Events: A Cohort Analysis. *Am. J. Respir. Crit. Care Med.* **2018**, *198*. [CrossRef] [PubMed]

12. Meier, C.R.; Jick, S.S.; Derby, L.E.; Vasilakis, C.; Jick, H. Acute respiratory-tract infections and risk of first-time acute myocardial infarction. *Lancet* **1998**, *351*, 1467–1471. [CrossRef]

13. Smeeth, L.; Thomas, S.L.; Hall, A.J.; Hubbard, R.; Farrington, P.; Vallance, P. Risk of myocardial infarction and stroke after acute infection or vaccination. *N. Engl. J. Med.* **2004**, *351*, 2611–2618. [CrossRef] [PubMed]

14. Clayton, T.C.; Thompson, M.; Meade, T.W. Recent respiratory infection and risk of cardiovascular disease: Case-control study through a general practicedatabase. *Eur. Heart J.* **2008**, *29*, 96–103. [CrossRef] [PubMed]

15. Chen, Y.-W.R.; Leung, J.M.; Sin, D.D. A Systematic Review of Diagnostic Biomarkers of COPD Exacerbation. *PLoS ONE* **2016**, *11*, e0158843. [CrossRef] [PubMed]

16. Hill, J.; Heslop, C.; Man, S.F.; Frohlich, J.; Connett, J.E.; Anthonisen, N.R.; Wise, R.A.; Tashkin, D.P.; Sin, D.D. Circulating surfactant protein-D and the risk of cardiovascular morbidity and mortality. *Eur. Heart J.* **2011**, *32*, 1918–1925. [CrossRef] [PubMed]

17. Van Eeden, S.F.; Sin, D.D. Chronic obstructive pulmonary disease: A chronic systemic inflammatory disease. *Respiration* **2008**, *75*, 224–238. [CrossRef] [PubMed]

18. Danesh, J.; Kaptoge, S.; Mann, A.G.; Sarwar, N.; Wood, A.; Angleman, S.B.; Wensley, F.; Higgins, J.P.T.; Lucy Lennon, G.E.; Eiriksdottir, G.; et al. Long-term interleukin-6 levels and subsequent risk of coronary heart disease: Two new prospective studies and a systematic review. *PLoS Med.* **2008**, *5*, e78. [CrossRef] [PubMed]

19. Danesh, J.; Wheeler, J.G.; Hirschfield, G.M.; Eda, S.; Eiriksdottir, G.; Rumley, A.; Lowe, G.D.; Pepys, M.B.; Gudnason, V. C-reactive protein and other circulating markers of inflammation in the prediction of coronary heart disease. *N. Engl. J. Med.* **2004**, *350*, 1387–1397. [CrossRef] [PubMed]

20. Vanhaverbeke, M.; Veltman, D.; Pattyn, N.; De Crem, N.; Gillijns, H.; Cornelissen, V.; Janssens, S.; Sinnaeve, P.R. CRP-reactive protein during and after myocardial infarction in relation to cardiac injuryand left ventricular function at follow-up Running head: CRP during and after myocardial infarction. *Clin. Cardiol* **2018**. [CrossRef] [PubMed]

21. Maclay, J.D.; McAllister, D.A.; Johnston, S.; Raftis, J.; McGuinnes, C.; Deans, A.; Newby, D.E.; Mills, N.L.; MacNee, W. Increased platelet activation in patients with stable and acute exacerbation of COPD. *Thorax* **2011**, *66*, 769–774. [CrossRef] [PubMed]

22. Malerba, M.; Clini, E.; Malagola, M.; Avanzi, G.C. Platelet activation as a novel mechanism of atherothrombotic risk in chronic obstructive pulmonary disease. *Expert Rev. Hematol.* **2013**, *6*, 475–483. [CrossRef] [PubMed]

23. Wedzicha, J.A.; Seemungal, T.A.; MacCallum, P.K.; Paul, E.A.; Donaldson, G.C.; Bhowmik, A.; Jeffries, D.J.; Meade, T.W. Acute exacerbations of chronic obstructive pulmonary disease are accompanied by elevations of plasma fibrinogen and serum IL-6 levels. *Thromb. Haemost.* **2000**, *84*, 210–215. [PubMed]

24. Meade, T.W.; Ruddock, V.; Stirling, Y.; Chakrabarti, R.; Miller, G.J. Fibrinolytic activity, clotting factors and long term incidence of ischaemic heart disease in the Northwick Park Heart Study. *Lancet* **1993**, *342*, 1076–1079. [CrossRef]

25. Perski, A.; Olsson, G.; Landou, C.; de Faire, U.; Theorell, T.; Hamsten, A. Minimum heart rate and coronary atherosclerosis: Independent relations to global severity and rate of progression of angiographic lesions in men with myocardial infarction at a young age. *Am. Heart J.* **1992**, *123*, 609–616. [CrossRef]

26. Heidland, U.E.; Strauer, B.E. Left ventricular muscle mass and elevated heart rate are associated with coronary plaque disruption. *Circulation* **2001**, *104*, 1477–1482. [CrossRef] [PubMed]

27. Hoiseth, A.D.; Omland, T.; Hagve, T.A.; Brekke, P.H.; Soyseth, V. Determinants of high-sensitivity cardiac troponin T during acute exacerbation of chronic obstructive pulmonary disease: A prospective cohort study. *BMC Pulm. Med.* **2012**, *12*, 22. [CrossRef] [PubMed]

28. Vlachopoulos, C.; Aznaouridis, K.; Stefanadis, C. Prediction of cardiovascular event sandall-cause mortality with arterial stiffness: A systematic review and meta-analysis. *J. Am. Coll. Cardiol.* **2010**, *55*, 1318–1327. [CrossRef] [PubMed]

29. Vlachopoulos, C.; Alexopoulos, N.; Stefanadis, C. Fast in the aorta, slow in the coronaries. *Cardiology* **2010**, *116*, 257–260. [CrossRef] [PubMed]

30. Patel, A.R.; Kowlessar, B.S.; Donaldson, G.C.; Mackay, A.J.; Singh, R.; George, S.N.; Garcha, D.S.; Wedzicha, J.A.; Hurst, J.R. Cardiovascular risk, myocardial injury, and exacerbations of chronic obstructive pulmonary disease. *Am. J. Respir. Crit. Care Med.* **2013**, *188*, 1091–1099. [CrossRef] [PubMed]

31. Stewart, A.G.; Waterhouse, J.C.; Howard, P. Cardiovascular autonomic nerve function in patients with hypoxaemic chronic obstructive pulmonary disease. *Eur. Respir. J.* **1991**, *4*, 1207–1214. [PubMed]

32. Rothnie, K.J.; Smeeth, L.; Herrett, E.; Pearce, N.; Hemingway, H.; Wedzicha, J.; Timmis, A.; Quint, J.K. Closing the mortality gap after a myocardial infarction in people with and without chronic obstructive pulmonary disease. *Heart* **2015**, *101*, 1103–1110. [CrossRef] [PubMed]

33. Thygesen, K.; Alpert, J.S.; White, H.D. Joint ESC/ACCF/AHA/WHF Task Force for the Redefinition of Myocardial Infarction. Universal Definition of Myocardial Infarction. *J. Am. Coll. Cardiol.* **2007**, *50*. [CrossRef] [PubMed]

34. Nordenskjöld, A.M.; Hammar, P.; Ahlström, H.; Bjerner, T.; Duvernoy, O.; Lindahl, B. Unrecognized myocardial infarction assessed by cardiac magnetic resonance imaging is associated with adverse long-term prognosis. *PLoS ONE* **2018**, *13*. [CrossRef] [PubMed]

35. Budoff, M.J.; Dowe, D.; Jollis, J.G.; Gitter, M.; Sutherland, J.; Halamert, E.; Scherer, M.; Bellinger, R.; Martin, A.; Benton, R.; et al. Diagnostic performance of 64-multidetector row coronary computed tomographic angiography for evaluation of coronary artery stenosis in individuals without known coronary artery disease: Results from the prospective multicenter ACCURACY (Assessment by Coronary Computed TomographicAngiographyofIndividualsUndergoingInvasiveCoronaryAngiography)trial. *J. Am. Coll. Cardiol.* **2008**, *52*, 1724–1732. [PubMed]

36. Budoff, M.J.; Nasir, K.; Kinney, G.L.; Hokanson, J.E.; Barr, R.G.; Steiner, R.; Nath, H.; Lopez-Garcia, C.; Black-Shinn, J.; Casaburi, R. Coronary Artery and Thoracic Calcium on Non-contrast Thoracic CT Scans: Comparison of Ungated and Gated Examinations in Patients from the COPD Gene Cohort. *J. Cardiovasc. Comput. Tomogr.* **2011**, *5*, 113–118. [CrossRef] [PubMed]

37. Pavasini, R.; d'Ascenzo, F.; Campo, G.; Biscaglia, S.; Ferri, A.; Contoli, M.; Papi, A.; Ceconi, C.; Ferrari, R. Cardiac troponin elevation predicts all-cause mortality in patients with acute exacerbation of chronic obstructive pulmonary disease: Systematic review and meta-analysis. *Int. J. Cardiol.* **2015**, *191*, 187–193. [CrossRef] [PubMed]

38. Søyseth, V.; Bhatnagar, R.; Holmedahl, N.H.; Neukamm, A.; Høiseth, A.D.; Hagve, T.-A.; Einvik, G.; Omland, T. Acute exacerbation of COPD is associated with four fold elevation of cardiac troponinT. *Epidemiology* **2013**, *99*, 122–126.

39. Buchan, A.; Bennett, R.; Coad, A.; Barnes, S.; Russell, R.; Manuel, A.R. The role of cardiac biomarkers for predicting left ventricular dysfunction and cardiovascular mortality in acute exacerbations of COPD. *Open Heart* **2015**, *2*, e000052. [CrossRef] [PubMed]

40. Marcun, R.; Sustic, A.; Brguljan, P.M.; Kadivec, S.; Farkas, J.; Kosnik, M.; Coats, A.J.; Anker, S.D.; Lainscak, M. Cardiac biomarkers predict outcome after hospitalization for an acute exacerbation of chronic obstructive pulmonary disease. *Int. J. Cardiol.* **2012**, *161*, 156–159. [CrossRef] [PubMed]

41. Harrison, M.T.; Short, P.; Williamson, P.A.; Singanayagam, A.; Chalmers, J.D.; Schembri, S. Thrombocytosis is associated with increased short and long term mortality after exacerbation of chronic obstructive pulmonary disease: A role for antiplatelet therapy? *Thorax* **2014**, *69*, 609–615. [CrossRef] [PubMed]

42. Pavasini, R.; Biscaglia, S.; d'Ascenzo, F.; Del Franco, A.; Contoli, M.; Zaraket, F.; Guerra, F.; Ferrari, R.; Campo, G. Antiplatelet treatment reduces all-cause mortality in COPD patients: A systematic review and meta-analysis. *COPD* **2016**, *13*, 509–514. [CrossRef] [PubMed]

43. Goto, Y.; Faridi, M.K.; Camargo, C.A.; Hasegawa, K. The association of aspirin use with severity of acute exacerbation of chronic obstructivepulmonary disease: Retrospective cohort study. *NPJ Prim. Care Respir. Med.* **2018**, *28*, 7. [CrossRef] [PubMed]

44. Schwameis, R.; Pils, S.; Weber, M.; Hagmann, M.; Zeitlinger, M.; Sauermann, R. Acetylic Salicylic Acid for the Treatment of Chronic Obstructive Pulmonary Disease: A Randomized, Double-Blind, Placebo-Controlled Trial. *Pharmacology* **2016**, *98*, 93–98. [CrossRef] [PubMed]

45. Domanski, M.J.; Krause-Steinrauf, H.; Massie, B.M.; Deedwania, P.; Follmann, D.; Kovar, D.; Murray, D.; Oren, R.; Rosenberg, Y.; Young, J.; et al. A comparative analysis of the results from 4 trials of beta-blocker therapy for heart failure: BEST, CIBIS-II, MERIT-HF, and COPERNICUS. *J. Card. Fail.* **2003**, *9*, 354–363. [CrossRef]

46. Puente-Maestu, L.; Calle, M.; Ortega-González, Á.; Fuster, A.; González, C.; Márquez-Martín, E.; Tirado-Conde, G. Multicentric study on the beta-blocker use and relation with exacerbations in COPD. *Respir. Med.* **2014**, *108*, 737–744. [CrossRef] [PubMed]

47. Quint, J.K.; Herrett, E.; Bhaskaran, K.; Timmis, A.; Hemingway, H.; Wedzicha, J.A.; Smeeth, L. Effect of beta blockers on mortality after myocardial infarction in adults with COPD: Population based cohort study of UK electronic healthcare records. *BMJ* **2013**, *347*, f6650. [CrossRef] [PubMed]

48. Salpeter, S.; Ormiston, T.; Salpeter, E. Cardioselective beta-blockers for chronic obstructive pulmonary disease. *Cochrane Database Syst. Rev.* **2005**, *4*, CD003566.

49. Bhatt, S.P.; Wells, J.M.; Kinney, G.L.; Washko, G.R., Jr.; Budoff, M.; Kim, Y.I.; Dransfield, M.T. β-Blockers are associated with a reduction in COPD exacerbations. *Thorax* **2015**, *71*, 8–14. [CrossRef] [PubMed]

50. Dransfield, M.T.; Rowe, S.M.; Johnson, J.E.; Bailey, W.C.; Gerald, L.B. Use of betablockers and the risk of death in hospitalized patients with acute exacerbations of COPD. *Thorax* **2008**, *63*, 301–305. [CrossRef] [PubMed]

51. Rutten, F.H.; Zuithoff, N.P.; Hak, E.; Grobbee, D.E.; Hoes, A.W. β-blockers may reduce mortality and risk of exacerbations in patients with chronic obstructive pulmonary disease. *Arch. Intern. Med.* **2010**, *170*, 880–887. [CrossRef] [PubMed]

52. Du, Q.; Sun, Y.; Ding, N.; Lu, L.; Chen, Y. Beta-blockers reduced the risk of mortality and exacerbation in patients with COPD: A meta-analysis of observational studies. *PLoS ONE* **2014**, *9*, e113048. [CrossRef] [PubMed]

53. Mortensen, E.M.; Copeland, L.A.; Pugh, M.J.; Restrepo, M.I.; de Molina, R.M.; Nakashima, B.; Anzueto, A. Impact of statins and ACE inhibitors on mortality after COPD exacerbations. *Respir. Res.* **2009**, *10*, 45. [CrossRef] [PubMed]

54. Mancini, G.B.; Etminan, M.; Zhang, B.; Levesque, L.E.; FitzGerald, J.M.; Brophy, J.M. Reduction of morbidity and mortality by statins, angiotensin-converting enzyme inhibitors, and angiotensin receptor blockers in patients with chronic obstructive pulmonary disease. *J. Am. Coll. Cardiol.* **2006**, *47*, 2554–2560. [CrossRef] [PubMed]

55. Criner, G.J.; Connett, J.E.; Aaron, S.D.; Albert, R.K.; Bailey, W.C.; Casaburi, R.; Cooper, A.D., Jr.; Curtis, J.L.; Dransfield, M.T.; Han, M.K.; et al. Simvastatin for the prevention of exacerbations in moderate-to-severe COPD. *N. Engl. J. Med.* **2014**, *370*, 2201–2210. [CrossRef] [PubMed]

56. Morgan, A.D.; Zakeri, R.; Quint, J.K. Defining the relationship between COPD and CVD: What are the implications for clinical practice? *Ther. Adv. Respir. Dis.* **2018**, *12*, 1–16. [CrossRef] [PubMed]

57. Wise, R.A.; Anzueto, A.; Cotton, D.; Dahl, R.; Devins, T.; Disse, B.; Dusser, D.; Joseph, E.; Kattenbeck, S.; Koenen-Bergmann, M.; et al. Tiotropium Respimat inhaler and the risk of death in COPD. *N. Engl. J. Med.* **2013**, *369*, 1491–1501. [CrossRef] [PubMed]

58. Lipson, D.A.; Barnhart, F.; Brealey, N.; Brooks, J.; Criner, G.J.; Day, N.C.; Dransfield, M.T.; Halpin, D.M.G.; Han, M.K.; Jones, C.L.; et al. Once-Daily Single-Inhaler Triple versus Dual Therapy in Patients with COPD. *N. Engl. J. Med.* **2018**, *378*, 1671–1680. [CrossRef] [PubMed]

59. Wang, M.T.; Liou, J.T.; Lin, C.W.; Tsai, C.L.; Wang, Y.H.; Hsu, Y.J.; Lai, J.H. Association of Cardiovascular Risk with Inhaled Long-Acting Bronchodilators in Patients with Chronic Obstructive Pulmonary Disease A Nested Case-Control Study. *JAMA Intern. Med.* **2018**, *178*, 229–238. [CrossRef] [PubMed]

12

Redox Biology of Right-Sided Heart Failure

Nataliia V. Shults, Oleksiy Melnyk, Dante I. Suzuki and Yuichiro J. Suzuki *

Department of Pharmacology and Physiology, Georgetown University Medical Center, 3900 Reservoir Road NW, Washington, DC 20007, USA; ns1015@georgetown.edu (N.V.S.); oleksiym@ymail.com (O.M.); dantealessiajustin@gmail.com (D.I.S.)
* Correspondence: ys82@georgetown.edu

Abstract: Right-sided heart failure is the major cause of death among patients who suffer from various forms of pulmonary hypertension and congenital heart disease. The right ventricle (RV) and left ventricle (LV) originate from different progenitor cells and function against very different blood pressures. However, differences between the RV and LV formed after birth have not been well defined. Work from our laboratory and others has accumulated evidence that redox signaling, oxidative stress and antioxidant regulation are important components that define the RV/LV differences. The present article summarizes the progress in understanding the roles of redox biology in the RV chamber-specificity. Understanding the mechanisms of RV/LV differences should help develop selective therapeutic strategies to help patients who are susceptible to and suffering from right-sided heart failure. Modulations of redox biology may provide effective therapeutic avenues for these conditions.

Keywords: antioxidants; redox; reactive oxygen species; right heart failure

1. Introduction

Patients with pulmonary hypertension and repaired congenital heart disease are at risk for developing right-sided heart failure [1–3]. However, the pathogenic mechanism of right heart failure is not well understood [4]. Much of the knowledge concerning the biology of the heart has been derived from the studies of the left ventricle (LV) and it has generally been assumed that the biology of the right ventricle (RV) is identical to that of the LV. However, some studies have revealed that mechanisms of right and left heart failure may be different. In the LV, concentric hypertrophy in response to systemic hypertension is often followed by the transition to dilation with eccentric cardiac hypertrophy and thinning of the ventricular wall. By contrast, in pulmonary hypertension, the concentrically hypertrophied RV appears to undergo failure, manifested by a well-known pathological observation of cor pulmonale [5,6]. Further, it is unclear whether therapies that were developed to treat LV failure really benefit patients with right-sided heart failure. Thus, understanding the differences between the RV and LV should contribute to the development of new therapeutic strategies.

Developmentally, LV and RV myocytes are derived from different precursor cells. Cells in the first heart field (primary heart field) contribute to the formation of the LV myocardium, whereas cells in the second heart field (anterior heart field) construct the RV myocardium [7–9]. Functionally, unlike the LV, the RV pumps the blood against a wide range of pressures throughout life (~100 mmHg in utero and ~10 mmHg after birth). However, the overall protein expression patterns of the adult RV and LV free walls were found to be remarkably similar [10]. Defining the subtle differences between the two ventricles may promote the development of therapeutic strategies that are tailored to specific pathologic conditions. Our laboratory previously identified some differences in protein expression between the RV and LV [11,12], as well as differentially regulated signal transduction pathways [12,13]. Notably, these studies revealed the importance of redox regulation in the RV to LV differences. This article summarizes our studies as well as ones by others, which describe redox biology of right-sided heart failure.

2. Oxidative Modifications in Right-Sided Heart Failure

In rats, the injection of an inhibitor of the vascular endothelial growth factor receptor (SU5416) plus stimuli such as hypoxia and ovalbumin immunization trigger pulmonary arterial hypertension [14,15] and right heart failure [16,17]. It was found that failing RVs in response to SU5416/ovalbumin-induced pulmonary hypertension are subjected to specific types of protein oxidation. Total protein S-glutathionylation, nitrotyrosine formation, and S-nitrosocysteine formation were found to be higher in the failing RV compared to control RV [17]. Mass spectrometry identified that these S-nitrotyrosinylated proteins include heat shock protein-90 and sarcoplasmic reticulum Ca^{2+}-ATPase, and S-glutathionylated proteins include heat shock protein-90 and NADH-ubiquinone oxidoreductase [17].

Total protein carbonylation was not altered in the RVs of rats with pulmonary hypertension compared with the controls [17]. However, our metabolomics analysis revealed that peptides that contain susceptible amino acids for carbonylation, that is, arginine, lysine, proline and threonine (as previously described by Berlett and Stadtman [18]), were lower in the RVs of pulmonary hypertensive rats than in controls [19]. Twenty-eight peptides were identified to be significantly decreased at least two-fold in the RVs of pulmonary hypertensive rats (Table 1). Notably, the Phe-Lys-Lys peptide was found to be more than 40-fold lower in the RVs of rats with pulmonary hypertension than in the RVs of healthy rats. Among these 28 peptides, 24 contained at least one carbonylation-susceptible amino acid. Among 112 amino acids within these 28 peptides, 51 amino acids (over 45%) were identified as carbonylation-susceptible amino acids that comprise four amino acids out of 20 (that is, 20%).

Table 1. Metabolomics studies identified peptides that are lower in right ventricles (RVs) of Sprague Dawley rats with pulmonary arterial hypertension (PAH) than in controls. $p < 0.05$ ($n = 10$). Most of the peptides contain carbonylation-susceptible amino acids (AAs) indicated in bold.

Peptides	Fold Difference (Control/PAH)	Total # of AAs	Carbonylation Susceptible AAs #	%
Glu Ile **Lys Pro**	4.8	4	2	50
Asp **Lys Lys Pro**	2.5	4	3	75
Lys Arg Thr Thr	2.2	4	4	100
Phe Gly **Arg Arg**	4.5	4	2	50
Ser Val **Lys Arg**	2.5	4	2	50
Lys Trp **Lys**	2.0	3	2	67
Lys Tyr Ile Glu	2.7	4	1	25
Ser Leu Leu Ser Phe	2.2	5	0	0
Asp Leu Phe **Arg**	2.4	4	1	25
Thr Thr Gly Leu Ile	2.8	5	2	40
Lys Tyr **Thr Arg**	2.5	4	3	75
Arg Ser **Lys Arg**	3.0	4	3	75
Trp Phe Trp	2.3	3	0	0
Asn **Arg** Phe **Lys**	2.8	4	2	50
His Ile Ile Val	3.1	4	0	0
Arg Lys Lys Cys	3.0	4	3	75
Asn **Arg** Phe **Lys**	3.2	4	2	50
Phe Ile Gln **Lys**	3.0	4	1	25
Ala **Arg** Tyr **Arg**	2.6	4	2	50
Ala Ala Ile **Lys**	4.8	4	1	25
Glu Phe **Pro** Trp	2.3	4	1	25
Phe **Thr Thr Thr**	2.2	4	3	75
Val **Arg** His **Arg**	2.6	4	2	50
Ile Ile Val Tyr	2.2	4	0	0
Pro Gln **Arg Thr**	3.0	4	3	75
Phe **Lys Lys**	41.7	4	2	50
Thr Thr Gly Leu Ile	2.5	4	2	50
Glu **Lys** Ala **Arg**	2.1	4	2	50

#: number.

3. RV-Specific Redox Regulation of GATA4 Gene Expression

GATA4, a major transcription factor in the regulation of cardiac hypertrophy [20], is activated through post-translational modification mechanisms in the LV [21]. In our previously studies [12], the RV GATA4 DNA binding activity was found to be increased in a rat model of pulmonary hypertension. However, this was not because of the post-translational activation of this protein, but due to increased gene transcription, since both protein and mRNA levels of GATA4 were also increased in response to pulmonary hypertension in the RV, but not in the LV [12]. Our laboratory cloned the *Gata4* promoter [22] and found that CBF/NF-Y binding to CCAAT box mediates the increased *GATA4* gene expression [12]. Annexin A1 was found to interact with CBF/NF-Y during pulmonary hypertension-mediated RV hypertrophy and negatively regulate CBF/NF-Y DNA binding [12]. Further, annexin A1 gets degraded in the RV, but not in the LV, in response to pulmonary hypertension, indicating that the activation of CBF/NF-Y-dependent *GATA4* gene transcription is through releasing the negative regulation by annexin A1 [12]. This RV-specific mechanism of GATA4 activation that is dependent on the activation of gene transcription may be defined by the difference in the expression levels of CBF/NF-Y as the RV has more CBF-B compared to the LV, while the annexin A1 levels were comparable between the two ventricles [12]. The finding that annexin A1 is involved in this mechanism of RV hypertrophy was of great interest in terms of redox signaling biology because our laboratory previously found a mechanism that involves the proteasome-dependent degradation of annexin A1 in response to protein carbonylation in smooth muscle cells [23]. Annexin A1 was found to be also carbonylated in response to pulmonary hypertension in the RV, but not in the LV [12]. As an RV-specific mechanism of cell signaling, our laboratory proposed the "oxidation/degradation pathway of signal transduction" involving carbonylation and subsequent degradation of annexin A1 by proteasomes that regulate CBF/NF-Y-dependent *GATA4* gene expression (Figure 1A) [12]. Table 2 summarizes a series of experimental observations that led to this proposed mechanism. The higher CBF/NF-Y-to-annexin A1 ratio allows for the increased sensitivity for the CBF/NF-Y activation as annexin A1 gets degraded, hence conferring the RV-specificity of this mechanism. Figure 1B depicts that, under low CBF/NF-Y-to annexin-A1 ratio, ROS-dependent annexin A1 degradation does not allow for efficient CBF/NY-Y activation to promote *GATA4* gene expression.

Table 2. List of experimental observations for the RV-specific mechanism of GATA4 activation regulated by redox signaling.

Pulmonary hypertension activates GATA4 DNA binding activity in the RV.
Pulmonary hypertension increases GATA4 protein expression in the RV.
Pulmonary hypertension increases *Gata4* mRNA expression in the RV.
The *Gata4* promoter contains a functionally important CCAAT box.
The CBF/NF-Y transcription factor regulates CCAAT box of the *Gata4* promoter.
CBF/NF-Y binds to annexin A1.
Pulmonary hypertension promotes the degradation of annexin A1.
The degradation of annexin A1 is regulated by metal-catalyzed oxidation of annexin A1.
The RV has higher CBF/NF-Y-to-annexin A1 ratio than the left ventricle (LV)

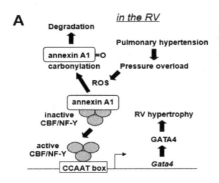

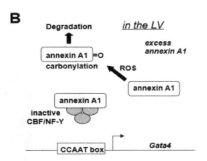

Figure 1. Proposed right ventricles (RV)-specific GATA4 activation mechanism. (**A**) Pulmonary hypertension produces reactive oxygen species (ROS) in the RV that in turn promote the carbonylation of annexin A1 protein. Carbonylation elicits the annexin A1 degradation by proteasomes, liberating CBF/NF-Y transcription factor that activates *Gata4* gene transcription [12]. (**B**) In the left ventricle (LV), the low CBF/NF-Y-to-annexin A1 ratio with excess annexin A1 does not allow for the efficient CBF/NF-Y activation.

It was also found that global cardiac ischemia/reperfusion injury results in reduced expression of GATA4 in the RV, but not in the LV [13]. Our laboratory previously established that GATA4 plays an important role in regulating the gene expression of an anti-apoptotic protein Bcl-x$_L$ in cardiomyocytes [24,25]. Consistently, the RV-specific downregulation of GATA4 by ischemia/reperfusion seems to reflect Bcl-x$_L$ gene expression, as global myocardial ischemia/reperfusion downregulated Bcl-x$_L$ in the RV, but not in the LV [13].

4. The RV-Specific Redox Regulation of Serotonin Signaling

Our laboratory also discovered that serotonin promoted protein carbonylation in the RV, but not in the LV [11]. RV and LV homogenates derivatized with 2,4-dinitrophenylhydrazine (DNPH) exhibit multiple carbonylated proteins. Perfusing the isolated rat heart with serotonin for 10 min increased carbonylation of various proteins in the RV, but not in the LV [11]. It was concluded that the mechanism of this RV/LV difference is because monoamine oxidase-A is less expressed in the RV [11]. Thus, the intracellular serotonin degradation action of monoamine oxidase-A may trigger serotonin-induced protein carbonylation in the RV.

5. Metabolomics Analysis to Define the Difference between the RV and LV

To investigate the possible differences between the adult RV and LV, metabolomics analysis was performed using RV and LV free wall tissues obtained from adult rats by examining molecules with mass less than 1000. While a majority of metabolites seem to be expressed at similar levels between the RV and LV, some molecules exhibited statistically significant difference between their levels in the two ventricles. From these data, four biologically relevant molecules that occur at different levels between the RV and LV were identified. Among them, the levels of (3*R*)-3-hydroxy-8′-apocarotenol

(Figure 2A) and coprocholic acid (Figure 2B) were found to be higher in the RV than in the LV. By contrast, 1alpha,25-dihydroxy-25,25-diphenyl-26,27-dinorvitamin D3 (Figure 2C) and neuromedin N (Figure 2D) were found to occur at lower levels in the RV compared to the LV. These identified molecules may exhibit redox properties. (3R)-3-hydroxy-8'-apocarotenol has potential to confer a similar activity as β-carotene. In addition, it possesses a hydroxyl group that may be redox active. Coprocholic acid and 1alpha,25-dihydroxy-25,25-diphenyl-26,27-dinorvitamin D3 also contain four and three hydroxyl groups, respectively.

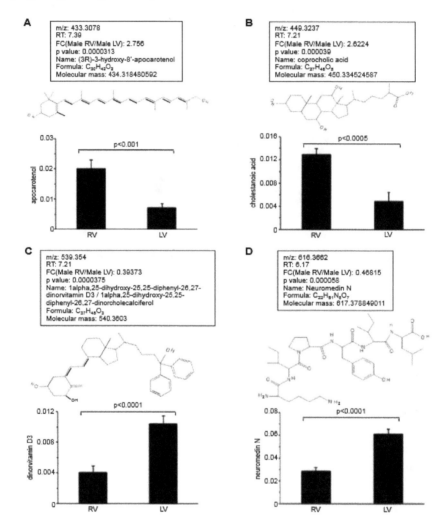

Figure 2. Notable metabolites differentially expressed between the RV and LV. The RV and LV wall tissues were dissected from male Sprague Dawley rats and subjected to metabolomics analysis ($n = 10$). The analysis of metabolomics data revealed 4 biologically notable molecules including (**A**) (3R)-3-hydroxy-8'-apocarotenol, (**B**) coprocholic acid, (**C**) 1alpha,25-dihydroxy-25,25-diphenyl-26, 27-dinorvitamin D3 and (**D**) neuromedin N that exhibited significant differences in the RV and LV. For each molecule, the experimental m/z values (which represent mass), retention time (RT), fold-change (FC) ratio of RV to LV, p-values, name of the molecule, empirical formula, mass of the molecule and the chemical structures are noted. Bar graphs represent means $\pm$ SEM of the intensity values obtained from mass spectra.

Neuromedin N and another larger peptide, neuromedin N, both elicit cell signaling by activating neurotensin receptors. Neuromedin N is a small peptide with six amino acids, Lys-Ile-Pro-Tyr-Ile-Leu, while neurotensin contains 13 amino acids, Glu-Leu-Tyr-Glu-Asn-Lys-Pro-Arg-Arg-Pro-Tyr-Ile-Leu. Interestingly, both peptides are relatively rich in carbonylation-susceptible amino acids described above.

33% of amino acids in neuromedin N and 38% in neurotensin are composed of carbonylation-susceptible amino acids.

To investigate the possible role of neurotensin/neuromedin N in right heart failure, immunohistochemistry experiments using the neurotensin/neuromedin N antibody were performed to compare the RVs of control rats to those of rats with right heart failure promoted by the injection of SU5416 plus chronic hypoxia that promotes severe pulmonary hypertension [26]. The examination of immunohistochemistry data revealed the occurrence of some RV myocytes that do not stain with the neurotensin/neuromedin N antibody. Figure 3A shows such observations from multiple animals. By contrast, the LV from pulmonary hypertension rats did not exhibit this phenomenon. Quantifications of the number of myocytes that did not stain with the neurotensin/neuromedin N antibody determined that the RVs of pulmonary hypertensive rats only exhibit such cells (Figure 3B). Thus, it appears that pressure overload to the RV in response to pulmonary hypertension modified some of cardiomyocytes so that they no longer express neurotensin or neuromedin N. In the context of redox biology, it would be interesting and potentially important to determine the carbonyl status of these peptides in the future.

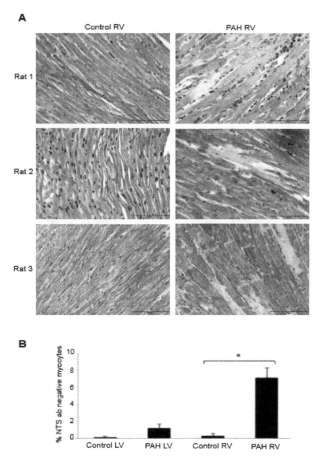

Figure 3. Neurotensin/neuromedin N expression in the heart of rats with pulmonary arterial hypertension (PAH). Male Sprague Dawley rats were subcutaneously injected with SU5416 (20 mg/kg body weight), maintained in hypoxia in a chamber set to maintain 10% O_2 [12,26] for three weeks and then in normoxia for 17 weeks [27,28]. Heart tissues were immersed in buffered 10% formalin, embedded in paraffin, cut and mounted on glass slides. Tissue sections were subjected to immunohistochemistry using the neurotensin/neuromedin N (NTS) antibody (catalog # MBS8505326; MyBioSource, Inc., San Diego, CA, USA). (**A**) Representative immunohistochemistry images of the RVs from 3 pairs of control and PAH animals. (**B**) The bar graph represents means ± SEM of % NTS antibody-negative cells in the LV and RV. * denotes values significantly different from each other at $p < 0.001$.

6. RV/LV Differences in Oxidative Stress and Antioxidant Defense

Studies of experimental animals and human patients revealed that the RV is more susceptible to the occurrence of oxidative stress than the LV in the setting of heart failure because the RV has weaker antioxidant-adaptive defense mechanisms [3,29,30].

In female Wistar rats, Schreckenberg et al. [29] found that the RV is subjected to higher oxidative stress as detected by dihydroethidium staining for superoxide and measurements of peroxynitrite using an enzyme-linked immunosorbent assay. Differential superoxide levels between the two ventricles may be due to varied expression of manganese superoxide dismutase. In this study, using nitric oxide deficiency as a model of heart failure, authors concluded that the RV cannot cope with oxidative stress because this ventricle lacks the ability to upregulate manganese superoxide dismutase.

In human heart failure patients, Borchi et al. [30] reported that NADPH oxidase-dependent production of superoxide is higher in the RV compared to the LV. Lipid peroxidation as assessed by measuring the levels of malondialdehyde was also higher in the RV of failing hearts compared to the LV. Taken together with their data on antioxidant enzyme activities, authors concluded that oxidative stress promotes antioxidant-adaptive responses more in the LV compared to the RV.

In children with tetralogy of Fallot, Chaturvedi et al. [31] observed RV oxidative stress after the surgical repair. These authors concluded that patients destined to develop acute RV dysfunction and log intensive care unit stays after tetralogy of Fallot repair suffer more oxidative stress. Reddy et al. [32] further reported that, in children with tetralogy of Fallot, the RV fails to adapt to hypoxic stress. In their study, the expression of glutathione peroxidase was found to be lower in the RV of patients with lower O_2 saturations.

7. Conclusions

The RV health is crucial to patients with pulmonary hypertension as well as with congenital heart disease including tetralogy of Fallot, pulmonary atresia, transposition of the great arteries and hypoplastic left heart syndrome. While the global RV and LV gene expression patterns and cell signaling mechanisms are similar, there are some subtle but crucial differences between RV and LV that may potentially define chamber-specific therapeutic strategies. Redox signaling, oxidative stress status and antioxidant regulation define important RV/LV differences. Further work focusing on these biological mechanisms may improve preventative and/or treatment strategies to help patients who are susceptible to developing right-sided heart failure. We hope that this article will promote further basic research concerning redox mechanisms of RV failure and possibly future clinical trials for the use of redox agents for the treatment of right-sided heart failure.

Author Contributions: Conceptualization, N.V.S. and Y.J.S.; Methodology, N.V.S. and Y.J.S.; Software, N.V.S., O.M., D.I.S. and Y.J.S.; Validation, N.V.S., O.M., D.I.S. and Y.J.S.; Formal Analysis, N.V.S., O.M., D.I.S. and Y.J.S.; Investigation, N.V.S., O.M., D.I.S. and Y.J.S.; Resources, Y.J.S.; Data Curation, N.V.S., O.M., D.I.S. and Y.J.S.; Writing–Original Draft Preparation, N.V.S. & Y.J.S.; Writing–Review & Editing, N.V.S., O.M., D.I.S. and Y.J.S.; Visualization, N.V.S., O.M., D.I.S. and Y.J.S.; Supervision, N.V.S. and Y.J.S.; Project Administration, Y.J.S.; Funding Acquisition, Y.J.S.

Acknowledgments: Authors would like to dedicate this work to the memory of six-year old Eloise Holland who suffered from right heart failure due to tetralogy of Fallot.

References

1. Konstam, M.A.; Kiernan, M.S.; Bernstein, D.; Bozkurt, B.; Jacob, M.; Kapur, N.K.; Kociol, R.D.; Lewis, E.F.; Mehra, M.R.; Pagani, F.D.; et al. Evaluation and Management of Right-Sided Heart Failure: A Scientific Statement from the American Heart Association. *Circulation* **2018**, *137*, e578–e622. [CrossRef] [PubMed]
2. Guimaron, S.; Guihaire, J.; Amsallem, M.; Haddad, F.; Fadel, E.; Mercier, O. Current knowledge and recent advances of right ventricular molecular biology and metabolism from congenital heart disease to chronic pulmonary hypertension. *BioMed Res. Int.* **2018**, *2018*, 1981568. [CrossRef] [PubMed]

3.   Reddy, S.; Bernstein, D. Molecular mechanisms of right ventricular failure. *Circulation* **2015**, *132*, 1734–1742. [CrossRef] [PubMed]

4.   Voelkel, N.F.; Quaife, R.A.; Leinwand, L.A.; Barst, R.J.; McGoon, M.D.; Meldrum, D.R.; Dupuis, J.; Long, C.S.; Rubin, L.J.; Smark, F.W.; et al. Right ventricular function and failure: The need to know more. Report of a National Heart, Lung and Blood Institute Working Group on Cellular and Molecular Mechanisms of Right Heart Failure. *Circulation* **2006**, *114*, 1883–1891. [CrossRef] [PubMed]

5.   Boxt, L.M. Radiology of the right ventricle. *Radiol. Clin. N. Am.* **1999**, *37*, 379–400. [CrossRef]

6.   Budev, M.M.; Arroliga, A.C.; Wiedemann, H.P.; Matthay, R.A. Cor pulmonale: An overview. *Semin. Respir. Crit. Care Med.* **2003**, *24*, 233–244. [PubMed]

7.   Zaffran, S.; Kelly, R.G.; Meilhac, S.M.; Buckingham, M.E.; Brown, N.A. Right ventricular myocardium derives from the anterior heart field. *Circ. Res.* **2004**, *95*, 261–268. [CrossRef] [PubMed]

8.   Verzi, M.P.; McCulley, D.J.; De Val, S.; Dodou, E.; Black, B.L. The right ventricle, outflow tract, and ventricular septum comprise a restricted expression domain within the secondary/anterior heart field. *Dev. Biol.* **2005**, *287*, 134–145. [CrossRef] [PubMed]

9.   Srivastava, D. Making or breaking the heart: From lineage determination to morphogenesis. *Cell* **2006**, *126*, 1037–1048. [CrossRef] [PubMed]

10. Suzuki, Y.J. Molecular basis of right ventricular hypertrophy and failure in pulmonary vascular disease. In *Textbook of Pulmonary Vascular Disease*; Yuan, J.X.J., Garcia, J.G.N., Hales, C.A., Archer, S.L., Rich, S., West, J.B., Eds.; Springer: New York, NY, USA, 2011; pp. 1305–1312.

11. Liu, L.; Marcocci, L.; Wong, C.M.; Park, A.M.; Suzuki, Y.J. Serotonin-mediated protein carbonylation in the right heart. *Free Radic. Biol. Med.* **2008**, *45*, 847–854. [CrossRef] [PubMed]

12. Park, A.; Wong, C.; Jelinkova, L.; Liu, L.; Nagase, H.; Suzuki, Y.J. Pulmonary hypertension-induced GATA4 activation in the right ventricle. *Hypertension* **2010**, *56*, 1145–1151. [CrossRef] [PubMed]

13. Zungu-Edmondson, M.; Suzuki, Y.J. Differential stress response mechanisms in right and left ventricles. *J. Rare Dis. Res. Treat.* **2016**, *1*, 39–45. [PubMed]

14. Taraseviciene-Stewart, L.; Kasahara, Y.; Alger, L.; Hirth, P.; Mc Mahon, G.; Waltenberger, J.; Voelkel, N.F.; Tuder, R.M. Inhibition of the VEGF receptor 2 combined with chronic hypoxia causes cell death-dependent pulmonary endothelial cell proliferation and severe pulmonary hypertension. *FASEB J.* **2001**, *15*, 427–438. [CrossRef] [PubMed]

15. Mizuno, S.; Farkas, L.; Al Husseini, A.; Farkas, D.; Gomez-Arroyo, J.; Kraskauskas, D.; Nicolls, M.R.; Cool, C.D.; Bogaard, H.J.; Voelkel, N.F. Severe pulmonary arterial hypertension induced by SU5416 and ovalbumin immunization. *Am. J. Respir. Cell Mol. Biol.* **2012**, *47*, 679–687. [CrossRef] [PubMed]

16. Bogaard, H.J.; Natarajan, R.; Henderson, S.C.; Long, C.S.; Kraskauskas, D.; Smithson, L.; Ockaili, R.; McCord, J.M.; Voelkel, N.F. Chronic pulmonary artery pressure elevation is insufficient to explain right heart failure. *Circulation* **2009**, *120*, 1951–1960. [CrossRef] [PubMed]

17. Wang, X.; Shults, N.V.; Suzuki, Y.J. Oxidative profiling of the failing right heart in rats with pulmonary hypertension. *PLoS ONE* **2017**, *12*, e0176887. [CrossRef] [PubMed]

18. Berlett, B.S.; Stadtman, E.R. Protein oxidation in aging, disease, and oxidative stress. *J. Biol. Chem.* **1997**, *272*, 20313–20316. [CrossRef] [PubMed]

19. Suzuki, Y.J.; Shults, N.V. Redox Signaling in the Right Ventricle. *Adv. Exp. Med. Biol.* **2017**, *967*, 315–323. [CrossRef] [PubMed]

20. Molkentin, J.D.; Olson, E.N. GATA4: A novel transcriptional regulator of cardiac hypertrophy? *Circulation* **1997**, *96*, 3833–3835. [PubMed]

21. Van Berlo, J.H.; Elrod, J.W.; Aronow, B.J.; Pu, W.T.; Molkentin, J.D. Serine 105 phosphorylation of transcription factor GATA4 is necessary for stress-induced cardiac hypertrophy in vivo. *Proc. Natl. Acad. Sci. USA* **2011**, *108*, 12331–12336. [CrossRef] [PubMed]

22. Suzuki, Y.J.; Nagase, H.; Wong, C.M.; Kumar, S.V.; Jain, V.; Park, A.M.; Day, R.M. Regulation of Bcl-x_L expression in lung vascular smooth muscle. *Am. J. Respir. Cell Mol. Biol.* **2007**, *36*, 678–687. [CrossRef] [PubMed]

23. Wong, C.M.; Cheema, A.K.; Zhang, L.; Suzuki, Y.J. Protein carbonylation as a novel mechanism in redox signaling. *Circ. Res.* **2008**, *102*, 310–318. [CrossRef] [PubMed]

24. Kitta, K.; Day, R.M.; Kim, Y.; Torregroza, I.; Evans, T.; Suzuki, Y.J. Hepatocyte growth factor induces GATA-4 phosphorylation and cell survival in cardiac muscle cells. *J. Biol. Chem.* **2003**, *278*, 4705–4712. [CrossRef] [PubMed]

13

Effect of Statin Therapy on Arterial Wall Inflammation Based on 18F-FDG PET/CT

Matteo Pirro [1], Luis E. Simental-Mendía [2], Vanessa Bianconi [1], Gerald F. Watts [3,4], Maciej Banach [5,6] and Amirhossein Sahebkar [7,8,9,]*

[1] Unit of Internal Medicine, Angiology and Arteriosclerosis Diseases, Department of Medicine, University of Perugia, 06129 Perugia, Italy; matteo.pirro@unipg.it (M.P.); v.bianconi.vb@gmail.com (V.B.)
[2] Biomedical Research Unit, Mexican Social Security Institute, Durango 34067, Mexico; luis_simental81@hotmail.com
[3] School of Medicine, Faculty of Health and Medical Sciences, University of Western Australia, Perth X2213, Australia; gerald.watts@uwa.edu.au
[4] Lipid Disorders Clinic, Cardiometabolic Services, Department of Cardiology, Royal Perth Hospital, Perth X2213, Australia
[5] Department of Hypertension, WAM University Hospital in Lodz, Medical University of Lodz, Zeromskiego 113, 93-338 Lodz, Poland; maciej.banach@umed.lodz.pl
[6] Polish Mother's Memorial Hospital Research Institute (PMMHRI), 93-338 Lodz, Poland
[7] Biotechnology Research Center, Pharmaceutical Technology Institute, Mashhad University of Medical Sciences, Mashhad 9177948564, Iran
[8] Neurogenic Inflammation Research Center, Mashhad University of Medical Sciences, Mashhad 9177948564, Iran
[9] School of Pharmacy, Mashhad University of Medical Sciences, Mashhad 9177948564, Iran
* Correspondence: sahebkara@mums.ac.ir;

Abstract: Aim. To evaluate by meta-analysis of interventional studies the effect of statin therapy on arterial wall inflammation. **Background.** Arterial exposure to low-density lipoprotein (LDL) cholesterol levels is responsible for initiation and progression of atherosclerosis and arterial wall inflammation. 18F-fluorodeoxyglucose Positron Emission Tomography-Computed Tomography (18F-FDG PET/CT) has been used to detect arterial wall inflammation and monitor the vascular anti-inflammatory effects of lipid-lowering therapy. Despite a number of statin-based interventional studies exploring 18F-FDG uptake, these trials have produced inconsistent results. **Methods.** Trials with at least one statin treatment arm were searched in PubMed-Medline, SCOPUS, ISI Web of Knowledge, and Google Scholar databases. Target-to-background ratio (TBR), an indicator of blood-corrected 18F-FDG uptake, was used as the target variable of the statin anti-inflammatory activity. Evaluation of studies biases, a random-effects model with generic inverse variance weighting, and sensitivity analysis were performed for qualitative and quantitative data assessment and synthesis. Subgroup and meta-regression analyses were also performed. **Results.** Meta-analysis of seven eligible studies, comprising 10 treatment arms with 287 subjects showed a significant reduction of TBR following statin treatment (Weighted Mean Difference (WMD): -0.104, $p = 0.002$), which was consistent both in high-intensity (WMD: -0.132, $p = 0.019$) and low-to-moderate intensity statin trials (WMD: -0.069, $p = 0.037$). Statin dose/duration, plasma cholesterol and C-reactive protein level changes, and baseline TBR did not affect the TBR treatment response to statins. **Conclusions.** Statins were effective in reducing arterial wall inflammation, as assessed by 18F-FDG PET/CT imaging. Larger clinical trials should clarify whether either cholesterol-lowering or other pleiotropic mechanisms were responsible for this effect.

Keywords: atherosclerosis; cholesterol; FDG; inflammation; PET; statins

---

1. Introduction

Atherosclerosis, the leading cause of cardiovascular (CV)-related deaths worldwide [1], is a disease process that is initiated, maintained and destabilized by an abnormal engagement of several cellular and molecular pathways of the inflammation cascade [2]. Exposure to elevated plasma low-density lipoprotein (LDL) cholesterol levels, either in the presence of or in the absence of additional CV risk factors, initiates and drives progressive lipid and inflammatory cell infiltration in the arterial wall [1,2], which may result in atherosclerotic plaque complications (e.g., erosion, rupture, etc.), ischemic-related organ injury and death [3,4].

Due to the recognized role of LDL cholesterol (LDL-C) in initiating and promoting atherosclerosis, followed by arterial wall inflammation [1,2], the anti-inflammatory effect of statins, as the most widely prescribed class of cholesterol-lowering drugs, has been largely explored [5–8]. Among a plethora of documented pleiotropic actions [9–14], there is accumulating evidence showing that statin therapy reduces inflammation in vitro, in experimental and clinical studies, though it is still debated whether it may depend on either cholesterol-lowering or pleiotropism [15]. Regardless of the mechanisms underlying the anti-inflammatory effects of statins, several circulating biomarkers of inflammation and acute phase reactants are down-regulated by statin treatment [7,15]. Despite low-grade systemic inflammation being frequently associated with atherosclerosis [16,17], the relationship with serum is sometimes contradictory [18–20], possibly suggesting that plasma biomarkers might not accurately reflect the degree of arterial wall inflammation. Hence, diagnostic tools that are more directly reflective of arterial inflammation have been sought.

One such method is 18F-fluorodeoxyglucose Positron Emission Tomography (18F-FDG PET) combined with computed tomography (CT), which has been used in both preclinical and clinical studies for the evaluation of inflammation in the arterial wall [18–22]. Over the last few years, significant technical progresses have been achieved in order to extend the CV applications of 18F-FDG PET/CT, which include improved image acquisition, measurements, and reconstruction protocols [23]. This has allowed a number of clinical trials to provide promising results of 18F-FDG PET/CT in detecting atherosclerotic plaque inflammation [18–20], discriminating stable from unstable plaques [24,25], predicting CV prognosis [26–29], and monitoring response to CV-related therapies [21,30,31].

In addition, 18F-FDG PET has been used to assess the impact of statin treatment on arterial wall inflammation in a few interventional studies [32–38]. In these studies [32–38], arterial 18F-FDG uptake was expressed as the Target-to-Background Ratio (TBR), that is a measure of the blood-normalized standardized uptake value (SUV). Since the reliability of TBR may be hampered by the low spatial resolution of PET, CT has been combined to improve 18F-FDG detection [21]. In these studies [32–38], the impact of different statins, at different doses, on inflammation of different arterial segments and in different clinical settings has been investigated. However, most of the studies have involved small numbers of patients, different clinical settings, varying statins with varying doses and treatment duration, different arterial segments, image acquisition/analysis, etc. Not surprisingly, the results of statin therapy on arterial wall inflammation using 18F-FDG PET/CT have been varied and inconclusive [32–38].

In order to overcome some of the inconsistencies, we carried out a systematic review and meta-analysis of previously reported trials with statins and 18F-FDG uptake, expressed as TBR.

2. Methods

2.1. Search Strategy

This study was designed according to the guidelines of the preferred reporting items for systematic reviews and meta-analysis (PRISMA) statement. PubMed-Medline, Scopus, ISI Web of Knowledge and Google Scholar databases were searched using the following search terms in titles and abstracts: (18F-fluorodeoxyglucose OR "18 F-fluorodeoxyglucose" OR FDG OR "18 F-FDG" OR "FDG-18 F" OR "18F-FDG" OR "FDG-18F" OR fluorodeoxyglucose OR "18 F FDG" OR "18F FDG" OR 18FDG OR "18 FDG") AND (atorvastatin OR simvastatin OR rosuvastatin OR lovastatin OR fluvastatin OR pravastatin OR pitavastatin). The wild-card term "*" was used to increase the sensitivity of the search strategy. The search was limited to articles published in English language. The literature was searched from inception to 19 January 2018.

2.2. Study Selection

Original studies were included if they met the following inclusion criteria: (i) being an interventional study with a statin treatment arm, (ii) investigating the impact of statin treatment on arterial wall inflammation based on the 18F-FDG PET/CT method, and (iii) presentation of arterial wall FDG uptake as TBR values (as a vein-normalized index) at baseline and after statin therapy or presenting the net change values. Exclusion criteria were: (i) non-clinical studies, (ii) non-interventional studies, e.g., observational studies with case-control, cross-sectional, or cohort designs, and (iii) lack of sufficient information on baseline or follow-up TBR values or presenting arterial wall FDG uptake as non-normalized indices.

2.3. Data Extraction

Eligible studies were reviewed and the following data were abstracted: (1) first author's name, (2) year of publication, (3) country where the study was performed, (4) study design, (5) number of treated subjects, (6) type of statin used, (7) statin dose, (8) duration of treatment, (9) age, gender and body mass index (BMI) of study participants, (10) baseline and follow-up TBR values, and (11) concentrations of plasma lipids, lipoproteins, and C-reactive protein (CRP).

2.4. Quality Assessment

The quality of involved studies in this meta-analysis was evaluated using the Cochrane criteria as previously described [39].

2.5. Quantitative Data Synthesis

Meta-analysis was conducted using Comprehensive Meta-Analysis (CMA) V2 software (Biostat, NJ, USA). A random-effects model (using DerSimonian-Laird method) and the generic inverse variance weighting method were used to compensate for the heterogeneity of studies in terms of study design, treatment protocol and the populations being studied [40]. Standard deviations (SDs) of the mean difference were calculated as follows: SD = square root $(SD_{post-treatment})^2 - (2R \times SD_{pre-treatment} \times SD_{post-treatment})$, assuming a correlation coefficient $(R) = 0.5$. Where standard error of the mean (SEM) was only reported, SD was estimated using the following formula: SD = SEM $\times$ sqrt (n), where n is the number of subjects. Heterogeneity was assessed quantitatively using Cochrane Q and I^2 statistic. Effect sizes were expressed as weighted mean difference (WMD) and 95% confidence interval (CI). If the outcome measures were reported in median and range (or 95% confidence interval [25]), mean and SD values were estimated using the method described by Wan et al. [41]. In order to evaluate the influence of each study on the overall effect size, a sensitivity analysis was conducted using the leave-one-out method (i.e., removing one study each time and repeating the analysis) [42,43]. Subgroup analyses were performed to evaluate the impact of treatment intensity on the estimated effect size and also to assess the effect size based on the TBR of most-diseased segment (MDS) of the index vessel.

2.6. Meta-Regression

As potential confounders of treatment response, duration of treatment, statin dose, mean changes in plasma levels of LDL-C and CRP, and baseline TBR were entered into a random-effects meta-regression model to explore their association with the estimated effect size on arterial wall inflammation.

2.7. Publication Bias

Evaluation of the funnel plot, Begg's rank correlation, and Egger's weighted regression tests were employed to assess the presence of publication bias in the meta-analysis. When there was an evidence of funnel plot asymmetry, potentially missing studies were imputed using the "trim and fill" method [44]. The number of potentially missing studies required to make the p-value non-significant was estimated using the "fail-safe N" method as another index of publication bias.

3. Results

Overall, 77 articles were found following the multi-database search. After screening of titles and abstracts, 16 articles were assessed in full text. Of these, nine were excluded because of a duplicate report ($n = 3$), not reporting TBR values ($n = 5$), and non-interventional study ($n = 1$). This left seven eligible articles for meta-analysis (Figure 1).

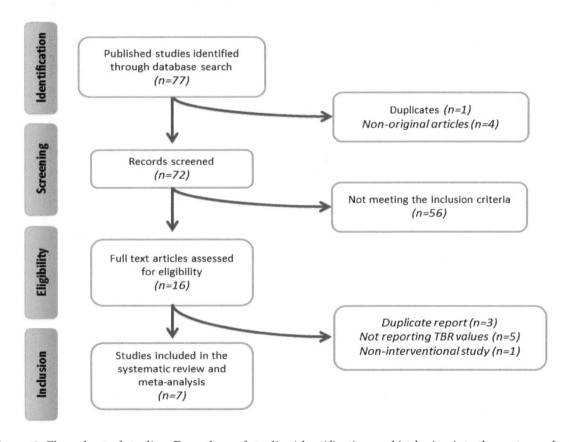

Figure 1. Flow chart of studies. Procedure of studies identification and inclusion into the meta-analysis.

3.1. Study Characteristics

Data were pooled from seven clinical trials comprising 10 treatment arms with 287 individuals. Of the selected studies, all reported whole vessel TBR of the index vessel. Aside from whole vessel TBR, three trials also reported TBR of the MDS of the index vessel. The included studies [32–38] used different types and doses of statins, and they were published between 2010 [33] and 2016 [36]. The range of treatment duration was from three months [32,35,36,38] to one year [34]. Study designs of included trials were open-label [32,33,36–38] and parallel group [34,35]. Selected studies enrolled subjects with atherosclerosis [32,38], hyperlipidemia [37], stable angina pectoris [33], HIV-infection [34], arterial inflammation [35], and ankylosing spondylitis [36]. The clinical and biochemical characteristics of the included clinical trials are presented in Table 1.

Table 1. Characteristics of studies included in the meta-analysis.

Author	Study Design	Target Population	Treatment Duration	n	Study Groups	Age (years)	Female (n, %)	BMI (kg/m²)	Total Cholesterol (mg/dL)	LDL Cholesterol (mg/dL)*	HDL Cholesterol (mg/dL)	Triglycerides (mg/dL)	C-reactive Protein (mg/L)	TBR in Index Vessel
Emami et al. (2015) [32]	Open-label trial	History of atherosclerosis	3 months	24 / 24	Atorvastatin 80 mg/day / Placebo	62.1 ± 5.9 / 62.8 ± 7.1	8 (33.3) / 6 (25)	ND / ND	ND / ND	92 ± 19 / 91 ± 24	53 ± 14 / 49 ± 11	ND / ND	1.0 (2.4)* / 1.6 (3.4)*	2.41 ± 0.33 / 2.50 ± 0.59
Ishii et al. (2010) [33]	Randomized, open-label trial	Japanese adults with stable angina pectoris	6 months	15 / 15	Atorvastatin 5 mg/day / Atorvastatin 20 mg/day	55 ± 10 / 53 ± 11	7 (46.7) / 5 (33.3)	ND / ND	234 ± 36 / 244 ± 25	150 ± 28 / 162 ± 20	48 ± 14 / 47 ± 13	170 ± 121 / 189 ± 81	1.0 ± 0.6 / 1.4 ± 0.9	Ascending aorta 1.11 ± 0.10 / 1.15 ± 0.14 Femoral artery 1.10 ± 0.16 / 1.12 ± 0.11
Lo et al. (2015) [34]	Randomized, double-blind, placebo-controlled	HIV-infected patients	1 year	19 / 21	Atorvastatin 40 mg/day / Placebo	52.2 ± 3.8 / 50.0 ± 5.6	4 (21) / 4 (19)	25.6 ± 2.9 / 25.8 ± 4.8	198.8 ± 37.9 / 192.2 ± 27.1	123.7 ± 36.7 / 124.9 ± 32.1	51.8 ± 19.3 / 50.7 ± 15.1	120.5 (97.4-204.6)* / 113.4 (92.1-135.5)*	0.8 (0.3-1.9)* / 1.1 (0.4-2.4)*	Aorta 2.08 ± 0.32 / 2.20 ± 0.37 Segment of aorta 2.18 ± 0.33 / 2.26 ± 0.37
Tawakol et al. (2013) [35]	Randomized, double-blind trial	Individuals with arterial inflammation	3 months	34 / 34	Atorvastatin 10 mg/day / Atorvastatin 80 mg/day	61 (53-68)* / 58.5 (53-68)*	8 (23.5) / 8 (23.5)	31.1 (26.9-32.5)* / 32 (26.7-35.5)*	176.5 (161-192)* / 178 (154-203)*	104 (86-118)* / 107.5 (85-129)*	49 (43-60)* / 44 (39-48)*	114.5 (78-182)* / 129 (87-179)*	ND / ND	MDS 2.34 (2.01-2.93)* / 2.48 (2.23-2.81)* WV 2.21 (2.02-2.49)* / 2.28 (2.06-2.52)*
van der Valk et al. (2016) [36]	Open-label trial	Patients with ankylosing spondylitis	3 months	18 / 20	Atorvastatin 40 mg/day / Control	46 ± 9 / 48 ± 7	6 (33.3) / 8 (40.0)	26 ± 4 / 26 ± 3	212.7 ± 48.7 / 207.3 ± 38.7	137.3 ± 44.5 / 124.1 ± 39.4	50.7 ± 15.5 / 65.7 ± 13.5	95.7 (70.9-167.4)* / 78.8 (41.6-128.4)*	5.0 (1.5-9.3)* / 1.1 (0.7-1.5)*	1.50 ± 0.14 / 1.37 ± 0.15
Watanabe et al. (2015) [37]	Randomized, open-label trial	Patients with hyperlipidemia	6 months	10 / 10	Pitavastatin 2 mg/day / Pravastatin 10 mg/day	68 ± 5 / 64 ± 11	2 (20) / 3 (30)	ND / ND	202 ± 67 / 225 ± 21	150 ± 21 / 142 ± 24	52 ± 12 / 54 ± 15	134 ± 35 / 167 ± 63	2.8 ± 4.1 / 1.7 ± 2.2	1.29 ± 0.22 / 1.19 ± 0.16
Wu et al. (2012) [38]	Open-label trial	Subjects with atherosclerosis	3 months	43	Atorvastatin 40 mg/day	54 ± 10	19 (44.1)	24.5 ± 3.2	199 ± 42	108 ± 36	45 ± 12	154 ± 70	1.2 ± 1.4	1.31 ± 0.21

Values are expressed as mean ± SD. * Mean (interquartile range). Abbreviations: ND, no data; BMI, body mass index; MDS, most-diseased segment; WV, whole vessel.

3.2. F18-FDG PET/CT Procedure

FDG-PET and contrast-enhanced CT imaging of the arteries was performed in different vessels. In this regard, Emami et al. [32] assessed the arterial FDG in the right carotid, left carotid, and aorta. Ishii et al. [33] evaluated the ascending aorta and the right and left femoral arteries. Lo et al. [34] measured FDG-PET of the aorta. Two studies [35,37] performed FDG-PET/CT imaging of the thoracic aorta and carotid arteries. Van der Valk et al. [36] assessed arterial wall inflammation in carotid arteries. Finally, Wu et al. [38] determined FDG uptake in several arterial segments, including the ascending aorta, arch, thoracic descending aorta, abdominal aorta, and bilaterial iliofemoral arteries.

3.3. Risk of Bias Assessment

With respect to the random sequence generation and allocation concealment, two trials exhibited high risk of bias [36,38]. Additionally, several studies had risk of bias for blinding of participants, personnel, and outcome assessors [32,33,36–38]. Nonetheless, all selected studies showed low risk of bias for incomplete outcome data and selective outcome reporting. Details of the risk of bias assessment are shown in Table 2.

Table 2. Quality of bias assessment of the included studies, according to the Cochrane guidelines.

Study	Sequence Generation	Allocation Concealment	Blinding of Participants, Personnel and Outcome Assessors	Incomplete Outcome Data	Selective Outcome Reporting	Other Sources of Bias
Emami et al. (2015) [32]	U	U	H	L	L	U
Ishii et al. (2010) [33]	U	L	H	L	L	U
Lo et al. (2015) [34]	L	L	L	L	L	L
Tawakol et al. (2013) [35]	U	U	U	L	L	U
van der Valk et al. (2016) [36]	H	H	H	L	L	U
Watanabe et al. (2015) [37]	U	U	H	L	L	U
Wu et al. (2012) [38]	H	H	H	L	L	U

L, low risk of bias; H, high risk of bias; U, unclear risk of bias.

3.4. Quantitative Data Synthesis

Meta-analysis of data from seven studies comprising 10 treatment arms suggested a significant reduction of arterial wall FDG uptake based on TBR index following treatment with statins (WMD: -0.104, 95% CI: -0.171, -0.038, $p = 0.002$; I^2: 89.32%) (Figure 2A). The effect size was robust in the leave-one-out sensitivity analysis (Figure 2B) and not mainly driven by any single study. Four studies comprising five treatment arms reported arterial MDS TBR, which showed a significant reduction by statin therapy (WMD: -0.186, 95% CI: -0.272, -0.100, $p < 0.001$; I^2: 61.71%) (Figure 3A). Subgroup analysis showed a significant reduction of arterial wall TBR with both high-intensity (WMD: -0.132, 95% CI: -0.242, -0.021, $p = 0.019$; I^2: 93.44%) and low-to-moderate-intensity (WMD: -0.069, 95% CI: -0.134, -0.004, $p = 0.037$; I^2: 64.93%) statin therapy (Figure 3B); however, there was no significant difference between the two subgroups ($p = 0.340$).

3.5. Meta-Regression

Random-effects meta-regression was performed to assess the impact of potential confounders on the effects of statin therapy on arterial wall inflammation. The results did not suggest a significant association between the impact of statins on TBR and treatment duration (slope: 0.005; 95% CI: -0.002, 0.01; $p = 0.138$), atorvastatin dose (slope: -0.001; 95% CI: -0.004, 0.002; $p = 0.512$), LDL-C change (slope: 0.004; 95% CI: -0.0002, 0.01; $p = 0.062$), CRP change (slope: 0.05; 95% CI: -0.01, 0.11; $p = 0.087$), and baseline TBR (slope: 0.023; 95% CI: -0.136, 0.181; $p = 0.779$) (Figure 4).

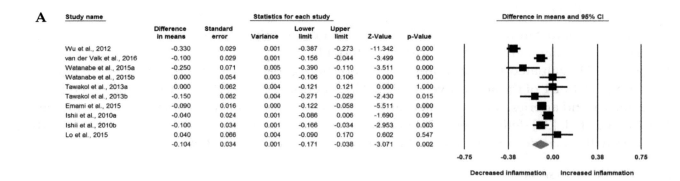

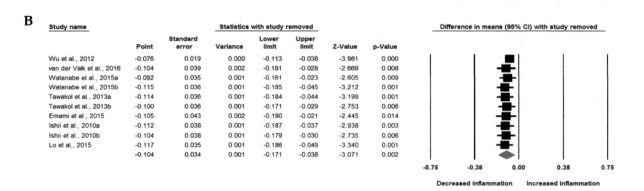

Figure 2. Impact of statin treatment on arterial wall fluorodeoxyglucose (FDG) uptake. Forest plot displaying weighted mean difference and 95% confidence intervals for the impact of statin therapy on arterial wall FDG uptake based on whole vessel target-to-background ratio (TBR) index (**A**). (**B**) shows the results of leave-one-out sensitivity analysis.

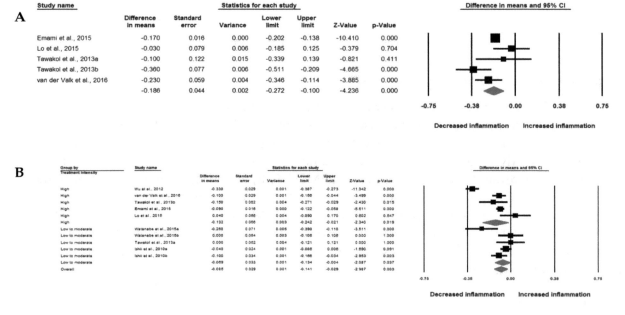

Figure 3. Impact of statin treatment on FDG uptake of the most diseased arterial segment. Forest plot displaying weighted mean difference and 95% confidence intervals for the impact of statin therapy on arterial wall FDG uptake based on the most diseased segment of vessel TBR (**A**). (**B**) shows the results of meta-analysis stratified according to the intensity (high versus low-to-moderate) of statin therapy.

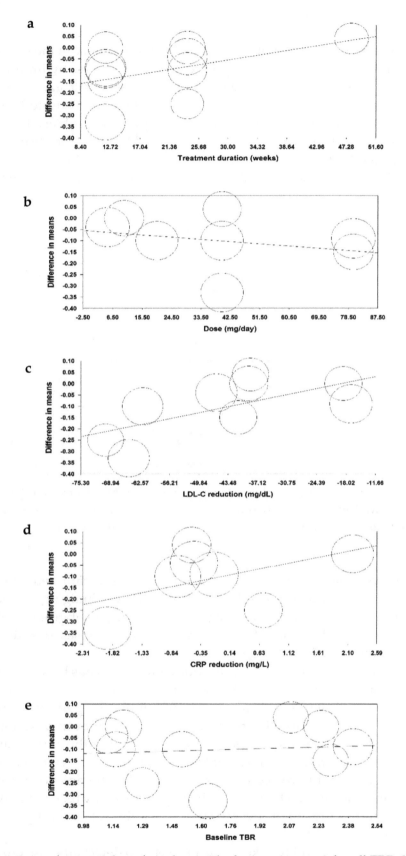

Figure 4. Associations of potential confounders with changes in arterial wall TBR. Meta-regression bubble plots of the association between mean changes in arterial wall TBR index with treatment duration (**a**), atorvastatin dose (**b**) and mean changes in plasma LDL-cholesterol (**c**), C-reactive protein (**d**), and baseline TBR (**e**). The size of each circle is inversely proportional to the variance of change.

3.6. Publication Bias

Visual inspection of Begg's funnel plots showed a slight asymmetry in the meta-analyses of statins' effects on arterial wall inflammation. This asymmetry was corrected by imputing one potentially missing study using "trim and fill" method, yielding a corrected effect size of −0.12 (95% CI: −0.18, −0.05) (Figure 5). Begg's rank correlation (tau = −0.11, z = 0.45, p = 0.655) and Egger's regression test (t = 0.02, df = 8, p = 0.988) did not suggest the presence of publication bias. The results of "fail-safe N" test suggested that 230 missing studies would be required to make the observed significant result non-significant. Given that for this meta-analysis we were able to identify seven eligible studies (with 10 treatment arms), it is far too unlikely that 230 studies were missed, thereby implying the lack of any significant publication bias.

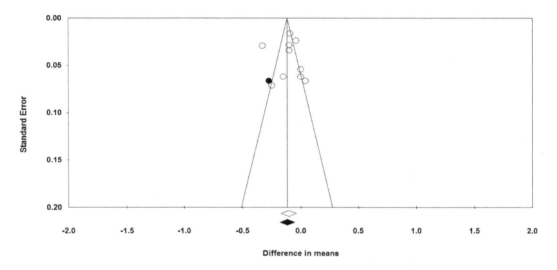

Figure 5. Publication biases. Funnel plot detailing publication bias in the studies reporting statin therapy on arterial wall FDG uptake based on whole vessel TBR index. Open and closed circles represent reported studies and potentially missing studies imputed using "trim and fill" method.

4. Discussion

In this meta-analysis, statin treatment resulted in a significant reduction of arterial wall inflammation, based on TBR measurement by 18F-FDG PET/CT imaging. Although the included clinical trials recruited only a limited number of patients for larger subgroup analyses and estimate of confounders, we did not find any significant influence of statin doses, duration of treatment, and cholesterol-lowering efficacy on TBR changes.

The pro-inflammatory role of increased LDL cholesterol levels has been documented by in vitro, experimental and clinical studies [1,2,45–47]. Additionally, statin-related cholesterol-lowering has been accompanied by the down-regulation of multiple pro-inflammatory pathways in atherogenesis [48]. Intriguingly, early anti-inflammatory effects of statins have often been described even before the reduction of plasma cholesterol levels occurs, thus suggesting that the anti-inflammatory effects of statins might be, at least in part, independent of their cholesterol-lowering action [15]. Irrespective of the mechanisms explaining the recognized ability of statin therapy to suppress inflammation, statin-related reduction of plasma CRP levels has been prospectively associated with atherosclerotic plaque regression [49] and reduction of several clinical meaningful CV end-points [50], though this has not been always confirmed [51].

Measurement of some plasma biomarkers may be useful to detect atherosclerosis-related systemic inflammation [52–55]; however, the same biomarkers may not accurately reflect the degree of the inflammatory burden within the arterial wall and, more specifically, in the atherosclerotic plaques. In this regard, the association between inflammation at the plasma and arterial wall levels was not always confirmed across the different studies [18–20]. Based on this background, several techniques have been proposed with the aim of detecting inflammation within the arterial wall and atherosclerotic plaques [23]. 18F-FDG PET/CT has been used for this purpose both in preclinical and clinical studies, with the progressive attempt to improve and standardize image acquisition and reconstruction protocols, as well as measurement of 18F-FDG uptake [18–31]. Overall, these studies have consistently demonstrated that 18F-FDG is taken up mostly by macrophages within the atherosclerotic plaques, albeit other cells (i.e., endothelial cells, vascular smooth muscle cells, neutrophils, lymphocytes) may participate in tracer uptake [21,22]. TBR, as a measure of SUV, demonstrated to be a reproducible index for quantification of 18F-FDG uptake in the inflamed arterial wall [21]. However, although TBR represents a useful tool for detecting arterial inflammation, it must be underlined that arterial 18F-FDG uptake is not necessarily atherosclerosis-related, but may be associated with other less frequent disease processes (e.g., giant cell arteritis, Takayasu arteritis, arterial grafts and aortic aneurysm infections, periaortitis, chemotherapy- or radiation-induced arterial inflammation, etc.) in the absence of atherosclerosis [56]. Regardless of this limitation, TBR was able to discriminate stable from unstable plaques (i.e., culprit lesions), as well as patients with stable angina from those with unstable angina [24,25]. In a retrospective study of 309 older subjects without history of cancer and coronary heart disease at baseline, ascending aorta TBR has been associated with coronary heart disease events [27]. Also, a few studies have revealed that arterial 18F-FDG uptake was prospectively associated with an unfavorable CV prognosis [26,28,29]. Hence, 18F-FDG PET/CT has been increasingly considered as a promising diagnostic and prognostic tool in the atherosclerosis-mediated CV disease field.

An additional use of 18F-FDG PET/CT is the monitoring of vascular wall inflammation during treatment of CV risk factors [21,30–38]. Few interventional studies in humans have reported the impact of statin treatment on arterial TBR values extracted from 18F-FDG PET/CT analysis [32–38]. In particular, seven studies (including 10 treatment arms) fulfilled the inclusion/exclusion criteria of this meta-analysis. Arterial TBR improved in 6 out of 10 arms [32,33,35–38], with the remaining four [33–35,37] showing unaltered TBR after statin treatment. Specifically, TBR of the thoracic aorta and carotid atherosclerotic plaques did not improve in one arm, including hyperlipidemic patients taking low-dose (10 mg/daily) pravastatin therapy [37]; in this study, not including a placebo-controlled arm, a modest 27% reduction of plasma LDL cholesterol level was observed along with a 2.29-fold increase in plasma CRP level. Two additional studies not including a placebo-controlled arm did not observe a significant arterial TBR change after low-dose atorvastatin treatment [33,35]. Specifically, only 5 mg/daily of atorvastatin has been used by Ishii et al [33]. Also, in the 10 mg/daily atorvastatin arm of the study by Tawakol et al. [35], 65% of patients received a statin before randomization to atorvastatin, thus limiting the ability of the low-dose atorvastatin 10 mg/daily to improve a baseline statin-influenced TBR value. This limitation was overcome, however, by atorvastatin 80 mg/daily in the second arm of the study by Tawakol et al. [35]. Finally, 40 mg/daily of atorvastatin was administered for one year in the study by Lo et al [34], but this was not sufficient to improve aortic TBR in HIV-infected patients receiving antiretroviral therapy, despite a significant 31% LDL cholesterol reduction and a three-fold decrease of plasma CRP level. However, as stated in Reference [34], technical issues compromised the possibility of reaching adequate statistical power to detect changes in the arterial wall inflammation. Regardless of the possible reasons explaining the failure of statin therapy in 4 out of 10 arms, it must be pointed out that: (1) overall, statin therapy significantly reduced arterial wall TBR, (2) neither duration/dose of statin treatment nor statin-related changes in plasma LDL cholesterol and CRP levels had a significant influence on the association between statin treatment and TBR improvement, and (3) unmeasured confounding variables or combinations of confounders might have interfered with the latter association, which was not tested in this meta-analysis.

There were some limitations for this meta-analysis. The overall sample size was relatively small, and populations differed in health status at baseline, statin preparations, doses, and duration of therapy, which limited the ability to draw direct conclusions, as well as the statistical power for additional subgroup and meta-regression analyses. However, it is worth noting that the present meta-analysis could provide a total population size that is considerably higher than the numbers recruited in each individual study, thus providing a more reliable conclusion. We also reported the presence of biases with respect to random sequence generation, allocation concealment, and blinding procedures in some studies, which may have reduced the quality of the results. Finally, heterogeneity of clinical settings and arterial segments examined by 18F-FDG PET/CT, in the absence of a larger sample size, have precluded the possibility to explore the impact of statin treatment in specific populations and arterial regions. Despite these potential limitations, statistical compensation for heterogeneity was performed, and the overall result of this meta-analysis was robust in sensitivity analysis.

In conclusion, our meta-analysis showed the significant anti-inflammatory effect of statin treatment at the arterial wall level; however, unresolved issues remain regarding the presumptive factors that either mediate or confound such an effect. Larger clinical trials are warranted to resolve this uncertainty and to verify whether the local anti-inflammatory effects of satins, as detected by arterial 18F-FDG PET/CT, might translate into favorable clinical outcomes. Moreover, given that most of the studies included in this analysis had a relatively short duration of follow-up, it remains to be established if the anti-inflammatory effects of statins, as assessed by 18F-FDG PET/CT, are enhanced over time and following prolonged exposure of arteries to low concentrations of LDL. It also remains to be investigated if the findings of 18F-FDG PET/CT are correlated with alterations of biomarkers of vascular inflammation, as well as circulating levels of pro-inflammatory cytokines in statin-treated subjects. Finally, biomimetic nanoparticles have recently emerged as potential tools for targeting and imaging of inflammation, e.g., through mimicking the interactions between cell adhesion molecules and selectins in the inflamed vascular site [57,58]. The use of these nanoparticles, with modalities like radioisotope imaging, magnetic resonance imaging, and ultrasound, could allow efficient monitoring of the anti-inflammatory action of statins and other lipid-lowering therapies on the arterial wall and could be confirmatory to 18F-FDG PET/CT findings as detailed in this study.

Acknowledgments: The authors thank Evan A. Stein for his valuable help in improving the manuscript.

References

1.   Roth, G.A.; Johnson, C.; Abajobir, A.; Abd-Allah, F.; Abera, S.F.; Abyu, G.; Ahmed, M.; Aksut, B.; Alam, T.; Alam, K.; et al. Global, Regional, and National Burden of Cardiovascular Diseases for 10 Causes, 1990 to 2015. *J. Am. Coll. Cardiol.* **2017**, *70*, 1–25. [CrossRef]

2.   Hansson, G.K. Inflammation and Atherosclerosis: The End of a Controversy. *Circulation* **2017**, *136*, 1875–1877. [CrossRef]

3.   Catapano, A.L.; Graham, I.; De Backer, G.; Wiklund, O.; Chapman, M.J.; Drexel, H.; Hoes, A.W.; Jennings, C.S.; Landmesser, U.; Pedersen, T.R.; et al. ESC Scientific Document Group. 2016 ESC/EAS Guidelines for the Management of Dyslipidaemias. *Eur. Heart J.* **2016**, *37*, 2999–3058. [CrossRef] [PubMed]

4.   Ference, B.A.; Ginsberg, H.N.; Graham, I.; Ray, K.K.; Packard, C.J.; Bruckert, E.; Hegele, R.A.; Krauss, R.M.; Raal, F.J.; Schunkert, H.; et al. Low-density lipoproteins cause atherosclerotic cardiovascular disease. 1. Evidence from genetic, epidemiologic, and clinical studies. A consensus statement from the European Atherosclerosis Society Consensus Panel. *Eur Heart J.* **2017**, *38*, 2459–2472. [CrossRef] [PubMed]

5.   Deshmukh, H.; Chasman, D.; Trompet, S.; Li, X.; Sun, F.; Hitman, G.; Colhoun, H. Meta-analysis of genome-wide association studies to assess C-reactive protein response to statin therapy. *Lancet* **2016**, *387*, S37. [CrossRef]

6.   Ridker, P.M.; Danielson, E.; Fonseca, F.A.; Genest, J.; Gotto, A.M., Jr.; Kastelein, J.J.; Koenig, W.; Libby, P.; Lorenzatti, A.J.; MacFadyen, J.G.; et al. Rosuvastatin to prevent vascular events in men and women with elevated C-reactive protein. *N. Engl. J. Med.* **2008'** *359*, 2195–2207. [CrossRef] [PubMed]

7.   Zhang, L.; Zhang, S.; Jiang, H.; Sun, A.; Wang, Y.; Zou, Y.; Ge, J.; Chen, H. Effects of statin therapy on inflammatory markers in chronic heart failure: A meta-analysis of randomized controlled trials. *Arch. Med. Res.* **2010**, *41*, 464–471. [CrossRef]

8. Bielecka-Dabrowa, A.; Mikhailidis, D.P.; Rizzo, M.; von Haehling, S.; Rysz, J.; Banach, M. The influence of atorvastatin on parameters of inflammation left ventricular function, hospitalizations and mortality in patients with dilated cardiomyopathy—5-year follow-up. *Lipids Health Dis.* **2013**, *12*, 47. [CrossRef] [PubMed]

9. Mohajeri, M.; Banach, M.; Atkin, S.L.; Butler, A.E.; Ruscica, M.; Watts, G.F.; Sahebkar, A. MicroRNAs: Novel Molecular Targets and Response Modulators of Statin Therapy. *Trends Pharmacol. Sci.* **2018**, *39*, 967–981. [CrossRef]

10. Bahrami, A.; Parsamanesh, N.; Atkin, S.L.; Banach, M.; Sahebkar, A. Effect of statins on toll-like receptors: A new insight to pleiotropic effects. *Pharmacol. Res.* **2018**, *135*, 230–238. [CrossRef]

11. Sahebkar, A.; Kotani, K.; Serban, C.; Ursoniu, S.; Mikhailidis, D.P.; Jones, S.R.; Ray, K.K.; Blaha, M.J.; Rysz, J.; Toth, P.P.; et al. Statin therapy reduces plasma endothelin-1 concentrations: A meta-analysis of 15 randomized controlled trials. *Atherosclerosis* **2015**, *241*, 433–442. [CrossRef] [PubMed]

12. Parizadeh, S.M.R.; Azarpazhooh, M.R.; Moohebati, M.; Nematy, M.; Ghayour-Mobarhan, M.; Tavallaie, S.; Rahsepar, A.A.; Amini, M.; Sahebkar, A.; Mohammadi, M.; et al. Simvastatin therapy reduces prooxidant-antioxidant balance: Results of a placebo-controlled cross-over trial. *Lipids* **2011**, *46*, 333–340. [CrossRef] [PubMed]

13. Serban, C.; Sahebkar, A.; Ursoniu, S.; Mikhailidis, D.P.; Rizzo, M.; Lip, G.Y.H.; Kees Hovingh, G.; Kastelein, J.J.P.; Kalinowski, L.; Rysz, J.; et al. A systematic review and meta-analysis of the effect of statins on plasma asymmetric dimethylarginine concentrations. *Sci. Rep.* **2015**, *5*, 9902. [CrossRef]

14. Sahebkar, A.; Serban, C.; Mikhailidis, D.P.; Undas, A.; Lip, G.Y.H.; Muntner, P.; Bittner, V.; Ray, K.K.; Watts, G.F.; Hovingh, G.K.; et al. Association between statin use and plasma d-dimer levels: A systematic review and meta-analysis of randomised controlled trials. *Thromb. Haemost.* **2015**, *114*, 546–557. [CrossRef] [PubMed]

15. Diamantis, E.; Kyriakos, G.; Quiles-Sanchez, L.V.; Farmaki, P.; Troupis, T. The Anti-Inflammatory Effects of Statins on Coronary Artery Disease: An Updated Review of the Literature. *Curr. Cardiol. Rev.* **2017**, *13*, 209–216. [CrossRef] [PubMed]

16. Buffon, A.; Biasucci, L.M.; Liuzzo, G.; D'Onofrio, G.; Crea, F.; Maseri, A. Widespread coronary inflammation in unstable angina. *N. Engl. J. Med.* **2002**, *347*, 5–12. [CrossRef] [PubMed]

17. Libby, P.; Ridker, P.M.; Hansson, G.K. Progress and challenges in translating the biology of atherosclerosis. *Nature* **2011**, *473*, 317–325. [CrossRef] [PubMed]

18. Duivenvoorden, R.; Mani, V.; Woodward, M.; Kallend, D.; Suchankova, G.; Fuster, V.; Rudd, J.H.; Tawakol, A.; Farkouh, M.E.; Fayad, Z.A. Relationship of serum inflammatory biomarkers with plaque inflammation assessed by FDG PET/CT: The dal-PLAQUE study. *JACC Cardiovasc. Imaging* **2013**, *6*, 1087–1094. [CrossRef] [PubMed]

19. Rudd, J.H.; Bansilal, S.; Machac, J.; Woodward, M.; Fuster, V. Relationships among regional arterial inflammation, calcification, risk factors, and biomarkers: A prospective fluorodeoxyglucose positron-emission tomography/computed tomography imaging study. *Circ. Cardiovasc. Imaging* **2009**, *2*, 107–115. [CrossRef] [PubMed]

20. Yang, S.J.; Kim, S.; Choi, H.Y.; Kim, T.N.; Yoo, H.J.; Seo, J.A.; Kim, S.G.; Kim, N.H.; Baik, S.H.; Choi, D.S.; et al. High-sensitivity C-reactive protein in the low- and intermediate-Framingham risk score groups: Analysis with 18F-fluorodeoxyglucose positron emission tomography. *Int. J. Cardiol.* **2013**, *163*, 277–281. [CrossRef] [PubMed]

21. Rosenbaum, D.; Millon, A.; Fayad, Z.A. Molecular imaging in atherosclerosis: FDG PET. *Curr. Atheroscler. Rep.* **2012**, *14*, 429–437. [CrossRef] [PubMed]

22. Tarkin, J.M.; Joshi, F.R.; Rajani, N.K.; Rudd, J.H. PET imaging of atherosclerosis. *Future Cardiol.* **2015**, *11*, 115–131. [CrossRef] [PubMed]

23. Huet, P.; Burg, S.; Le Guludec, D.; Hyafil, F.; Buvat, I. Variability and uncertainty of 18F-FDG PET imaging protocols for assessing inflammation in atherosclerosis: Suggestions for improvement. *J. Nucl. Med.* **2015**, *56*, 552–559. [CrossRef]

24. Dilsizian, V.; Jadvar, H. Science to Practice: Does FDG Differentiate Morphologically Unstable from Stable Atherosclerotic Plaque? *Radiolog* **2017**, *283*, 1–3. [CrossRef]

25. Rogers, I.S.; Nasir, K.; Figueroa, A.L.; Cury, R.C.; Hoffmann, U.; Vermylen, D.A.; Brady, T.J.; Tawakol, A. Feasibility of FDG imaging of the coronary arteries: Comparison between acute coronary syndrome and stable angina. *JACC Cardiovasc. Imaging* **2010**, *3*, 388–397. [CrossRef] [PubMed]

26. Figueroa, A.L.; Abdelbaky, A.; Truong, Q.A.; Corsini, E.; MacNabb, M.H.; Lavender, Z.R.; Lawler, M.A.; Grinspoon, S.K.; Brady, T.J.; Nasir, K.; et al. Measurement of arterial activity on routine FDG PET/CT images improves prediction of risk of future CV events. *JACC Cardiovasc. Imaging* **2013**, *6*, 1250–1259. [CrossRef] [PubMed]

27. Iwatsuka, R.; Matsue, Y.; Yonetsu, T.; O'uchi, T.; Matsumura, A.; Hashimoto, Y.; Hirao, K. Arterial inflammation measured by 18F-FDG-PET-CT to predict coronary events in older subjects. *Atherosclerosis* **2018**, *268*, 49–54. [CrossRef]

28. Marnane, M.; Merwick, A.; Sheehan, O.C.; Hannon, N.; Foran, P.; Grant, T.; Dolan, E.; Moroney, J.; Murphy, S.; O'rourke, K.; et al. Carotid plaque inflammation on 18F-fluorodeoxyglucose positron emission tomography predicts early stroke recurrence. *Ann. Neurol.* **2012**, *71*, 709–718. [CrossRef]

29. Rominger, A.; Saam, T.; Wolpers, S.; Cyran, C.C.; Schmidt, M.; Foerster, S.; Nikolaou, K.; Reiser, M.F.; Bartenstein, P.; Hacker, M. 18F-FDG PET/CT identifies patients at risk for future vascular events in an otherwise asymptomatic cohort with neoplastic disease. *J. Nucl. Med.* **2009**, *50*, 1611–1620. [CrossRef] [PubMed]

30. Van Wijk, D.F.; Sjouke, B.; Figueroa, A.; Emami, H.; van der Valk, F.M.; MacNabb, M.H.; Hemphill, L.C.; Schulte, D.M.; Koopman, M.G.; Lobatto, M.E.; et al. Nonpharmacological lipoprotein apheresis reduces arterial inflammation in familial hypercholesterolemia. *J. Am. Coll. Cardiol.* **2014**, *64*, 1418–1426. [CrossRef]

31. Xu, J.; Nie, M.; Li, J.; Xu, Z.; Zhang, M.; Yan, Y.; Feng, T.; Zhao, X.; Zhao, Q. Effect of pioglitazone on inflammation and calcification in atherosclerotic rabbits: An 18F-FDG-PET/CT in vivo imaging study. *Herz* **2017**, *43*, 733–740. [CrossRef]

32. Emami, H.; Vucic, E.; Subramanian, S.; Abdelbaky, A.; Fayad, Z.A.; Du, S.; Roth, E.; Ballantyne, C.M.; Mohler, E.R.; Farkouh, M.E.; et al. The effect of BMS-582949, a P38 mitogen-activated protein kinase (P38 MAPK) inhibitor on arterial inflammation: A multicenter FDG-PET trial. *Atherosclerosis* **2015**, *240*, 490–496. [CrossRef] [PubMed]

33. Ishii, H.; Nishio, M.; Takahashi, H.; Aoyama, T.; Tanaka, M.; Toriyama, T.; Tamaki, T.; Yoshikawa, D.; Hayashi, M.; Amano, T.; et al. Comparison of atorvastatin 5 and 20 mg/d for reducing F-18 fluorodeoxyglucose uptake in atherosclerotic plaques on positron emission tomography/computed tomography: A randomized, investigator-blinded, open-label, 6-month study in Japanese adults scheduled for percutaneous coronary intervention. *Clin. Ther.* **2010**, *32*, 2337–2347. [CrossRef] [PubMed]

34. Lo, J.; Lu, M.T.; Ihenachor, E.J.; Wei, J.; Looby, S.E.; Fitch, K.V.; Oh, J.; Zimmerman, C.O.; Hwang, J.; Abbara, S.; et al. Effects of statin therapy on coronary artery plaque volume and high-risk plaque morphology in HIV-infected patients with subclinical atherosclerosis: A randomised, double-blind, placebo-controlled trial. *Lancet HIV* **2015**, *2*, e52–e63. [CrossRef]

35. Tawakol, A.; Fayad, Z.A.; Mogg, R.; Alon, A.; Klimas, M.T.; Dansky, H.; Subramanian, S.S.; Abdelbaky, A.; Rudd, J.H.; Farkouh, M.E.; et al. Intensification of statin therapy results in a rapid reduction in atherosclerotic inflammation: Results of a multicenter fluorodeoxyglucose-positron emission tomography/computed tomography feasibility study. *J. Am. Coll. Cardiol.* **2013**, *62*, 909–917. [CrossRef] [PubMed]

36. Van der Valk, F.M.; Moens, S.J.; Verweij, S.L.; Strang, A.C.; Nederveen, A.J.; Verberne, H.J.; Nurmohamed, M.T.; Baeten, D.L.; Stroes, E.S. Increased arterial wall inflammation in patients with ankylosing spondylitis is reduced by statin therapy. *Ann. Rheum. Dis.* **2016**, *75*, 1848–1851. [CrossRef]

37. Watanabe, T.; Kawasaki, M.; Tanaka, R.; Ono, K.; Kako, N.; Saeki, M.; Onishi, N.; Nagaya, M.; Sato, N.; Miwa, H.; et al. Anti-inflammatory and morphologic effects of pitavastatin on carotid arteries and thoracic aorta evaluated by integrated backscatter trans-esophageal ultrasound and PET/CT: A prospective randomized comparative study with pravastatin (EPICENTRE study). *Cardiovasc. Ultrasound* **2015**, 13. [CrossRef]

38. Wu, Y.W.; Kao, H.L.; Huang, C.L.; Chen, M.F.; Lin, L.Y.; Wang, Y.C.; Lin, Y.H.; Lin, H.J.; Tzen, K.Y.; Yen, R.F.; et al. The effects of 3-month atorvastatin therapy on arterial inflammation, calcification, abdominal adipose tissue and circulating biomarkers. *Eur. J. Nucl. Med. Mol. Imaging* **2012**, *39*, 399–407. [CrossRef]

39. Green, S.; Higgins, J. (Eds.) *Cochrane Handbook for Systematic Reviews of Interventions*; Version 5.0.2; The Cochrane Collaboration: London, UK, 2009.

40. Sutton, A.J.; Abrams, K.R.; Jones, D.R.; Jones, D.R.; Sheldon, T.A.; Song, F. *Methods for Meta-Analysis in Medical Research*; J. Wiley: Hoboken, NJ, USA, 2000.

41. Wan, X.; Wang, W.; Liu, J.; Tong, T. Estimating the sample mean and standard deviation from the sample size, median, range and/or interquartile range. *BMC Med. Res. Methodol.* **2014**, *14*, 135. [CrossRef]

42. Sahebkar, A.; Simental-Mendía, L.E.; Watts, G.F.; Serban, M.C.; Banach, M. Comparison of the effects of fibrates versus statins on plasma lipoprotein(a) concentrations: A systematic review and meta-analysis of head-to-head randomized controlled trials. *BMC Med.* **2017**, *15*, 22. [CrossRef]

43. Sahebkar, A. Does PPARγ2 gene Pro12Ala polymorphism affect nonalcoholic fatty liver disease risk? Evidence from a meta-analysis. *DNA Cell Biol.* **2013**, *32*, 188–198. [CrossRef] [PubMed]

44. Duval, S.; Tweedie, R. Trim and fill: A simple funnel-plot-based method of testing and adjusting for publication bias in meta-analysis. *Biometrics* **2000**, *56*, 455–463. [CrossRef] [PubMed]

45. Paciullo, F.; Fallarino, F.; Bianconi, V.; Mannarino, M.R.; Sahebkar, A.; Pirro, M. PCSK9 at the crossroad of cholesterol metabolism and immune function during infections. *J. Cell. Physiol.* **2017**, *232*, 2330–2338. [CrossRef] [PubMed]

46. Pirro, M.; Bianconi, V.; Paciullo, F.; Mannarino, M.R.; Bagaglia, F.; Sahebkar, A. Lipoprotein(a) and inflammation: A dangerous duet leading to endothelial loss of integrity. *Pharm. Res.* **2017**, *119*, 178–187. [CrossRef] [PubMed]

47. Pirro, M.; Schillaci, G.; Savarese, G.; Gemelli, F.; Mannarino, M.R.; Siepi, D.; Bagaglia, F.; Mannarino, E. Attenuation of inflammation with short-term dietary intervention is associated with a reduction of arterial stiffness in subjects with hypercholesterolaemia. *Eur. J. Cardiovasc. Prev. Rehabil.* **2004**, *11*, 497–502. [CrossRef] [PubMed]

48. Montecucco, F.; Mach, F. Update on statin-mediated anti-inflammatory activities in atherosclerosis. *Semin. Immunopathol.* **2009**, *31*, 127–142. [CrossRef]

49. Nissen, S.E.; Tuzcu, E.M.; Schoenhagen, P.; Crowe, T.; Sasiela, W.J.; Tsai, J.; Orazem, J.; Magorien, R.D.; O'shaughnessy, C.; Ganz, P. Statin therapy, LDL cholesterol, C-reactive protein, and coronary artery disease. *N. Engl. J. Med.* **2005**, *352*, 29–38. [CrossRef] [PubMed]

50. Ridker, P.M.; Cannon, C.P.; Morrow, D.; Rifai, N.; Rose, L.M.; McCabe, C.H.; Pfeffer, M.A.; Braunwald, E. C-reactive protein levels and outcomes after statin therapy. *N. Engl. J. Med.* **2005**, *352*, 20–28. [CrossRef]

51. Yousuf, O.; Mohanty, B.D.; Martin, S.S.; Joshi, P.H.; Blaha, M.J.; Nasir, K.; Blumenthal, R.S.; Budoff, M.J. High-sensitivity C-reactive protein and cardiovascular disease: A resolute belief or an elusive link? *J. Am. Coll. Cardiol.* **2013**, *62*, 397–408. [CrossRef]

52. Krintus, M.; Kozinski, M.; Kubica, J.; Sypniewska, G. Critical appraisal of inflammatory markers in cardiovascular risk stratification. *Crit. Rev. Clin. Lab. Sci.* **2014**, *51*, 263–279. [CrossRef]

53. Mannarino, E.; Pirro, M. Endothelial injury and repair: A novel theory for atherosclerosis. *Angiology* **2008**, *59*, 69S–72S. [CrossRef] [PubMed]

54. St-Pierre, A.C.; Bergeron, J.; Pirro, M.; Cantin, B.; Dagenais, G.R.; Després, J.P.; Lamarche, B. Effect of plasma C-reactive protein levels in modulating the risk of coronary heart disease associated with small, dense, low-density lipoproteins in men (The Quebec Cardiovascular Study). *Am. J. Cardiol.* **2003**, *91*, 555–558. [CrossRef]

55. Wang, J.; Tan, G.J.; Han, L.N.; Bai, Y.Y.; He, M.; Liu, H.B. Novel biomarkers for cardiovascular risk prediction. *J. Geriatr. Cardiol.* **2017**, *14*, 135–150. [PubMed]

56. Chrapko, B.E.; Chrapko, M.; Nocuń, A.; Stefaniak, B.; Zubilewicz, T.; Drop, A. Role of 18F-FDG PET/CT in the diagnosis of inflammatory and infectious vascular disease. *Nucl. Med. Rev.* **2016**, *19*, 28–36. [CrossRef] [PubMed]

57. Chacko, A.M.; Hood, E.D.; Zern, B.J.; Muzykantov, V.R. Targeted Nanocarriers for Imaging and Therapy of Vascular Inflammation. *Curr. Opin. Colloid Interface Sci.* **2011**, *16*, 215–227. [CrossRef] [PubMed]

58. Jin, K.; Luo, Z.; Zhang, B.; Pang, Z. Biomimetic nanoparticles for inflammation targeting. *Acta Pharm. Sin. B* **2018**, *8*, 23–33. [CrossRef] [PubMed]

14

Outcome of Robot-Assisted Bilateral Internal Mammary Artery Grafting via Left Pleura in Coronary Bypass Surgery

Chieh-Jen Wu [1,2], Hsin-Hung Chen [3,4], Pei-Wen Cheng [3,4], Wen-Hsien Lu [5,6],
Ching-Jiunn Tseng [3,5] and Chi-Cheng Lai [7,8,*]

[1]   Cardiovascular Center, Kaohsiung Veterans General Hospital, Kaohsiung 813, Taiwan; cjwu@vghks.gov.tw
[2]   Graduate Institute of Clinical Medicine, College of Medicine, Kaohsiung Medical University,
      Kaohsiung 807, Taiwan
[3]   Department of Medical Education and Research, Kaohsiung Veterans General Hospital, Kaohsiung 813,
      Taiwan; shchen0910@gmail.com (H.-H.C.); peiwen420@gmail.com (P.-W.C.); cjtseng@vghks.gov.tw (C.-J.T.)
[4]   Yuh-Ing Junior College of Health Care & Management, Kaohsiung 821, Taiwan
[5]   School of Medicine, National Yang-Ming University, Taipei 112, Taiwan; whlu@vghks.gov.tw
[6]   Department of Pediatrics, Kaohsiung Veterans General Hospital, Kaohsiung 813, Taiwan
[7]   Department of Cardiology, Kaohsiung Municipal United Hospital, Kaohsiung 804, Taiwan
[8]   Department of Biological Sciences, National Sun Yat-Sen University, Kaohsiung 804, Taiwan
*   Correspondence: llccheng@vghks.gov.tw;

Abstract: Studies are extremely limited for the investigation of the clinical outcome of da Vinci robot-assisted bilateral internal mammary artery (BIMA) grafting in coronary artery bypass grafting (CABG) surgery. This study aimed to explore the short-term outcome of da Vinci robot-assisted BIMA grafting through the left pleural space. Relevant data were collected from patients with multi-vessel coronary artery disease receiving two kinds of CABG: a group of patients receiving da Vinci robot-assisted CABG with BIMA grafting, and another group of patients receiving sternotomy CABG with BIMA grafting. Primary endpoints, which included cardiovascular and renal endpoints, were analyzed between the groups using the chi-square test, analysis of variance test, and Kaplan–Meier analysis. Compared with the conventional group ($n = 22$), the robotic group ($n = 22$) had a significantly longer operation time (12.7 ± 1.7 vs. 8.5 ± 1.5 hours; $p < 0.01$) and a marginally lower mean of serum creatinine at baseline (1.2 ± 0.3 vs. 2.0 ± 1.7 mg/dL; $p = 0.04$). Primary endpoints (5, 22.7% vs. 12, 54.5%; $p = 0.03$) and renal endpoints (1, 4.5% vs. 7, 31.8%; $p = 0.02$) at six months were significantly reduced in the robotic group compared with the conventional group. There were no differences in cardiovascular endpoints at six months between the groups (1, 4.5% vs. 0; $p = 1.00$). The data showed that da Vinci robot-assisted BIMA grafting was safe, with equal cardiovascular events and lowered renal events at six months, as compared to conventional sternotomy BIMA grafting, despite the longer procedure time. The short-term study suggests that da Vinci robot-assisted BIMA grafting may be considered a favorable surgical option for patients with severe coronary artery disease.

Keywords: bilateral internal mammary artery; coronary artery disease; coronary artery bypass grafting; da Vinci; sternotomy; outcome

1. Introduction

International guidelines recommend coronary artery bypass grafting (CABG) surgery as a treatment option in patients with left main disease and/or multi-vessel coronary artery disease (CAD) [1–3]. Conventional CABG surgery requires sternotomy, which generates a long mid-sternal wound scar and potentiates sternal wound infection, particularly in patients receiving bilateral internal mammary artery (BIMA) grafting [4–6]. On the other hand, numerous studies have documented the clinical benefit of BIMA grafting, including prolonged graft patency [7,8], lowered adverse cardiovascular events [8,9], and improved survival [9–13]. A conflicting result obtained from a registry study showed that BIMA grafting was not associated with better outcomes compared with single internal mammary artery grafting [14]. In order to minimize surgical trauma and avoid sternotomy, a robot-assisted technique using a da Vinci operator system (Intuitive Surgical, Mountain View, CA, USA) was introduced into the field of CABG surgery. A few studies showed that robotic CABG surgeries had favorable cardiovascular outcomes [15–18]. In addition, a meta-analysis of 16 pooled studies exhibited that there were significantly fewer renal failure events in robot-assisted endoscopic CABG, as compared to conventional CABG [19]. However, no studies have reported on the composite endpoints of cardiovascular and renal events between da Vinci robot-assisted BIMA grafting and conventional BIMA grafting. Therefore, this retrospective study was designed to investigate the primary endpoints of cardiovascular and renal events between the two patient groups with severe CAD receiving robot-assisted BIMA graft via the left pleura or conventional sternotomy BIMA grafting. The present results were expected to elucidate the short-term primary outcome and help guide surgical decision in patients with severe CAD.

2. Materials and Methods

2.1. Study Design and Patient Selection

The study was a single-center, retrospective, non-randomized, and non-controlled observational study based upon the analysis of the database of a single medical center, and was designed to detect the differences in adverse events between two patient groups: Group 1 of patients receiving da Vinci robot-assisted CABG with BIMA grafting via left pleura and Group 2 of patients receiving conventional sternotomy CABG with BIMA grafting. Consecutively collected patients were those who had been angiographically diagnosed with left main disease and/or multi-vessel CAD, and thereafter received two kinds of CABG surgeries. They were matched by age. For both groups, femoral artery and vein cannulations were performed for the preparation of cardiopulmonary bypass with systemic heparinization. Beating heart CABG with BIMA skeletonization and mobilization was routinely conducted in all patients, with an on- or off-pump according to the patient's hemodynamic status and the operator's discretion. A radial artery (RA) or great saphenous vein (GSV) was harvested as a conduit with the right internal mammary artery (RIMA) for anastomosis of the left circumflex artery (LCX) and of the right coronary artery (RCA). The procedures of the two kinds of CABG surgeries are detailed below. Patients were excluded if they received an urgent CABG, received a hybrid of percutaneous coronary intervention (PCI) and CABG, received left internal mammary artery (LIMA) grafting or RIMA grafting alone, presented with ST-segment elevation myocardial infarction, or had previously been enrolled in another clinical study. All patients received a daily dose of 100 mg aspirin indefinitely, in combination with a daily dose 75 mg clopidogrel as dual antiplatelet therapy with an expected duration of at least one year after the index surgeries. Clinical follow-up was scheduled in hospital, three months, and six months after discharge for data collection. Primary endpoints consisted of a composite of cardiovascular and renal endpoints. Relevant data were recorded for patient characteristics, clinical presentations, and adverse events during the follow-up period. All patients in the two groups were thoroughly informed about the procedure preoperatively and provided written consent. The study protocol had been examined and approved by the committee of the hospital. The present study was performed in accordance with the Declaration of Helsinki and local regulatory guidelines.

2.2. Da Vinci Robot-Assisted CABG with BIMA Grafting via Left Pleura

Each beating-heart da Vinci robot-assisted CABG with unilateral BIMA grafting was performed with an on- or off-cardiopulmonary pump according to a patient's hemodynamic status by an experienced team led by a well-trained CABG surgeon with more than 15 years of CABG surgery experience. After general anesthesia and aseptic procedures, a double-lumen was intubated for single right-lung or bilateral low-volume ventilation in order to mobilize the BIMA grafts. A BIMA graft was mobilized through the left pleura using the da Vinci robot-assisted operation system, with the left chest elevated at approximately 30 degrees and with the patient in supine position. The chest cavity was insufflated with carbon dioxide to expand the surgical space. An RIMA was first mobilized through the left pleural and pre-mediastinal space with two-lung low-volume ventilation. Then, an LIMA was mobilized with single right-lung ventilation. The vessels were anastomosed by direct-vision through a left thoracotomy in the second intercostal space with a surgical wound of about 6–12 cm in length. The mobilized LIMA was anastomosed with the left anterior descending artery (LAD); the RA or GSV served as an additional conduit for connection with the RIMA and for anastomoses of the LCX-obtuse marginal branch (LCX-OM) and/or the RCA-posterior descending artery (RCA-PDA).

2.3. Conventional Sternotomy CABG with BIMA Grafting

Patients received a full mid-sternotomy for conventional CABG surgeries with BIMA grafting. The mobilized BIMA and harvested RA or GSV in each patient were anastomosed with native coronary arteries by direct-vision through a mid-sternal exposed surgical wound of about 20–30 cm in length. Similar to the da Vinci robot surgery, the RA or GSV served as an additional conduit for connection with RIMA and for anastomoses with LCX-OM and/or RCA-PDA. All patients in the two groups were treated and monitored postoperatively at the intensive care unit.

2.4. Definitions

Adverse events in hospitals were defined as wound infection, severe blood loss requiring blood transfusion, pleural effusion, pulmonary edema, and pneumonia. The definition of CAD was coronary stenosis exceeding 50% in diameter of an adjacently normal segment. Estimated glomerular filtration rate (eGFR) was calculated using the modification of diet in renal disease equation. The definition of CKD stages was according to stratified values of eGFR recommended by the guidelines [20]. Consumed units of packed red blood cells or fresh frozen plasma were defined as the sum of the blood units used in hospital. Each operator determined the use of an intra-aortic balloon pump (IABP) according the hemodynamics in the peri-operative period. Myocardial infarction (MI) was defined according to the clinical symptoms, the level of serum troponin I >5 µg/L, new eletrocardiographic changes, or echocardiographic evidence of new regional wall motion abnormality. Operation room time was defined as the time interval between the patient's arrival at the operation room and the patient's departure from the recovery room.

2.5. Primary Endpoints at Six Months

Primary endpoints in the study included cardiovascular and renal endpoints. Cardiovascular endpoints including all-cause mortality, non-fatal MI, repeated revascularization, and non-fatal hemorrhagic and ischemic stroke; renal endpoints included a rise of serum creatinine >0.5 mg/dL above the baseline value, creatinine doubling (at least a 100% raise from the basal level of serum creatinine), and occurrence of CKD stage 4 or 5. An endpoint event was confirmed by two independent physicians according to the clinical symptoms and signs, laboratory data, electrocardiographic findings, and/or diagnostic images. The follow-up period was six months.

2.6. Statistical Analysis

All variables were statistically analyzed using SPSS software version 22 (SPSS Inc., Chicago, IL, USA). All categorical data and rates are displayed as numbers (percentages), and the continuous data are shown as means ± standard deviation. Baseline and outcome data between the groups were compared using chi-square test (χ^2) or Fisher exact test for categorical variables, and the analysis of variance test for continuous variables. Kaplan–Meier analysis with log-rank test was used to detect differences in cumulative event-free survival at six months between the two groups. A p value < 0.05 with two-sided 95% confidence interval was considered statistically significant for all tests. Analysis was conducted as time to the first event involving primary endpoints, without double counting of events.

3. Results

3.1. Patient Demographic and Characteristic Data

Data for a total of 44 patients were collected from November 2010 to January 2016 (Figure 1). In this cohort, 22 patients with left main disease and/or multi-vessel CAD received da Vinci robot-assisted CABG with BIMA grafting through the left pleura. The 22 age-matched patients received conventional sternotomy CABG with BIMA grafting. Figure 2A,B show endoscopically mobilized BIMA and the minimal surgical scars after robot-assisted surgery. Figure 2C,D show a large sternotomy wound and BIMA anastomosed with coronary arteries, and a larger surgical scar after conventional sternotomy surgery. The operation time was significantly longer in robotic CABG as compared with sternotomy CABG (12.7 ± 1.7 vs. 8.5 ± 1.5 h; p < 0.01). The mean serum creatinine at baseline was marginally lower in robotic CABG compared with sternotomy CABG (1.2 ± 0.3 vs. 2.0 ± 1.7 mg/dL; p = 0.04), whereas the mean eGFR was identical between groups (57.9 ± 31.5 vs. 65.4 ± 13.6 mL/min/1.73 m^2; p = 0.32). The baseline characteristics of the two groups are shown in Table 1.

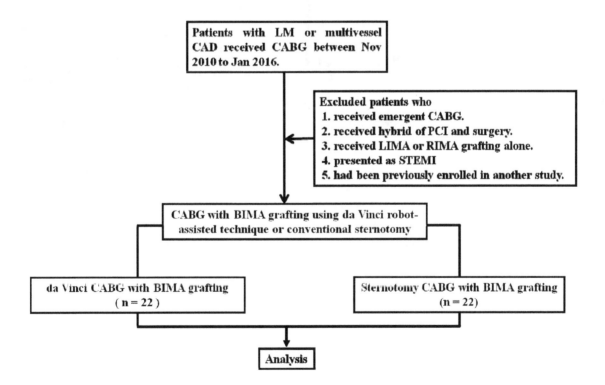

Figure 1. The patient flow chart. LM = left main; CABG = coronary artery bypass grafting; CAD = coronary artery disease; PCI = percutaneous coronary intervention; LIMA = left internal mammary artery; RIMA = right internal mammary artery; STEMI = ST-segment elevation myocardial infarction; BIMA = bilateral internal mammary artery.

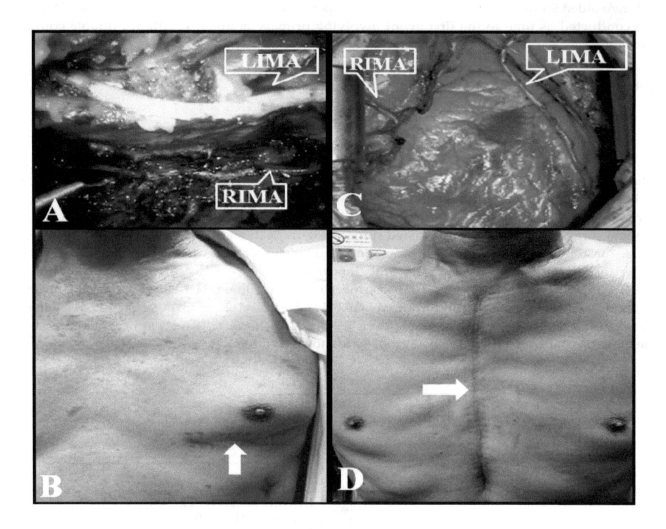

Figure 2. Wound healing in robotic and conventional sternotomy-assisted bilateral internal mammary artery grafting via the left pleura in coronary artery bypass grafting surgery. (**A**) Endoscopy shows that the left internal mammary artery (LIMA) (upper) and the right internal mammary artery (RIMA) (lower) were mobilized using the da Vinci operator system. (**B**) Surgical wounds (white arrows) of da Vinci robot-assisted CABG are small. (**C**) Finished anastomoses of LIMA (right) and RIMA (left) with coronary arteries are displayed in an explored sternal area of a sternotomy CABG. (**D**) A long mid-sternal wound scar (white arrow) is shown in a patient who had received a sternotomy CABG.

Table 1. Baseline characteristics between two surgical modalities.

	Da Vinci Robotic Surgery (n = 22)	Sternotomy Surgery (n = 22)	p Value
Male	20 (90.9)	21 (95.5)	1.00
Age (years)	61.2 ± 12.0	62.9 ± 10.5	0.63
Body mass index (kg/m^2)	26.9 ± 4.0	27.3 ± 3.2	0.70
Risk factors for CAD			
Diabetes mellitus	11 (50.0)	10 (45.5)	1.00
Hypertension	17 (77.3)	18 (81.8)	1.00
Dyslipidemia	13 (59.1)	12 (54.5)	1.00
Hyperuricemia	1 (4.5)	0 (0)	1.00
Drug allergy	5 (22.7)	1 (4.5)	0.19
Alcohol drinking	6 (23.7)	1 (4.5)	0.95
Cigarette smoking	10 (45.5)	11 (50.0)	1.00
Family history of CVD	8 (36.4)	2 (9.1)	0.03
CAD condition			
LM	10 (45.5)	13 (59.1)	0.55
TVD	17 (77.3)	20 (90.9)	0.41
DVD	5 (22.7)	2 (9.1)	0.41
Grafting conduit			
BIMA	22 (100.0)	22 (100.0)	1.00
Radial artery	19 (86.4)	19 (86.4)	1.00
GSV	3 (13.6)	3 (13.6)	1.00
Anastomosis number	3.0 ± 0.6	3.4 ± 0.7	0.34
On pump	10 (45.5)	16 (72.7)	0.12
On pump time (min)	123.9 ± 96.2	131.4 ± 59.8	0.81
Operation room time (h)	12.7 ± 1.7	8.5 ± 1.5	<0.01
Biomarkers at admission			
Hemoglobin (g/dL)	13.7 ± 1.6	12.7 ± 2.4	0.11
Creatinine (mg/dL)	1.2 ± 0.3	2.0 ± 1.7	0.04
eGFR (mL/min/1.73 m^2)	65.4 ± 13.6	57.9 ± 31.5	0.32
CKD stage			0.11
I/II	15 (68.2)	10 (45.5)	
III	7 (31.8)	7 (31.8)	
IV	0 (0)	3 (13.6)	
V	0 (0)	2 (9.1)	

Continuous data are presented as mean ± standard deviation; category data are presented as number (percentage); CABG = coronary artery bypass grafting; BMI = body mass index; CAD = coronary artery disease; CVD = cardiovascular disease; LM = left main; TVD = triple vessel disease; DVD = double vessel disease; LIMA = left internal mammary artery; RIMA = right internal mammary artery; eGFR = estimated glomerular filtration rate; CKD = chronic kidney disease.

3.2. In-Hospital Adverse Events

In-hospital adverse events did not differ between the groups ($p > 0.05$), except for a significantly lower incidence of CKD stages 4 and 5 in patients who received da Vinci robot-assisted CABG with BIMA grafting (1, 4.5% vs. 10, 45.4%, respectively; $p < 0.01$). In-hospital cardiovascular events were equal between the two groups, including death, non-fatal MI, repeated revascularization, and non-fatal stroke ($p > 0.05$). The adverse events in hospital are outlined in Table 2.

Table 2. Adverse events in hospital between two surgical modalities.

	Da Vinci Robotic Surgery (n = 22)	Sternotomy Surgery (n = 22)	p Value
Hospital stay (days)	21.0 ± 8.8	24.4 ± 14.0	0.34
ICU stay (days)	4.8 ± 3.5	5.0 ± 3.3	0.90
Ventilator weaning (days)	2.2 ± 1.8	2.3 ± 2.3	0.94
Renal events			
CKD stages IV/V	1 (4.5)	10 (22.7)	<0.01
Creatinine change >0.5 mg/dL	5 (22.7)	7 (31.8)	0.50
Doubling creatinine (mg/dL)	1 (4.8)	3 (13.6)	0.61
eGFR (mL/min/1.73 m^2) *	58.5 ± 22.1	45.5 ± 31.6	0.12
Hemodialysis	0 (0)	1 (4.5)	1.00
The lowest hemoglobin (g/dL)	11.9 ± 1.5	12.1 ± 1.5	0.57
Blood transfusion (U)			
FFP	5.3 ± 3.8	3.8 ± 4.3	0.28
PRBC	2.1 ± 2.0	1.4 ± 2.2	0.30
Adverse events	4 (18.2)	5 (27.8)	0.70
Death	0 (0)	0 (0)	1.00
Myocardial infarction	0 (0)	0 (0)	1.00
Stroke	0 (0)	0 (0)	1.00
Wound infection	1 (4.5)	1 (5.6)	1.00
Pneumonia	1 (4.5)	0 (0)	1.00
Pleural effusion	1 (4.5)	2 (11.1)	1.00
Post-operation IABP	2 (9.1)	3 (13.6)	1.00

Continuous data are presented as mean ± standard deviation; category data are presented as number (percentage); CABG = coronary artery bypass grafting; CKD = chronic kidney disease; eGFR = estimated glomerular filtration rate; FFP = fresh frozen plasma; PRBC = packed red blood cells; ICU = intensive care unit; eGFR * = indicate the lowest value of eGFR in hospital; IABP = intra-aortic balloon pump.

3.3. Primary Endpoints at Six Months

Primary endpoints at six months were significantly reduced in robotic CABG compared with sternotomy CABG (5, 22.7% vs. 12, 54.5%; $p = 0.03$) (Table 3). The finding was reinforced by the Kaplan–Meier analysis ($p = 0.03$ by log-rank test) (Figure 3). The significant reduction was mainly contributed by the fewer renal events in robotic surgery (1 vs. 7; $p = 0.02$). The cumulative rates of cardiovascular endpoints at six months were identical, including all-cause mortality (0 vs. 0; $p = 1.0$), non-fatal MI (0 vs. 1; $p = 1.0$), and non-fatal stroke (0 vs. 0; $p = 1.0$).

Table 3. Clinical outcomes at six months between two surgical modalities.

	Da Vinci Robotic Surgery (n = 22)	Sternotomy Surgery (n = 22)	p Value
Finished six months follow-up	19 (86.5)	21 (95.5)	
Primary endpoints	5 (22.7)	12 (54.5)	0.03
Cardiovascular events	1 (4.5)	0 (0)	1.00
Mortality	0 (0)	0 (0)	1.00
Myocardial infarction	1 (4.5)	0 (0)	1.00
Stoke	0 (0)	0 (0)	1.00
Renal events	1 (4.5)	7 (31.8)	0.02
CKD stages IV/V	0 (0)	7 (31.8)	0.02
Creatinine doubling	0 (0)	1 (4.5)	1.00
Creatinine change >0.5 mg/dL	1 (4.5)	5 (22.7)	0.18
Hemodialysis	0 (0)	1 (4.5)	1.00
eGFR (mL/min/1.73 m^2)	72.1 ± 19.0	56.9 ± 34.0	0.08
Re-hospitalization *	4 (18.2)	6 (27.3)	0.47

Continuous data are presented as mean ± standard deviation; category data are presented as number (percentage); CABG = coronary artery bypass grafting; * = re-hospitalizations due to any cause; primary endpoint = all-cause mortality, myocardial infarction, stock, CKD stages IV/V, and creatinine change >0.5 mg/dL.

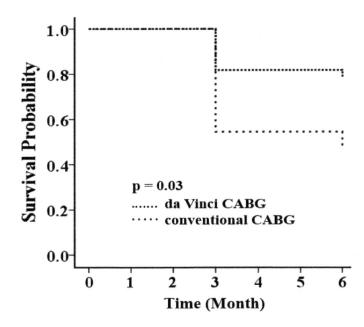

Figure 3. Kaplan–Meier survival analysis shows a significant reduction in the cumulative incidence of the composite of cardiovascular and renal endpoints at six months ($p = 0.03$ by log-rank test), including all-cause mortality, non-fatal myocardial infarction, repeated revascularization, non-fatal stroke, the presence of chronic kidney disease stage 4 or 5, creatinine doubling, and a raise of the baseline creatinine >0.5 mg/dL in patients receiving da Vinci CABG as compared with those receiving conventional CABG. CABG = coronary artery bypass grafting.

4. Discussion

The study generated three major findings: (1) primary endpoints were significantly reduced in patients receiving da Vinci robot-assisted BIMA grafting via the left pleura at six months, as compared with patients receiving sternotomy CABG with BIMA grafting; (2) the significant reduction in primary endpoints was contributed by the fewer renal events in robotic CABG. Cardiovascular endpoints were equal between the groups; (3) robotic CABG compared with conventional CABG had smaller surgical wounds but longer operation times, and identical hospital and ICU stay. The da Vinci robot-assisted CABG with BIMA grafting via the left pleura is considered a new surgical treatment option for patients with severe CAD.

Robotic CABG had a significant reduction in the rate of primary cardiovascular and renal endpoints as compared to sternotomy CABG. The relatively better renal function at baseline in da Vinci robot-assisted CABG with BIMA grafting may partially account for the significant reduction in adverse renal events in hospital and at six months. Renal dysfunction was reported to independently predict post-CABG adverse events, such as mortality and/or morbidity [21–23], and advanced renal diseases [24,25]. Compared with robotic CABG with BIMA grafting, the poorer renal function in conventional CABG possibly resulted in renal deterioration after CABG surgeries. In addition, the finding was consistent with the result obtained from a meta-analysis of 16 pooled studies which showed that robot-assisted CABG versus conventional CABG was associated with fewer renal failure events [19]. Furthermore, renal function may be preserved in off-pump CABG surgeries [26], despite the equality of cardiopulmonary pump use observed between the groups. A shorter elapsed time from coronary angiography until off-pump CABG was also reported to deteriorate renal function [27]. Nevertheless, the reason why there were fewer renal events in robotic CABG versus conventional CABG remains unclear. The finding needs to be further confirmed.

On the other hand, the two groups had identical rates of adverse cardiovascular events in hospital and at six months. The finding implicated that the da Vinci robot-assisted unilateral BIMA grafting was not inferior to the conventional BIMA grafting in terms of short-term cardiovascular outcome.

Furthermore, the data displayed satisfactory results with freedom from subsequent wound infection and post-operative ischemic stroke. A few trials indicated that BIMA harvesting may lead to a decline in blood supply to the sternum and increase the risk of sternal wound infection [4–6]. A BIMA graft-sparing aortic clamp and aortic anastomosis may reduce the risk of peri-operative ischemic stroke [8,17].

The present results disclosed that robotic CABG compared with conventional CABG had longer operation times but without longer ICU and hospital stays, and ventilation times. Similar to conventional BIMA mobilization, robot-assisted BIMA mobilization requires a longer procedure time [28,29], especially in RIMA mobilization through the left pleural and pre-mediastinal space. Unilateral BIMA grafting minimizes the surgical wounds but prolongs the operation times. The robot-assisted operation time may be shortened through collaborative team-work in a learning-curve manner [28]. This will increase operator comfort, reduce fatigue, and allow patients receiving da Vinci robot-assisted CABG with BIMA grafting to have safer interventional procedures, therefore greatly improving patient outcomes [30].

Several limitations have to be emphasized: (1) as the study had few case numbers, low event rates, short follow-up, and primary selection bias, its results should be interpreted with caution; (2) the heterogeneity at baseline and unmeasured confounders between the two different surgeries may have affected the outcomes; (3) other factors, such as hemodynamics, angiographically-proven coronary lesions, and systolic function at baseline, that differed between the two groups could have potentially influenced the outcomes, as these were not investigated in the study; (4) in the study, it was not mandatory to routinely check coronary angiograms to survey the graft patency.

In conclusion, the data showed that da Vinci robot-assisted CABG with left-pleural BIMA grafting compared with conventional sternotomy CABG with BIMA grafting did not increase in-hospital and short-term cardiovascular events but possibly lowered adverse renal events. The study suggests that the robot-assisted CABG with left-pleural BIMA grafting can be considered a new surgical option for patients with severe CAD. Further larger studies are needed to investigate long-term outcomes.

Author Contributions: The study was conceived and designed by C.-J.W., H.-H.C., P.-W.C., and C.-C.L. conducted most of the experiments with assistance from W.-H.L., and C.-J.T. The paper was written by C.-C.L., with contributions from H.-H.C. and C.-J.W.

Acknowledgments: This study was supported by the Kaohsiung Veterans General Hospital. We would like to thank participating assistants for their contribution in conducting the statistical analysis, including Tina Wu and Chung Jung Chang of the cardiovascular center of Kaohsiung Veterans General Hospital.

References

1.   Task Force, M.; Montalescot, G.; Sechtem, U.; Achenbach, S.; Andreotti, F.; Arden, C.; Budaj, A.; Bugiardini, R.; Crea, F.; Cuisset, T.; et al. 2013 ESC guidelines on the management of stable coronary artery disease: The task force on the management of stable coronary artery disease of the European society of cardiology. *Eur. Heart J.* **2013**, *34*, 2949–3003.

2.   Yates, M.T.; Soppa, G.K.; Valencia, O.; Jones, S.; Firoozi, S.; Jahangiri, M. Impact of European Society of Cardiology and European Association for Cardiothoracic Surgery Guidelines on Myocardial Revascularization on the activity of percutaneous coronary intervention and coronary artery bypass graft surgery for stable coronary artery disease. *J. Thorac. Cardiovasc. Surg.* **2014**, *147*, 606–610.

3.   Fihn, S.D.; Blankenship, J.C.; Alexander, K.P.; Bittl, J.A.; Byrne, J.G.; Fletcher, B.J.; Fonarow, G.C.; Lange, R.A.; Levine, G.N.; Maddox, T.M.; et al. 2014 ACC/AHA/AATS/PCNA/SCAI/STS focused update of the guideline for the diagnosis and management of patients with stable ischemic heart disease: A report of the american college of cardiology/american heart association task force on practice guidelines, and the american association

for thoracic surgery, preventive cardiovascular nurses association, society for cardiovascular angiography and interventions, and society of thoracic surgeons. *J. Thorac. Cardiovasc. Surg.* **2015**, *149*, e5–e23. [PubMed]

4. He, G.W.; Ryan, W.H.; Acuff, T.E.; Bowman, R.T.; Douthit, M.B.; Yang, C.Q.; Mack, M.J. Risk factors for operative mortality and sternal wound infection in bilateral internal mammary artery grafting. *J. Thorac. Cardiovasc. Surg.* **1994**, *107*, 196–202. [PubMed]

5. Deo, S.V.; Shah, I.K.; Dunlay, S.M.; Erwin, P.J.; Locker, C.; Altarabsheh, S.E.; Boilson, B.A.; Park, S.J.; Joyce, L.D. Bilateral Internal Thoracic Artery Harvest and Deep Sternal Wound Infection in Diabetic Patients. *Ann. Thorac. Surg.* **2013**, *95*, 862–869. [CrossRef] [PubMed]

6. Dai, C.; Lu, Z.; Zhu, H.; Xue, S.; Lian, F. Bilateral Internal Mammary Artery Grafting and Risk of Sternal Wound Infection: Evidence from Observational Studies. *Ann. Thorac. Surg.* **2013**, *95*, 1938–1945. [CrossRef] [PubMed]

7. Weiss, A.J.; Zhao, S.; Tian, D.H.; Taggart, D.P.; Yan, T.D. A meta-analysis comparing bilateral internal mammary artery with left internal mammary artery for coronary artery bypass grafting. *Ann. Cardiothorac. Surg.* **2013**, *2*, 390–400. [PubMed]

8. Glineur, D.; Papadatos, S.; Grau, J.B.; Shaw, R.E.; Kuschner, C.E.; Aphram, G.; Mairy, Y.; Vanbelighen, C.; Etienne, P.Y. Complete myocardial revascularization using only bilateral internal thoracic arteries provides a low-risk and durable 10-year clinical outcome. *Eur. J. Cardio-Thorac. Surg.* **2016**, *50*, 735–741. [CrossRef]

9. Kinoshita, T.; Asai, T.; Suzuki, T.; Kambara, A.; Matsubayashi, K. Off-Pump Bilateral Versus Single Skeletonized Internal Thoracic Artery Grafting in High-Risk Patients. *Circulation* **2011**, *124*, S130–S134. [CrossRef] [PubMed]

10. Kinoshita, T.; Asai, T.; Suzuki, T. Off-pump bilateral skeletonized internal thoracic artery grafting in patients with chronic kidney disease. *J. Thorac. Cardiovasc. Surg.* **2015**, *150*, 315–321. [CrossRef] [PubMed]

11. Pettinari, M.; Sergeant, P.; Meuris, B. Bilateral internal thoracic artery grafting increases long-term survival in elderly patients. *Eur. J. Cardiothorac. Surg.* **2015**, *47*, 703–709. [CrossRef]

12. Galbut, D.L.; Kurlansky, P.A.; Traad, E.A.; Dorman, M.J.; Zucker, M.; Ebra, G. Bilateral internal thoracic artery grafting improves long-term survival in patients with reduced ejection fraction: A propensity-matched study with 30-year follow-up. *J. Thorac. Cardiovasc. Surg.* **2012**, *143*, 844–853. [CrossRef]

13. Puskas, J.D.; Sadiq, A.; Vassiliades, T.A.; Kilgo, P.D.; Lattouf, O.M. Bilateral Internal Thoracic Artery Grafting Is Associated with Significantly Improved Long-Term Survival, Even Among Diabetic Patients. *Ann. Thorac. Surg.* **2012**, *94*, 710–715. [CrossRef]

14. Dalén, M.; Ivert, T.; Holzmann, M.J.; Sartipy, U. Bilateral versus Single Internal Mammary Coronary Artery Bypass Grafting in Sweden from 1997–2008. *PLoS ONE* **2014**, *9*, e86929. [CrossRef]

15. Yang, M.; Wu, Y.; Wang, G.; Xiao, C.; Zhang, H.; Gao, C. Robotic Total Arterial Off-Pump Coronary Artery Bypass Grafting: Seven-Year Single-Center Experience and Long-Term Follow-Up of Graft Patency. *Ann. Thorac. Surg.* **2015**, *100*, 1367–1373. [CrossRef]

16. Gong, W.; Cai, J.; Wang, Z.; Chen, A.; Ye, X.; Li, H.; Zhao, Q. Robot-assisted coronary artery bypass grafting improves short-term outcomes compared with minimally invasive direct coronary artery bypass grafting. *J. Thorac. Dis.* **2016**, *8*, 459–468. [CrossRef]

17. Ishikawa, N.; Watanabe, G.; Tomita, S.; Yamaguchi, S.; Nishida, Y.; Iino, K. Robot-Assisted Minimally Invasive Direct Coronary Artery Bypass Grafting. *ThoraCAB Circ. J.* **2014**, *78*, 399–402. [CrossRef]

18. Canale, L.S.; Bonatti, J. Mammary artery harvesting using the Da Vinci Si robotic system. *Rev. Bras. Cir. Cardiovasc.* **2014**, *29*, 107–109. [CrossRef]

19. Wang, S.; Zhou, J.; Cai, J.-F. Traditional coronary artery bypass graft versus totally endoscopic coronary artery bypass graft or robot-assisted coronary artery bypass graft-meta-analysis of 16 studies. *Eur. Rev. Med. Pharmacol. Sci.* **2014**, *18*, 790–797.

20. Inker, L.A.; Astor, B.C.; Fox, C.H.; Isakova, T.; Lash, J.P.; Peralta, C.A.; Tamura, M.K.; Feldman, H.I. KDOQI US Commentary on the 2012 KDIGO Clinical Practice Guideline for the Evaluation and Management of CKD. *Am. J. Kidney Dis.* **2014**, *63*, 713–735. [CrossRef]

21. Marui, A.; Okabayashi, H.; Komiya, T.; Tanaka, S.; Furukawa, Y.; Kita, T.; Kimura, T.; Sakata, R.; CREDO-Kyoto Investigators. Impact of occult renal impairment on early and late outcomes following coronary artery bypass grafting. *Interact. Cardiovasc. Thorac. Surg.* **2013**, *17*, 638–643. [CrossRef]

22. Cooper, W.A.; O'Brien, S.M.; Thourani, V.H.; Guyton, R.A.; Bridges, C.R.; Szczech, L.A.; Petersen, R.; Peterson, E.D. Impact of renal dysfunction on outcomes of coronary artery bypass surgery: Results from the society of thoracic surgeons national adult cardiac database. *Circulation* **2006**, *113*, 1063–1070. [CrossRef] [PubMed]

23. Hillis, G.S.; Croal, B.L.; Buchan, K.G.; El-Shafei, H.; Gibson, G.; Jeffrey, R.R.; Millar, C.G.; Prescott, G.J.; Cuthbertson, B.H. Renal function and outcome from coronary artery bypass grafting: Impact on mortality after a 2.3-year follow-up. *Circulation* **2006**, *113*, 1056–1062. [CrossRef] [PubMed]

24. Rydén, L.; Sartipy, U.; Evans, M.; Holzmann, M.J. Acute Kidney Injury After Coronary Artery Bypass Grafting and Long-Term Risk of End-Stage Renal Disease. *Circulation* **2014**, *130*, 2005–2011. [CrossRef] [PubMed]

25. Brown, J.R.; Cochran, R.P.; Leavitt, B.J.; Dacey, L.J.; Ross, C.S.; MacKenzie, T.A.; Kunzelman, K.S.; Kramer, R.S.; Hernandez, F., Jr.; Helm, R.E.; et al. Multivariable Prediction of Renal Insufficiency Developing After Cardiac Surgery. *Circulation* **2007**, *116*, 139–143. [CrossRef]

26. Hayashida, N.; Teshima, H.; Chihara, S.; Tomoeda, H.; Takaseya, T.; Hiratsuka, R.; Shoujima, T.; Takagi, K.; Kawara, T.; Aoyagi, S. Does Off-Pump Coronary Artery Bypass Grafting Really Preserve Renal Function? *Circ. J.* **2002**, *66*, 921–925. [CrossRef]

27. Ji, Q.; Mei, Y.; Wang, X.; Feng, J.; Wusha, D.; Cai, J.; Zhou, Y. Effect of Elapsed Time from Coronary Angiography Until Off-Pump Coronary Artery Bypass Surgery on Postoperative Renal Function. *Circ. J.* **2012**, *76*, 2356–2362. [CrossRef]

28. Wiedemann, D.; Bonaros, N.; Schachner, T.; Weidinger, F.; Lehr, E.J.; Vesely, M.; Bonatti, J. Surgical problems and complex procedures: Issues for operative time in robotic totally endoscopic coronary artery bypass grafting. *J. Thorac. Cardiovasc. Surg.* **2012**, *143*, 639–647. [CrossRef] [PubMed]

29. Bolotin, G.; Scott, W.W., Jr.; Austin, T.C.; Charland, P.J.; Kypson, A.P.; Nifong, L.W.; Salleng, K.; Chitwood, W.R., Jr. Robotic skeletonizing of the internal thoracic artery: Is it safe? *Ann. Thorac. Surg.* **2004**, *77*, 1262–1265. [CrossRef] [PubMed]

30. Ragosta, M.; Singh, K.P. Robotic-Assisted Percutaneous Coronary Intervention: Rationale, Implementation, Case Selection and Limitations of Current Technology. *J. Clin. Med.* **2018**, *7*, 23. [CrossRef] [PubMed]

15

Predictors for Target Vessel Failure after Recanalization of Chronic Total Occlusions in Patients Undergoing Surveillance Coronary Angiography

Martin Geyer [1,*,†], Johannes Wild [1,2,†], Marc Hirschmann [1], Zisis Dimitriadis [1], Thomas Münzel [1,3], Tommaso Gori [1,3] and Philip Wenzel [1,2,3,*]

[1]   Center for Cardiology, Cardiology I, University Medical Center Mainz of the Johannes Gutenberg-University Mainz, Langenbeckstr. 1, 55131 Mainz, Germany; Johannes.wild@unimedizin-mainz.de (J.W.); marc.hirschmann@icloud.com (M.H.); zisis.dimitriadis@unimedizin-mainz.de (Z.D.); tmuenzel@uni-mainz.de (T.M.); tommaso.gori@unimedizin-mainz.de (T.G.)

[2]   Center for Thrombosis and Hemostasis, University Medical Center Mainz of the Johannes Gutenberg-University Mainz, Langenbeckstr 1, 55131 Mainz, Germany

[3]   German Center for Cardiovascular Research (DZHK), Partner Site Rhine Main, Langenbeckstr. 1, 55131 Mainz, Germany

*   Correspondence: martin.geyer@unimedizin-mainz.de (M.G.); wenzelp@uni-mainz.de (P.W.);

†   M.G. and J.W. contributed equally and should both be considered as first authors.

Abstract: (1) Background: Knowledge about predictors for the long-time patency of recanalized chronic total coronary occlusions (CTOs) is limited. Evidence from invasive follow-up in the absence of acute coronary syndrome (routine surveillance coronary angiography) is scarce. (2) Methods: In a monocentric-retrospective analysis, we obtained baseline as well as periprocedural data of patients undergoing routine invasive follow-up. We defined target vessel failure (TVF) as a combined primary endpoint, consisting of re-occlusion, restenosis, and target vessel revascularization (TVR). (3) Results: We included 93 consecutive patients (15.1% female) from October 2013 to May 2018. After a follow-up period of 206 ± 129 days (median 185 (IQR 127–237)), re-occlusion had occurred in 7.5%, restenosis in 11.8%, and TVR in 5.4%; the cumulative incidence of TVF was 15.1%. Reduced TIMI-flow immediately after recanalization (OR for TVR: 11.0 (95% CI: 2.7–45.5), $p = 0.001$) as well as female gender (OR for TVR: 11.0 (95% CI: 2.1–58.5), $p = 0.005$) were found to be predictive for pathological angiographic findings at follow-up. Furthermore, higher blood values of high-sensitive troponin after successful revascularization were associated with all endpoints. Interestingly, neither the J-CTO score nor the presence of symptoms at the follow-up visit could be correlated to adverse angiographic results. (4) Conclusions: In this medium-sized cohort of patients with surveillance coronary angiography, we were able to identify reduced TIMI flow and female gender as the strongest predictors for future TVF.

Keywords: chronic total occlusion; target vessel failure; re-occlusion; surveillance coronary angiography

1. Introduction

Coronary chronic total occlusion (CTO) is defined as either absent or minimal antegrade coronary blood flow diagnosed by coronary angiography that had existed for >12 weeks [1]. According to registry data, this distinct subtype of coronary artery disease has a prevalence of up to 20% of all invasive coronary diagnostics [2]. Nevertheless, expert opinion on the optimal treatment strategy (conservative, interventional, or surgical) is still controversial. According to contemporary data on clinical practice, only about one third of all patients with a CTO are treated by revascularization (percutaneous coronary intervention (PCI) or coronary artery bypass grafting surgery (CABG)) [2]. In contrast to non-CTO PCIs with a procedural success rate of 98%, interventional CTO procedures are more complex and have a significantly lower periprocedural revascularization rate of 60% to 70% in non-specialized centers [2,3], which can exceed 90% in highly specialized units [4,5]. As a tool to assess and grade lesion difficulty as well as predicting successful guidewire crossing within 30 min in interventional recanalization, the J-CTO (Multicenter CTO Registry in Japan) score was developed and validated. The presence of five specific lesion characteristics in CTO vessels that are known to hamper revascularization success (blunt stump, occlusion length > 20 mm, calcification, vessel bending > 45 degrees, and previously failed PCI) are assigned to one point each and summarized [6]. Vessel revascularization in CTO lesions has been associated with clinical improvement of angina and a prognostic benefit regarding a lower rate of subsequent myocardial infarction and longer survival in clinical registries [7–10]. However, evidence on long-term angiographic results as well as potential predictors for vessel patency and re-occlusion post CTO-PCI is scarce. Results from other registries imply that a higher pre-interventional J-CTO score—beyond acute success—might have an impact on an increased probability for future adverse events [11,12]. Thus, the objectives of this study were (i) to investigate the incidence of long-term target vessel failure (re-occlusion, restenosis, and target vessel revascularization) as assessed by invasive follow-up in an all-comer retrospective monocentric analysis, and (ii) to identify potential predictors of future target vessel failure after successful CTO recanalization, including the J-CTO score.

2. Methods

Data of all patients consecutively treated with successful PCI for CTO-lesions in our center between October 2013 to September 2017 that had an elective control coronary angiography until May 2018 were included in this retrospective analysis. Surveillance angiography after a follow-up period of 3 to 12 months was routinely recommended after successful recanalization of a CTO vessel in accordance with the guidelines for high-risk lesions [13]. Patients primarily undergoing urgent invasive control for acute coronary syndrome at a follow-up instead of the elective control coronary angiography were excluded from the analysis. From October 2013 to September 2017, recanalization of CTO lesions by PCI was successfully performed in 201 cases in our center. For this retrospective analysis, data of 100 patients of this cohort with an invasive follow-up in our center were available (49.8%). Seven patients were excluded because of either an extremely long latency from the index procedure to follow-up ($n = 3$) and/or because of acute coronary syndrome as an indication for repeated invasive coronary angiography ($n = 5$) in order to prevent potential bias by findings not solely grounded on previously recommended routine control. All subjects were adult individuals (≥ 18 years) with pre-existing fluoroscopic evidence of a chronically occluded coronary vessel. The choice of the interventional approach (antegrade vs. retrograde recanalization, radial or femoral access) and material for intervention at the index visit (e.g., guiding catheters, guidewires, PCI balloons, and stents) was subject to the discretion of the operator.

Patients' characteristics, clinical features (angina pectoris: Defined as chest discomfort as classified by Canadian Cardiovascular Society (CCS) class >2; symptoms: Defined as the presence of angina pectoris CCS class >2 and/or dyspnea NYHA (New York Heart Association) class >1; echocardiographic baseline parameters; proof of vitality of the region of the CTO), comorbidities, cardiovascular risk factors, as well as features of the PCI procedure (e.g., treated vessel, dose of contrast dye and radiation, fluoroscopy and procedural duration, J-CTO score and its subfactors (lesion entry, length, bending, and previously failed PCI attempt) of the lesion, number and length of used stent material), periprocedural levels of biomarkers (e.g., high-sensitive troponin I, creatinine, C-reactive protein), and clinical and angiographic findings at the invasive follow-up visit were gathered and analyzed. For a detailed protocol to quantify the J-CTO score, see [6]. Adipositas was defined as BMI (Body mass index) ≥ 30 kg/m^2, according to the WHO definition. Renal impairment was defined as a glomerular filtration rate < 60 mL/min*1.73m^2. The grade of a potential restenosis at the follow-up coronary angiography was retrospectively reassessed and the diameter loss in comparison to the reference vessel diameter was quantified in a semi-automatic manner by the Quantitative Coronary Analysis (QCA) tool (Philips Healthcare, Andover, MA, USA) for this study. Additionally, TIMI flow—as defined by the Thrombolysis in Myocardial Infarction Trial, quantified in Grades 0–3—was recorded semi-quantitatively for the time points directly after the index procedure and at the follow-up visit.

The primary endpoints of the retrospective analysis of our patient cohort study were defined as follows:

(1) Re-occlusion: Defined as TIMI flow grade 0, as assessed by fluoroscopy of the treated vessel at the timepoint of surveillance coronary angiography.

(2) Restenosis: Defined as the recurrence of lumen loss >50% in the CTO vessel as quantified retrospectively by QCA (including re-occlusion).

(3) Target vessel failure (TVF): Defined as a combined endpoint by the presence of re-occlusion, restenosis, or target vessel revascularization (defined as a necessity for a repeated PCI within the former CTO vessel).

We compared baseline parameters and values of clinical, fluoroscopic, and laboratory findings during index hospitalization (CTO PCI procedure) and at the timepoint of invasive follow-up and assigned patients to groups dependent on the presence of each singular endpoint as well as the combined endpoint at the time of follow-up surveillance coronary angiography. Continuous variables are presented as a mean ± standard deviation or as a median and interquartile range and categorial variables are expressed as percentages. Continuous variables found not to follow a normal distribution when tested with the modified Kolmogorov–Smirnov test (Lilliefors test) and Shapiro–Wilk-test were compared using the Wilcoxon matched-pairs signed rank test or the Wilcoxon–Mann–Whitney test for comparison between each two groups. Normally distributed continuous variables were compared using the Students' t-test and categorical variables with Fisher's exact or Chi^2 test, as appropriate.

Logistic regression analyses were performed in order to identify potential predictors for the occurrence of endpoints. Odds ratios (ORs) are given with the corresponding 95% confidence intervals (CIs). Logistic regressions were calculated by a univariate and a multivariate model, which was adjusted for age, diabetes, hyperlipidemia, smoking, hypertension, and a positive family history of cardiovascular disease. Receiver operating characteristics (ROCs) curves were calculated for the sensitivity and specificity of the J-CTO score to predict each individual endpoint, and the areas under the curve (AUC) are presented with the corresponding 95% CI. p values < 0.05 (two-sided) were considered to be statistically significant. Statistical analysis was conducted using SPSS software version 24 (SPSS Inc., Chicago, IL, USA).

Since the study involved only an anonymized, retrospective analysis of diagnostic standard data, ethics approval was not required according to German law.

3. Results

At the time of the index procedure, the 93 patients included in our analysis had a mean age of 65.6 ± 11.0 years old, 15.1% of them were female, and they had been symptomatic (angina or dyspnea) before intervention in 81.7% of the cases. The predominant target vessel for CTO intervention was the right coronary artery in 54.8% of the cases and the mean J-CTO score was 1.49 ± 1.09. Most predominant cardiovascular risk factors comprised arterial hypertension (79.6%), smoking (57.0%), and hyperlipidemia (59.1%) as well as a history of previous PCI (74.2%). A detailed overview of the baseline characteristics of all included subjects is displayed in Table 1. A mean of 2.2 ± 1.1 stents were implanted over an average lesion length of 56.6 ± 30.5 mm. One patient (1.1%) received treatment with a drug-eluting balloon alone without additional stent implantation; in all other patients, second-generation drug-eluting stents or scaffolds (in 76 cases (82.8%), everolimus-eluting stents (EESs); in 4 cases (4.3%), biolimus eluting stents; in 9 cases (9.7%), everolimus-eluting bioresorbable vascular scaffolds (BVSs), and in 3 cases (3.2%), a combination of EESs and BVSs) were used to treat the lesion. No patient was treated by POBA (plain old balloon angioplasty). Three patients (3.2%) encountered periinterventional acute renal failure, and one patient (1.1%) had relevant bleeding at the site of vascular access; in all other patients, no relevant major adverse events during the index visit were recorded. In total, 95.7% (n = 89) of the recanalizations were performed via the antegrade approach and primary vascular access was via the radial artery in 62.4% of cases (n = 58). In accordance with the guidelines [8], 89.2% (83 patients) were treated with dual anti-platelet therapy alone, and 10 cases (10.8%) with a combination of antiplatelet therapy and an oral anticoagulant. The time elapsed from the index procedure to invasive follow-up was, on average, 206 ± 129 days (median 185 (IQR 127–237 days)).

Table 1. Baseline characteristics (n = 93).

Parameter	n (%)	Mean ± SD	Median (IQR)
Age at procedure (years)		65.6 ± 11.0	66.5 (58.2/74.6)
female gender	14 (15.1%)		
Angina before intervention	53 (57.0%)		
Symptoms before intervention	76 (81.7%)		
multivessel disease	80 (86.0%)		
previous CABG	10 (10.8%)		
previous PCI	70 (74.2%)		
Diabetes	31 (33.3%)		
Smoking	53 (57.0%)		
Hyperlipidemia	55 (59.1%)		
Family history of CAD	24 (25.8%)		
arterial hypertension	74 (79.6%)		
peripheral artery disease	9 (9.7%)		
cerebral artery disease	8 (8.6%)		
renal insufficiency	6 (6.4%)		
hyperthyroidism	13 (14.0%)		
weight (KG)		90.2 ± 20.3	87.3 (78.0/100.8)
height (meters)		1.74 ± 0.10	1.76 (1.68/1.80)
Body mass index (kg/m^2)		25.8 ± 4.8	24.9 (22.8/28.4)
Adipositas	14 (21.2%)		
mean LVEF (%)		50.5 ±9.6	55.0 (45.0/55.0)
reduced LVEF at baseline	19 (29.7%)		
proof of vitality of CTO region prior to intervention	52 (57.8%)		
CTO vessel			
LAD	19 (20.4%)		
LCX	23 (24.7%)		
RCA	51 (54.8%)		
J-CTO Score		1.49 ± 1.09	1.0 (1.0/2.0)
Components of the J-CTO Score			
Entry	27 (29.0%)		
Calcification	47 (50.5%)		
Bending > 45°	25 (26.9%)		
Lesion Length > 20 mm	29 (31.2%)		
Retry Lesion	12 (12.9%)		

Abbreviations: CABG: coronary artery bypass grafting, PCI: percutaneous coronary intervention, CTO: chronic total occlusion, LVEF: left ventricular ejection fraction. LAD: left anterior descending artery, LCX: left circumflex artery, RCA: right coronary artery. IQR: Interquartile Range, SD: standard deviation.

We compared patients' clinical and periinterventional characteristics, including gender, coronary vascular risk factors, renal impairment, left ventricular ejection fraction, duration and cumulative fluoroscopy dose, stent length and number, periinterventional biomarkers, and symptoms, at baseline and follow-up for each individual endpoint, and the cumulative endpoint. The incidence of re-occlusion was low (7.5%, n = 7) and re-stenosis of the former CTO lesion (including re-occlusion) was observed in 11.8% (n = 11). In five patients (5.4%), TVR was performed (two patients with treatment within the former CTO lesion, in three patients with de novo stenosis adjacent to the former CTO lesion). Thus, the incidence of the combined endpoint TVF was 15.1% (n = 14). Detailed results are presented in Table 2 (for enhanced results, see Supplementary Materials Table S1).

Table 2. Patients' baseline, periprocedural, and follow-up characteristics stratified for endpoints.

	Re-Occlusion			Restenosis			TVF		
	Re-Occlusion (n = 7)	No Re-Occlusion (n = 86)	p-Value	Restenosis (n = 11)	No Restenosis (n = 82)	p-Value	TVF (n = 14)	No TVF (n = 79)	p-Value
Baseline parameters									
female gender	28.6	14.0	0.283	36.4	12.2	0.058	35.7	11.3	0.034
Age at procedure	65.1 ± 6.9	65.6 ± 11.3	0.843	65.6 ± 7.5	65.6 ± 11.5	0.988	60.6 ± 13.4	66.5 ± 10.4	0.063
Reduced LVEF	20.0	30.5	1.000	22.2	30.9	0.713	30.0	29.6	1.000
LVEF baseline	51.8 ± 6.6	50.4 ± 9.8	0.923	51.0 ± 6.4	50.5 ± 10.0	0.667	50.4 ± 6.4	50.6 ± 10.1	0.466
Angina at baseline	57.1	57.0	1.000	54.5	57.3	1.000	50.0	58.2	0.574
Symptoms at baseline	100	80.2	0.342	100.0	79.3	0.206	92.9	79.7	0.453
Body Mass Index	23.6 ± 2.1	25.9 ± 4.9	0.356	23.1 ± 2.7	26.1 ± 4.9	0.130	23.8 ± 4.8	26.1 ± 4.8	0.158
J-CTO Score	1.86 ± 1.07	1.47 ± 1.09	0.307	1.55 ± 1.21	1.49 ± 1.08	0.843	1.60 ± 1.82	1.49 ± 1.05	0.889
J-CTO Score ≥ 3	28.6	22.1	0.654	37.5	22.0	0.707	28.6	21.5	0.511
Periprocedural characteristics									
CTO vessel									
- LAD	28.6	19.8		18.2	20.7		14.3	21.5	
- LCx	42.9	23.3		27.3	24.4		28.6	24.1	
- RCA	28.6	57.0	0.332	54.5	54.9	0.969	57.1	54.40	0.811
Reduced TIMI-flow post intervention	100.0	8.1	<0.001	90.9	4.9	<0.001	71.4	5.1	<0.001
Stent length (mm)	36.3 ± 41.1	58.3 ± 29.2	0.044	38.2 ± 36.2	59.1 ± 29.0	0.020	43.0 ± 35.9	59.0 ± 29.0	0.042
Stent number	1.6 ± 1.6	2.2 ± 1.0	0.065	1.6 ± 1.4	2.2 ± 1.0	0.040	1.9 ± 1.3	2.2 ± 1.0	0.183
Fluoroscopy dose (cgy*dm)	8062 ± 4148	7363 ± 6308	0.351	7547 ± 4697	7398 ± 6352	0.677	7134 ± 4324	7465 ± 6449	0.830
Fluoroscopy time (min)	29.6 ± 18.0	26.0 ± 15.9	0.570	30.8 ± 18.8	25.7 ± 15.6	0.388	30.2 ± 18.0	25.6 ± 15.6	0.347
Duration (total) (min)	165.1 ± 26.8	123.8 ± 44.8	0.006	154.6 ± 44.0	123.2 ± 44.0	0.013	144.4 ± 45.7	123.8 ± 44.4	0.056
Contrast volume (mL)	277.4 ± 159.4	240.7 ± 103.1	0.662	279.2 ± 141.2	238.8 ± 102.4	0.372	263.8 ± 132.2	239.9 ± 103.2	0.576
Periinterventional CK (u/L)	178.3 ± 141.2	116.0 ± 94.9	0.276	132.7 ± 120.8	118.8 ± 96.6	0.929	123.5 ± 108.9	119.9 ± 98.9	0.802
High-sensitive Troponin I periinterventional (pg/mL)	1'26.3 ± 1560.6	412.0 ± 1391.4	0.013	771.4 ± 1255.7	420.7 ± 1425.5	0.013	662.4 ± 1124.7	425.5 ± 1451.3	0.044
Creatinine periinterventional (mg/dL)	0.93 ± 0.11	1.16 ± 0.97	0.412	0.96 ± 0.14	1.17 ± 0.99	0.636	0.96 ± 0.13	1.18 ± 1.01	0.580
CrP periinterventional (mg/L)	37.0 ± 59.5	7.77 ± 15.7	0.238	23.6 ± 47.7	8.1 ± 16.4	0.712	21.8 ± 45.6	8.1 ± 16.5	0.685
Symptoms at follow-up									
Angina	28.6	32.5	1.000	36.4	31.6	0.741	35.7	31.6	0.763
Symptoms	42.9	53.4	0.704	54.5	52.4	1.000	50.0	53.2	1.000

values presented as percentages or mean values ± SD. Abbreviations: LVEF: left ventricular ejection fraction, CTO: chronic total occlusion, LAD: left anterior descending artery, LCx: left circumflex artery, RCA: right coronary artery, CrP: c-reactive protein, CK: creatin kinase. TVF: Target Vessel Failure.

When comparing baseline characteristics as well as periprocedural factors of the index procedure of patients encountering endpoints to those without adverse outcomes at the time of follow-up, we identified several parameters with statistically significant differences between the patient groups. Patients with reduced TIMI flow of the target vessel directly at the end of the index procedure were statistically significantly overrepresented in the groups encountering each of the endpoints. We observed a significantly greater incidence of re-occlusion (100% vs. 8.1%, $p < 0.001$), restenosis (90.9% vs. 4.9%, $p < 0.001$), and the combined endpoint (71.4% vs. 5.1%, $p < 0.001$). Furthermore, the patients reaching the endpoints had higher periprocedural levels of high-sensitive troponin I (1126.3 ± 1560.6 vs. 412.0 ± 1391.4, $p = 0.006$ for re-occlusion, 771.4 ± 1255.7 vs. 420.7 ± 1425.5, $p = 0.013$ for restenosis, and 662.4 ± 1124.7 vs. 425.5 ± 1451.3, $p = 0.044$ for TVF), and the cumulative length of implanted stents was significantly shorter (36.3 ± 41.1 vs. 58.3 ± 29.2, $p = 0.044$ for re-occlusion, 38.2 ± 36.2 vs. 59.1 ± 29.0 mm, $p = 0.020$ for restenosis, 43.0 ± 35.9 vs. 59.0 ± 29.0 mm, $p = 0.042$ for TVF). Other factors with statistically significant differences between the groups encountering endpoints were a lower number of implanted stents for restenosis, as well as a longer cumulative duration of the CTO index procedure both for re-occlusion and restenosis. Patients with female gender were significantly overrepresented in the target vessel failure group at follow-up (35.7% vs. 11.3%, $p = 0.034$)—a similar trend could also be observed for restenosis and re-occlusion, although this did not reach statistical significance (for details, see Table 2).

We performed logistic regression analyses to assess the odds ratios of independent predictors for each individual endpoint, including TVF, and adjusted those further for general cardiovascular risk factors (age, diabetes, hyperlipidemia, smoking, hypertension, and family history of cardiovascular disease) in a multivariate model. The results are presented in Table 3 (for further detailed calculations, see online Supplementary Materials Table S1). Individual factors as potential predictors for TVF comprised—as expected—reduced TIMI flow at the end of the index procedure all endpoints for re-occlusion (OR: 20.36 (95% CI: 3.21–129.00), $p = 0.001$), restenosis (OR: 21.29 (95% CI: 4.28–105.97), $p < 0.01$), and the combined endpoint/TVF (OR: 11.00 (95% CI: 2.66–45.45), $p = 0.001$). Female gender proved to be a predictor for the occurrence of restenosis (OR: 8.88 (95% CI: 1.58–49.89), $p = 0.013$) as well as target vessel failure (OR: 11.03 (95% CI: 2.08–58.47), $p = 0.005$). Of note, a lower BMI was assessed to be predictive regarding the endpoints of restenosis (OR: 0.73 (95% CI: 0.55–0.98), $p = 0.037$) and TVF (OR: 0.80 (95% CI: 0.65–0.99), $p = 0.037$).

The J-CTO score at the index procedure as well as the presence of its singular factors could not be correlated with the later occurrence of any of the singular endpoints or TVF. Neither was there any statistically significant difference between the groups reaching the endpoints and those without adverse events, nor were any ORs statistically significant (Figure 1). In order to further determine the sensitivity and specificity to predict each individual end point by the J-CTO score, we computed ROC curves. The AUC for re-occlusion was calculated as 0.61 (95% CI 0.40–0.82), for restenosis as 0.52 (95% CI 0.32–0.71), and for TVF as 0.51 (95% CI 0.33–0.70) (see online Supplementary Materials Figure S1), further documenting that the J-CTO score could not predict later adverse outcomes in our cohort. Interestingly, the presence of typical angina pectoris and/or dyspnea at the time of follow-up did also not have any correlation with the co-incidence of re-occlusion, restenosis, or TVR (see Table 2).

Table 3. Multivariate regression analysis (odds ratios) for re-occlusion, restenosis, and TVF.

	Re-Occlusion		Restenosis		TVF	
	OR (95% CI)	p-Value	OR (95% CI)	p-Value	OR (95% CI)	p-Value
Baseline parameters						
female gender	3.77 (0.54–26.43)	0.182	8.88 (1.58–49.89)	0.013	11.03 (2.08–58.47)	0.005
Age at procedure	0.99 (0.91–1.08)	0.822	1.00 (0.93–1.07)	0.995	0.95 (0.90–1.01)	0.080
Reduced LVEF	0.43 (0.04–5.09)	0.426	0.49 (0.08–3.10)	0.449	0.70 (0.13–3.87)	0.680
LVEF baseline	1.92 (0.91–1.16)	0.713	1.01 (0.92–1.10)	0.895	1.00 (0.92–1.09)	0.956
Angina at baseline	0.96 (0.19–4.79)	0.957	0.78 (0.20–2.97)	0.712	0.70 (0.21–2.40)	0.704
Symptoms at baseline	not calculable		not calculable		8.65 (0.62–121.31)	0.109
Body Mass Index	0.79 (0.57–1.09)	0.147	0.73 (0.55–0.98)	0.037	0.80 (0.65–0.99)	0.037
J-CTO-Score	1.42 (0.64–3.16)	0.394	1.03 (0.54–1.95)	0.929	1.11 (0.62–1.98)	0.728
J-CTO Score ≥ 3	1.40 (0.21–8.99)	0.721	1.26 (0.27–5.84)	0.768	1.35 (0.33–5.45)	0.676
Periprocedural characteristics						
CTO vessel						
-LAD						
-LCx						
-RCA	0.50 (0.18–1.38)	0.180	0.98 (0.37–2.14)	0.797	0.97 (0.43–2.19)	0.936
Reduced TIMI-flow post intervention	20.36 (3.21–129.00)	0.001	21.29 (4.28–105.97)	<0.001	11.00 (2.66–45.45)	0.001
Stent length (mm)	0.97 (0.94–1.00)	0.081	0.98 (0.95–1.00)	0.051	0.98 (0.95–1.00)	0.060
Stent number	0.52 (0.21–1.29)	0.156	0.58 (0.28–1.17)	0.125	0.70 (0.38–1.29)	0.255
Fluoroscopy dose (cgy*dm)	1.00 (1.00–1.00)	0.748	1.00 (1.00–1.00)	0.871	1.00 (1.00–1.00)	0.868
Fluoroscopy time (min)	1.02 (0.97–1.07)	0.470	1.02 (0.99–1.07)	0.233	1.03 (0.99–1.06)	0.185
Duration (total) (min)	1.02 (1.00–1.04)	0.025	1.02 (1.00–1.03)	0.030	1.01 (1.00–1.03)	0.056
Contrast volume (mL)	1.00 (1.00–1.01)	0.287	1.00 (1.00–1.01)	0.200	1.00 (1.00–1.03)	0.486
Periinterventional CK (u/L)	1.01 (1.00–1.01)	0.153	1.00 (0.99–1.01)	0.757	1.00 (0.99–1.01)	0.973
High-sensitive Troponin I periinterventional (pg/mL)	1.00 (1.00–1.00)	0.286	1.00 (1.00–1.00)	0.247	1.00 (1.00–1.00)	0.459
Creatinine periinterventional (mg/dL)	0.07 (0.00–8.94)	0.284	0.12 (0.00–4.57)	0.256	0.22 (0.01–5.91)	0.366
CrP periinterventional (mg/L)	1.03 (1.00–1.06)	0.049	1.02 (1.00–1.05)	0.067	1.02 (1.00–1.04)	0.103
Symptoms at follow-up						
Angina	0.75 (0.13–4.45)	0.750	1.24 (0.30–5.07)	0.762	0.99 (0.28–3.59)	0.992
Symptoms	0.69 (0.14–3.36)	0.642	1.27 (0.34–4.71)	0.723	0.92 (0.28–3.01)	0.891

Abbreviations: LVEF: left ventricular ejection fraction, CTO: chronic total occlusion, LAD: left anterior descending artery, LCx: left circumflex artery, RCA: right coronary artery, CrP: c-reactive protein, CK: creatin kinase. TVF: Target Vessel Failure.

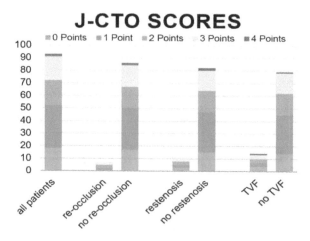

Figure 1. Distribution of the J-CTO score in all patients in the groups reaching endpoints. J-CTO scores were calculated for the whole study group and stratified for all single endpoints and the combined endpoint. In our study, the distribution of J-CTO scores did not differ significantly between groups (for details, see the text).

4. Discussion

Over the last years, percutaneous recanalization procedures of CTO lesions have been introduced into daily clinical practice in most PCI centers. Successful intervention in CTO lesions has been attributed to clinical as well as prognostic benefit [7–9]. Yet, follow-up data, including invasive control coronary angiography, as well as evidence on potential predictors for long-term success are rare.

The key findings of this retrospective study are as follows: In a monocentric retrospective analysis with routinely recommended invasive follow-up of intermediate to difficult CTO lesions (mean J-CTO score 1.49 ± 1.09), re-occlusion rates tended to be low. Yet, the incidence of adverse findings, like restenosis, target lesion revascularization, and the combined endpoint target vessel failure, was moderate but still relevant. Of all clinical parameters entered in the analysis, reduced TIMI flow of the target vessel at the end of the index procedure was the strongest predictor of the endpoints at the follow-up visit. Furthermore, patients with higher periinterventional levels of high-sensitive troponin I as well as a shorter cumulative length of implanted stents were overrepresented in the groups with a later occurrence of adverse events at the timepoint of surveillance coronary angiography. Female patients were at a higher risk for TVF. Interestingly, the pre-procedural J-CTO score was not predictive of the occurrence of later restenosis, re-occlusion, or TLV in our cohort.

Other retrospective analyses have aimed to identify potential predictors for later cardiac adverse events in cohorts of patients that underwent PCI for CTO lesions. In a retrospective analysis of 249 patients with a mean (non-invasive) follow-up of 19.8 ± 13.1 months, a higher J-CTO score was found to be associated with a higher rate of major adverse cardiovascular events (MACEs) [11]. Although the baseline characteristics in this cohort were mainly comparable (age 63 ± 11 years vs. 65.6 ± 11.0 years in our study, 70.3% vs. 84.9% male, right coronary artery as the target vessel in 49.4% vs. 54.8%, J-CTO score 1.8 ± 1.0 vs. 1.49 ± 1.09), the study design was distinctly different, which might account for the controversial findings. The follow-up was also survey based without surveillance coronary angiography and the endpoints were also determined differently by MACEs (cardiovascular or unknown cause of death, myocardial infarction, TVR by PCI or CABG). In another large European multi-center retrospective analysis of a total of 1395 patients with a mean follow-up of 23 months, female sex, high J-CTO score ≥ 3, and prior PCI as well as reduced left ventricular function were found to be correlated with a higher incidence of MACEs [12].

In our analysis, we identified female gender as a risk factor for TVF. Although some registries generated evidence that women derive the same benefit from CTO-PCI as men in regard to clinical benefit [14], female gender was found to be a predictor of PCI-related complications as well as MACEs in other retrospective studies too [12,15,16]. The reason for this observation remains unclear but may include differences in the hormonal status between men and women. Yet, this finding might strengthen the recommendation on optimal patient pre-selection. This should comprise of routine use of non-invasive testing for myocardial ischemia prior to recanalization attempts, especially in female patients who appear to be at elevated risk for future TVF.

Only a very few studies have assessed the mechanisms and predictors of target vessel failure in CTO patients. In a prospective multicenter noninferiority trial comparing the use of a sirolimus-Eluting stent (SES) to an Everolimus-eluting stent (EES) on 330 patients with total coronary occlusions, the incidence of re-occlusion (2.2% in the SES vs. 1.4% in the EES group) and re-stenosis (8.0% vs. 2.1%) was distinctly lower than in our study group [17]. The follow-up rate was high, with 85% in comparison to nearly 50% in our study. Yet, a less strict definition of total coronary occlusion (estimated duration of occlusion $\geq$ 4 weeks) was utilized for this trial, which might partially account for the different findings. In a monocentric retrospective Korean registry on 235 patients with PCI for CTO with an invasive follow-up rate of 61.3% after 6 months, a longer occlusion length was found to be predictive for a higher incidence of TVR [16].

In our PCI center from which we recruited the study population, surveillance invasive follow-up was routinely recommended but only opted for in nearly 50% of the individuals. According to European Guidelines [13], follow-up coronary angiography might be routinely performed in high-risk coronary setups. The strategy of routine invasive follow-up is discussed controversially because of limited evidence and—in contrast to the situation in Europe—American guidelines abstain from a recommendation [18]. One prospective randomized multicenter study in Japan ((Randomized Evaluation of Routine Follow-up Coronary Angiography after Percutaneous Coronary Intervention Trial) ReACT Trial) on 700 patients could not find evidence of a clinical benefit for a general angiographic follow-up at least in a normal risk patient cohort [19]. Of course, it remains controversial whether CTO-PCIs resemble a high-risk PCI collective (not further explained in the European guidelines) and, furthermore, an impact on further clinical benefit by this strategy of an early invasive follow-up and treatment of probably non-symptomatic re-stenosis remains hypothetic up to now. Nevertheless, our study provides evidence that surveillance coronary angiography might be justified after recanalization of CTO lesions, especially in the presence of specific factors predictive of TVF. Clinical findings, such as ongoing symptoms alone, with definite exclusion of acute coronary syndrome, might not be helpful to stratify patients at risk of potential TVF.

Some limitations of our study merit consideration: First, the design is a monocentric retrospective analysis with a mid-term follow-up. Due to the observational nature of the study, the follow-up rate was only 49.8%, which might further account for a potential selection bias, which has to be taken into account in the interpretation of our results. BVS were used for treatment in some cases, which are not available anymore. Although routine surveillance invasive follow-up was recommended in all patients, symptomatic individuals could be overrepresented at the follow-up visit, as the prevalence of angina pectoris and dyspnea at the time of follow-up was higher in comparison to other registries [12]. Indication for TVR was based on individual assessment of the interventional operator and not mandatorily grounded on further non-invasive or invasive evaluation of the stenosis (e.g., measurement of fractional flow reserve, intracoronary imaging like optical coherence tomography or intravascular ultrasound) and a potential clinical and prognostic benefit of these interventions has not been studied. Larger prospective randomized studies with defined protocol, including intracoronary imaging or flow measurements, for surveillance coronary angiography would be desirable. Furthermore, patients with female gender were relevantly underrepresented (15.1%), yet at a comparable extent to most published CTO registries [11,12,14–16].

5. Conclusions

In this retrospective monocentric cohort of patients undergoing routine follow-up coronary angiography after CTO recanalization, we found evidence that reduced TIMI flow at the end of the index procedure as well as female gender could be predictors of later angiographic adverse outcome (TVF). Furthermore, patients with a shorter cumulative length of implanted stents and higher periinterventional levels of high-sensitive troponin I were overrepresented in the group of patients encountering re-occlusion, restenosis, and TVF at the timepoint of invasive follow-up. In contrast to other registers, we could not prove any correlation between the initial J-CTO score of the treated CTO lesion and the later occurrence of any of the endpoints. Remarkably, symptoms at the time of follow-up coronary angiography could not be attributed to adverse angiographic results. Based on the still relevant rate of TVF, even in populations of intermediate lesion complexity, such as ours, routine invasive follow-up after CTO procedures appears to be justified and should rather be guided by the presence of risk predictors, and not by the occurrence of angina (with the exception of acute coronary syndrome). Thus, our present work might stress a potential beneficial value of routine surveillance coronary angiography after CTO interventions, especially for females and patients with reduced TIMI flow at the end of the index procedure.

Author Contributions: Conceptualization, M.G., J.W. and P.W.; methodology, M.G. and P.W.; validation, M.G. and P.W.; formal analysis, M.G., M.H., T.G. and P.W.; resources, M.G., T.M., Z.D. and P.W.; data curation, M.G., J.W. and M.H.; writing—original draft preparation, M.G.; writing—review and editing, P.W., T.G., Z.D. and T.M.; supervision and project administration, P.W. and T.M. All authors have read and agreed to the published version of the manuscript.

Acknowledgments: This work contains results that are part of the doctoral thesis of Marc Hirschmann. T.M., T.G. and P.W. are PIs of the DZHK (German Center for Cardiovascular Research), Partner Site Rhine-Main, Mainz, Germany.

References

1.   Strauss, B.H.; Shuvy, M.; Wijeysundera, H.C. Revascularization of Chronic Total Occlusions. *J. Am. Coll. Cardiol.* **2014**, *64*, 1281–1289. [CrossRef] [PubMed]

2.   Fefer, P.; Knudtson, M.L.; Cheema, A.N.; Galbraith, P.D.; Osherov, A.B.; Yalonetsky, S.; Gannot, S.; Samuel, M.; Weisbrod, M.; Bierstone, D.; et al. Current perspectives on coronary chronic total occlusions: The Canadian Multicenter Chronic Total Occlusions Registry. *J. Am. Coll. Cardiol.* **2012**, *59*, 991–997. [CrossRef] [PubMed]

3.   Rathore, S.; Matsuo, H.; Terashima, M.; Kinoshita, Y.; Kimura, M.; Tsuchikane, E.; Nasu, K.; Ehara, M.; Asakura, Y.; Katho, O.; et al. Procedural and in-hospital outcomes after percutaneous coronary interventions for chronic total occlusion of coronary arteries 2002 to 2008: Impact of novel guidewire techniques. *J. Am. Coll. Cardiol. Intv.* **2009**, *2*, 489–497. [CrossRef] [PubMed]

4.   Brilakis, E.S.; Banerjee, S.; Karmpaliotis, D.; Lombardi, W.L.; Tsai, T.T.; Shunk, K.A.; Kennedy, K.F.; Spertus, J.A.; Holmes, D.R., Jr.; Grantham, J.A. Procedural outcomes of chronic total occlusion percutaneous coronary intervention. A report from the NCDR (national cardiovascular data registry). *J. Am. Coll. Cardiol. Intv.* **2015**, *8*, 245–253. [CrossRef] [PubMed]

5.   Christopoulos, G.; Karmpaliotis, D.; Alaswad, K.; Yeh, R.W.; Jaffer, F.A.; Wyman, R.M.; Lombardi, W.L.; Menon, R.V.; Grantham, J.A.; Kandzari, D.E.; et al. Application and outcomes of a hybrid approach to chronic total occlusion percutaneous coronary intervention in a contemporary multicenter US registry. *Int. J. Cardiol.* **2015**, *98*, 222–228. [CrossRef] [PubMed]

6.   Morino, Y.; Abe, M.; Morimoto, T.; Kimura, T.; Hayashi, Y.; Muramatsu, T.; Ochiai, M.; Noguchi, Y.; Kato, K.; Shibata, Y.; et al. Predicting successful guidewire crossing through chronic total occlusion of native coronary lesions within 30 minutes. *J. Am. Coll. Cardiol. Intv.* **2011**, *4*, 213–221. [CrossRef] [PubMed]

7.   Hoye, A.; van Domburg, R.T.; Sonnenschein, K.; Serruys, P.W. Percutaneous coronary interventions for chronic total occlusions: The Thoraxcenter experience 1992–2002. *Eur. Heart J.* **2005**, *26*, 2630–2636. [CrossRef] [PubMed]

8.   Suero, J.A.; Marso, S.P.; Jones, P.G.; Laster, S.B.; Huber, K.C.; Giorgi, L.V.; Johnson, W.L.; Rutherford, B.D. Procedural outcomes and long-term survival among patients undergoing percutaneous coronary intervention of a chronic total occlusion in native coronary arteries: A 20-year experience. *J. Am. Coll. Cardiol.* **2001**, *38*, 409–414. [CrossRef]

9. George, S.; Cockburn, J.; Clayton, T.C.; Ludman, P.; Cotton, J.; Spratt, J.; Redwood, S.; de Belder, M.; de Belder, A.; Hill, J.; et al. Long-term follow-up of elective chronicl total coronary occlusion angioplasty. *J. Am. Coll. Cardiol.* **2014**, *64*, 235–243. [CrossRef] [PubMed]

10. Jones, D.A.; Rathod, K.S.; Pavlidis, A.N.; Gallagher, S.M.; Astroulakis, Z.; Lim, P.; Sirker, A.; Knight, C.J.; Dalby, M.C.; Malik, I.S.; et al. Outcomes after chronic total occlusion percutaneous coronary interventions: An observational study of 5496 patients from the Pan-London CTO Cohort. *Coron. Artery Dis.* **2018**, *29*, 557–563. [CrossRef] [PubMed]

11. Forounzandeh, F.; Suh, J.; Stahl, E.; Ko, Y.A.; Lee, S.; Joshi, U.; Sabharwal, N.; Almuwaqqat, Z.; Gandhi, R.; Lee, H.S.; et al. Performance of J-CTO and PROGRESS CTO-Scores in predicting angiographic success and long-term outcomes of percutaneous coronary interventions for chronic total occlusions. *Am. J. Cardiol.* **2018**, *121*, 14–20. [CrossRef] [PubMed]

12. Galassi, A.R.; Sianos, G.; Werner, G.S.; Escaned, J.; Tomasello, S.D.; Boukhris, M.; Castaing, M.; Büttner, J.H.; Bufe, A.; Kalnins, A.; et al. Retrograde recanalization of chronic total occlusions in Europe. *J. Am. Coll. Cardiol.* **2015**, *65*, 2388–2400. [CrossRef] [PubMed]

13. Neumann, F.J.; Sousa-Uva, M.; Ahlsson, A.; Alfonso, F.; Banning, A.P.; Benedetto, U.; Byrne, R.A.; Collet, J.P.; Falk, V.; Head, S.J.; et al. 2018 ESC/EACTS Guidelines on myocardial revascularization. *Eur. Heart J.* **2019**, *40*, 87–165. [CrossRef] [PubMed]

14. Pershad, A.; Gulati, M.; Karmpaliotis, D.; Moses, J.; Nicholson, W.J.; Nugent, K.; Tang, Y.; Sapontis, J.; Lombardi, W.; Grantham, J.A.; et al. A sex stratified outcome analysis from the OPEN-CTO registry. *Catheter. Cardiovasc. Interv.* **2019**, *93*, 1041–1047. [CrossRef]

15. Toma, A.; Stähli, B.E.; Gick, M.; Ferenc, M.; Mashayekhi, K.; Buettner, H.J.; Neumann, F.J.; Gebhard, C. Temporal changes in outcomes of women and men undergoing percutaneous coronary intervention for chronic total occlusion: 2005–2013. *Clin. Res. Cardiol.* **2018**, *107*, 449–459. [CrossRef]

16. Ahn, J.; Rha, S.W.; Choi, B.; Choi, S.Y.; Byun, J.K.; Mashaly, A.; Abdelshafi, K.; Park, Y.; Jang, W.Y.; Kim, W.; et al. Impact of chronic total occlusion length on six-month angiographic and 2-year clinical outcomes. *PLoS ONE* **2018**, *13*, 30198571. [CrossRef] [PubMed]

17. Teeuwen, K.; van der Schaaf, R.; Adraenssens, T.; Koolen, J.J.; Smits, C.; Henriques, J.P.S.; Vermeersch, P.H.; Tjon Joe Gin, R.M.; Schölzel, B.E.; Kelder, J.C.; et al. Randomized multicenter trial investigating angiographic outcomes of hybrid sirolimus-eluting stents with biodegradable polymer compared with everolimus-eluting stents with durable polymer in chronic total occlusions. *J. Am. Coll. Cardiol. Intervn.* **2017**, *10*, 133–143. [CrossRef] [PubMed]

18. Levine, G.N.; Bates, E.R.; Blankenship, J.C.; Bailey, S.R.; Bittl, J.A.; Cercek, B.; Chambers, C.E.; Ellis, S.G.; Guyton, R.A.; Hollenberg, S.M.; et al. 2011 ACCF/AHA/SCAI Guideline for percutaneous coronary intervention: Executive summary. *Circulation* **2011**, *124*, 2474–2609. [CrossRef]

19. Shiomi, H.; Morimoto, T.; Kitaguchi, S.; Nakagawa, Y.; Ishii, K.; Haruna, Y.; Takamisawa, I.; Motooka, M.; Nakao, K.; Matsuda, S.; et al. The ReACT Trial. Randomized evaluation of routine follow-up coronary angiography after percutaneous coronary intervention trial. *J. Am. Coll. Cardiol. Intv.* **2017**, *10*, 109–117. [CrossRef] [PubMed]

Permissions

List of Contributors

José Miguel Rivera-Caravaca and Francisco Marín
Department of Cardiology, Hospital Clínico Universitario Virgen de la Arrixaca, University of Murcia, Instituto Murciano de Investigación Biosanitaria (IMIB-Arrixaca), CIBERCV, 30120 Murcia, Spain

Raúl Teruel-Montoya and Vicente Vicente
Department of Hematology and Medical Oncology, Hospital General Universitario Morales Meseguer, University of Murcia, Centro Regional de Hemodonación, Instituto Murciano de Investigación Biosanitaria (IMIB-Arrixaca), 30003 Murcia, Spain CIBERER (U765), 30003 Murcia, Spain

Laura Zapata-Martínez, Nuria García-Barberá, Vanessa Roldán, Rosa Cifuentes-Riquelme, José Antonio Crespo-Matas, Ascensión María de los Reyes-García, Sonia Águila, María Piedad Fernández-Pérez, Laura Reguilón-Gallego, Constantino Martínez and Rocío González-Conejero
Department of Hematology and Medical Oncology, Hospital General Universitario Morales Meseguer, University of Murcia, Centro Regional de Hemodonación, Instituto Murciano de Investigación Biosanitaria (IMIB-Arrixaca), 30003 Murcia, Spain

Ramez Morcos, Joel Casale, Rupesh Manam and Vikram Patel
Department of Internal Medicine, Florida Atlantic University, Boca Raton, FL 33431, USA

Haider Al Taii and Priya Bansal
Department of Cardiovascular Diseases, Florida Atlantic University, Boca Raton, FL 33431, USA

Anthony Cioci and Michael Kucharik
College of Medicine, Florida Atlantic University, Boca Raton, FL 33431, USA

Arjun Malhotra
University of Miami, Coral Gables, FL 33124, USA

Brijeshwar Maini
Tenet Florida & Department of Cardiovascular Diseases, Florida Atlantic University, Boca Raton, FL 33431, USA

José Ramón López-Mínguez and Juan Manuel Nogales-Asensio
Cardiology Department, Interventional Cardiology Section, Hospital Universitario de Badajoz, 06080 Badajoz, Spain

Eduardo Infante De Oliveira
Cardiology Department, Interventional Cardiology Section, Hospital de Santa María, 1649-028 Lisbon, Portugal

Lino Santos
Cardiology Department, Interventional Cardiology Section, Centro Hospitalario de Vila Nova de Gaia, 4430-999 Vila Nova de Gaia Oporto, Portugal

Rafael Ruiz-Salmerón
Cardiology Department, Interventional Cardiology Section, Hospital Virgen de la Macarena, 41009 Seville, Spain

Dabit Arzamendi-Aizpurua
Cardiology Department, Interventional Cardiology Section, Hospital Santa Creu i San Pau, 08041 Barcelona, Spain

Marco Costa
Cardiology Department, Interventional Cardiology Section, Centro Hospitalar e Universitário de Coimbra, 3004-561 Coimbra, Portugal

Hipólito Gutiérrez-García
Cardiology Department, Interventional Cardiology Section, Hospital Clínico de Valladolid, 47003 Valladolid, Spain

Jose Antonio Fernández-Díaz
Cardiology Department, Interventional Cardiology Section, Hospital Puerta de Hierro, Majadahona, 28222 Madrid, Spain

Xavier Freixa
Cardiology Department, Interventional Cardiology Section, Hospital Clínic de Barcelona, 08036 Barcelona, Spain

Ignacio Cruz-González
Cardiology Department, Interventional Cardiology Section, Hospital Universitario de Salamanca, 37007 Salamanca, Spain

Raúl Moreno
Cardiology Department, Interventional Cardiology Section, Hospital La Paz, 28046 Madrid, Spain

Andrés Íñiguez-Romo
Cardiology Department, Interventional Cardiology Section, Hospital Álvaro Cunqueiro, 36213 Vigo, Pontevedra, Spain

Fernando Alfonso-Manterola
Cardiology Department, Interventional Cardiology Section, Hospital La Princesa, IIS-IP, CIBER-CV, Universidad Autónoma de Madrid, 28006 Madrid, Spain

Rabea Asleh and Jon R. Resar
Division of Cardiology, Department of Medicine, Johns Hopkins University School of Medicine, Baltimore, MD 21205, USA

Jacek Kubica
Department of Cardiology and Internal Medicine, Nicolaus Copernicus University, Collegium Medicum, 85067 Bydgoszcz, Poland

Mirosław Gozdek
Department of Cardiology and Internal Medicine, Nicolaus Copernicus University, Collegium Medicum, 85067 Bydgoszcz, Poland
Thoracic Research Centre, Nicolaus Copernicus University, Collegium Medicum in Bydgoszcz, Innovative Medical Forum, 85067 Bydgoszcz, Poland

Kamil Zieliński
Thoracic Research Centre, Nicolaus Copernicus University, Collegium Medicum in Bydgoszcz, Innovative Medical Forum, 85067 Bydgoszcz, Poland
Department of Cardiology, Warsaw Medical University, 02091Warsaw, Poland

Michał Pasierski
Thoracic Research Centre, Nicolaus Copernicus University, Collegium Medicum in Bydgoszcz, Innovative Medical Forum, 85067 Bydgoszcz, Poland
Clinical Department of Cardiac Surgery, Central Clinical Hospital of the Ministry of Interior and Administration, Centre of Postgraduate Medical Education, 02607 Warsa, Poland

Piotr Suwalski
Clinical Department of Cardiac Surgery, Central Clinical Hospital of the Ministry of Interior and Administration, Centre of Postgraduate Medical Education, 02607 Warsa, Poland

Mariusz Kowalewski
Thoracic Research Centre, Nicolaus Copernicus University, Collegium Medicum in Bydgoszcz, Innovative Medical Forum, 85067 Bydgoszcz, Poland
Clinical Department of Cardiac Surgery, Central Clinical Hospital of the Ministry of Interior and Administration, Centre of Postgraduate Medical Education, 02607 Warsa, Poland
Department of Cardio-Thoracic Surgery, Heart and Vascular Centre, Maastricht University Medical Centre, 6229 HX Maastricht, The Netherlands

Roberto Lorusso
Department of Cardio-Thoracic Surgery, Heart and Vascular Centre, Maastricht University Medical Centre, 6229 HX Maastricht, The Netherlands

Matteo Matteucci
Department of Cardio-Thoracic Surgery, Heart and Vascular Centre, Maastricht University Medical Centre, 6229 HX Maastricht, The Netherlands
Department of Cardiac Surgery, Circolo Hospital, University of Insubria, 21100 Varese, Italy

Dario Fina
Department of Cardio-Thoracic Surgery, Heart and Vascular Centre, Maastricht University Medical Centre, 6229 HX Maastricht, The Netherlands
Department of Cardiology, IRCCS Policlinico San Donato, University of Milan, 20097 Milan, Italy

Federica Jiritano
Department of Cardio-Thoracic Surgery, Heart and Vascular Centre, Maastricht University Medical Centre, 6229 HX Maastricht, The Netherlands
Department of Cardiac Surgery, University Magna Graecia of Catanzaro, 88100 Catanzaro, Italy

Paolo Meani
Department of Cardio-Thoracic Surgery, Heart and Vascular Centre, Maastricht University Medical Centre, 6229 HX Maastricht, The Netherlands
Department of Intensive Care Unit, Maastricht University Medical Centre (MUMC+), 6229 HX Maastricht, The Netherlands

Giuseppe Maria Raffa and Michele Pilato
Department for the Treatment and Study of Cardiothoracic Diseases and Cardiothoracic Transplantation, IRCCS-ISMETT (Instituto Mediterraneo per i Trapianti e Terapie ad alta specializzazione), 90127 Palermo, Italy

Pietro Giorgio Malvindi
Wessex Cardiothoracic Centre, University Hospital Southampton, Southampton SO16 6YD, UK

Domenico Paparella
GVM Care & Research, Department of Cardiovascular Surgery, Santa Maria Hospital, 70124 Bari, Italy
Department of Emergency and Organ Transplant, University of Bari Aldo Moro, 70121 Bari, Italy

Artur Słomka
Thoracic Research Centre, Nicolaus Copernicus University, Collegium Medicum in Bydgoszcz, Innovative Medical Forum, 85067 Bydgoszcz, Poland
Chair and Department of Pathophysiology, Nicolaus Copernicus University, Collegium Medicum, 85067 Bydgoszcz, Poland

Dariusz Jagielak
Department of Cardiac Surgery, Gdańsk Medical University, 80210 Gdańsk, Poland

Ronny R. Buechel
Department of Nuclear Medicine, Cardiac Imaging, University Hospital Zurich, University of Zurich, 8091 Zurich, Switzerland

Helen Kovari
Division of Infectious Diseases and Hospital Epidemiology, University of Zurich, 8091 Zurich, Switzerland

Dima A. Hammoud
Center for Infectious Disease Imaging, Radiology and Imaging Sciences, National Institutes of Health, Bethesda, MD 20892, USA

Sahar Avazzadeh, Shauna McBride and Leo. R Quinlan
Physiology and Human Movement Laboratory, CÚRAM SFI Centre for Research in Medical Devices, School of Medicine, Human biology building, National University of Ireland (NUI) Galway, H91 TK33 Galway, Ireland

Barry O'Brien and Ken Coffey
AtriAN Medical Limited, Unit 204, NUIG Business Innovation Centre, Upper Newcastle, H91 TK33 Galway, Ireland

Martin O'Halloran
Translational Medical Devise Lab (TMD Lab), Lambe Institute of Translational Research, University College Hospital Galway, H91 ERW1 Galway, Ireland

Adnan Elahi
Translational Medical Devise Lab (TMD Lab), Lambe Institute of Translational Research, University College Hospital Galway, H91 ERW1 Galway, Ireland
Electrical & Electronic Engineering, School of Engineering, National University of Ireland Galway, H91 TK33 Galway, Ireland

Alan Soo
Department of Cardiothoracic Surgery, University Hospital Galway, Saolta Hospital HealthCare Group, H91 YR71 Galway, Ireland

Sandro Ninni and Gilles Lemesle
CHU Lille, Department of Cardiology, University of Lille, F-59000 Lille, France
Institut Pasteur de Lille, U1011, F-59000 Lille, France

Thibaud Meurice
Hôpital Privé Le Bois, 59003 Lille, France

Olivier Tricot
Centre Hospitalier de Dunkerque, 59240 Dunkerque, France

Nicolas Lamblin and Christophe Bauters
CHU Lille, Department of Cardiology, University of Lille, F-59000 Lille, France
Institut Pasteur de Lille, U1167, F-59000 Lille, France

Emilija Miskinyte, Jennifer Erley, Seyedeh Mahsa Zamani, Radu Tanacli and Rolf Gebker
Department of Internal Medicine/Cardiology, German Heart Center Berlin, 13353 Berlin, Germany

Paulius Bucius
Department of Internal Medicine/Cardiology, German Heart Center Berlin, 13353 Berlin, Germany
Department of Cardiology, Medical Academy, Lithuanian University of Health Sciences, 50161 Kaunas, Lithuania

Tomas Lapinskas
Department of Cardiology, Medical Academy, Lithuanian University of Health Sciences, 50161 Kaunas, Lithuania

Christian Stehning
Philips Healthcare, 22335 Hamburg, Germany

Christopher Schneeweis
Klinik für Kardiologie und Internistische Intesivmedizin, Krankenhaus der Augustinerinnen, 50678 Köln, Germany

Sebastian Kelle and Burkert Pieske
Department of Internal Medicine/Cardiology, German Heart Center Berlin, 13353 Berlin, Germany
DZHK (German Centre for Cardiovascular Research), Partner Site Berlin, 10785 Berlin, Germany
Department of Internal Medicine/Cardiology, Charité Campus Virchow Clinic, 13353 Berlin, Germany

Volkmar Falk
DZHK (German Centre for Cardiovascular Research), Partner Site Berlin, 10785 Berlin, Germany
Department of Cardiothoracic Surgery, German Heart Center Berlin, 13353 Berlin, Germany

Natalia Solowjowa
Department of Cardiothoracic Surgery, German Heart Center Berlin, 13353 Berlin, Germany

Gianni Pedrizzetti
Department of Engineering and Architecture, University of Trieste, 34127 Trieste, Italy

Tommaso Gori and Thomas Münzel
Zentrum für Kardiologie, University Medical Center, Johannes Gutenberg University Mainz, 55131 Mainz, Germany
German Centre for Cardiovascular Research, partner site Rhine Main, 55131 Mainz, Germany
Center for Cardiology, Cardiology I, University Medical Center Mainz of the Johannes Gutenberg-University Mainz, Langenbeckstr. 1, 55131 Mainz, Germany

Stephan Achenbach
Department of Cardiology, Friedrich-Alexander University Erlangen-Nürnberg, 91054 Erlangen, Germany

Thomas Riemer
IHF GmbH-Institut für Herzinfarktforschung, 67063 Ludwigshafen, Germany

Julinda Mehilli
Department of Cardiology, Munich University Clinic, LMU, 80539 Munich, Germany
German Centre for Cardiovascular Research, partner site Munich Heart Alliance, 80539 Munich, Germany

Holger M. Nef
Department of Cardiology, University of Giessen, Medizinische Klinik I, 35392 Giessen, Germany

Christoph Naber
Klinik für Kardiologie und Angiologie, Elisabeth-Krankenhaus, 45138 Essen, Germany

Gert Richardt
Herzzentrum, Segeberger Kliniken GmbH, 23795 Bad Segeberg, Germany

Jochen Wöhrle
Department of Internal Medicine II, University of Ulm, 89081 Ulm, Germany

Ralf Zahn
Abteilung für Kardiologie, Herzzentrum Ludwigshafen, 67063 Ludwigshafen, Germany

Till Neumann
Department of Cardiology, University of Essen, 45138 Essen, Germany

Johannes Kastner
Department of Cardiology, University of Vienna Medical School, 1090 Wien, Austria

Axel Schmermund
Bethanien Hospital, 60389 Frankfurt, Germany

Christian Hamm
Department of Cardiology, University of Giessen, Medizinische Klinik I, 35392 Giessen, Germany
Department of Cardiology, Kerckhoff Heart and Thorax Center, 61231 Bad Nauheim, Germany

Isabella C. Schoepf and Philip E. Tarr
University Department of Medicine and Infectious Diseases Service, Kantonsspital Baselland, University of Basel, 4101 Bruderholz, Switzerland

Ronny R. Buechel
Department of Nuclear Medicine, Cardiac Imaging, University Hospital Zurich, University of Zurich, 8091 Zurich, Switzerland

Matteo Pirro and Vanessa Bianconi
Unit of Internal Medicine, Angiology and Arteriosclerosis Diseases, Department of Medicine, University of Perugia, 06129 Perugia, Italy

Luis E. Simental-Mendía
Biomedical Research Unit, Mexican Social Security Institute, Durango 34067, Mexico

Gerald F. Watts
School of Medicine, Faculty of Health and Medical Sciences, University of Western Australia, Perth X2213, Australia
Lipid Disorders Clinic, Cardiometabolic Services, Department of Cardiology, Royal Perth Hospital, Perth X2213, Australia

Maciej Banach
Department of Hypertension, WAM University Hospital in Lodz, Medical University of Lodz, Zeromskiego 113, 93-338 Lodz, Poland
Polish Mother's Memorial Hospital Research Institute (PMMHRI), 93-338 Lodz, Poland

Amirhossein Sahebkar
Biotechnology Research Center, Pharmaceutical Technology Institute, Mashhad University of Medical Sciences, Mashhad 9177948564, Iran
Neurogenic Inflammation Research Center, Mashhad University of Medical Sciences, Mashhad 9177948564, Iran
School of Pharmacy, Mashhad University of Medical Sciences, Mashhad 9177948564, Iran

Chieh-Jen Wu
Cardiovascular Center, Kaohsiung Veterans General Hospital, Kaohsiung 813, Taiwan
Graduate Institute of Clinical Medicine, College of Medicine, Kaohsiung Medical University, Kaohsiung 807, Taiwan

Hsin-Hung Chen and Pei-Wen Cheng
Department of Medical Education and Research, Kaohsiung Veterans General Hospital, Kaohsiung 813, Taiwan
Yuh-Ing Junior College of Health Care & Management, Kaohsiung 821, Taiwan

Ching-Jiunn Tseng
Department of Medical Education and Research, Kaohsiung Veterans General Hospital, Kaohsiung 813, Taiwan
School of Medicine, National Yang-Ming University, Taipei 112, Taiwan

Wen-Hsien Lu
School of Medicine, National Yang-Ming University, Taipei 112, Taiwan
Department of Pediatrics, Kaohsiung Veterans General Hospital, Kaohsiung 813, Taiwan

Chi-Cheng Lai
Department of Cardiology, Kaohsiung Municipal United Hospital, Kaohsiung 804, Taiwan
Department of Biological Sciences, National Sun Yat-Sen University, Kaohsiung 804, Taiwan

Martin Geyer, Marc Hirschmann and Zisis Dimitriadis
Center for Cardiology, Cardiology I, University Medical Center Mainz of the Johannes Gutenberg-University Mainz, Langenbeckstr. 1, 55131 Mainz, Germany

Johannes Wild
Center for Cardiology, Cardiology I, University Medical Center Mainz of the Johannes Gutenberg-University Mainz, Langenbeckstr. 1, 55131 Mainz, Germany
Center for Thrombosis and Hemostasis, University Medical Center Mainz of the Johannes Gutenberg-University Mainz, Langenbeckstr 1, 55131 Mainz, Germany

Philip Wenzel
Center for Cardiology, Cardiology I, University Medical Center Mainz of the Johannes Gutenberg-University Mainz, Langenbeckstr. 1, 55131 Mainz, Germany
Center for Thrombosis and Hemostasis, University Medical Center Mainz of the Johannes Gutenberg-University Mainz, Langenbeckstr 1, 55131 Mainz, Germany
German Center for Cardiovascular Research (DZHK), Partner Site Rhine Main, Langenbeckstr. 1, 55131 Mainz, Germany

Index

Printed in the USA
CPSIA information can be obtained
at www.ICGtesting.com
JSHW051403091023
49903JS00006B/260